Minimally Invasive Pancreatoduodenectomy in Cancer

Springer Nature More Media App

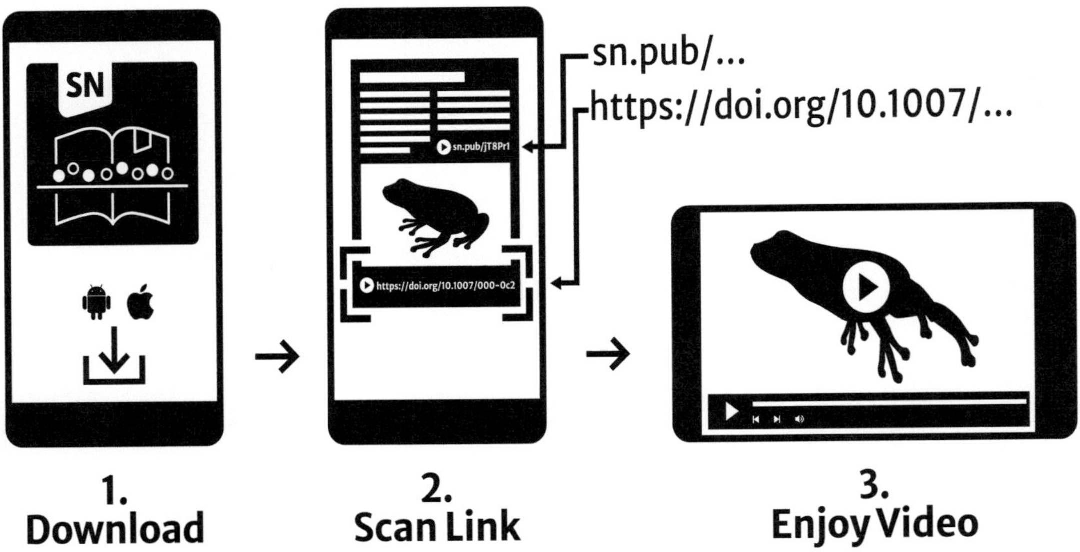

Support: customerservice@springernature.com

Benedetto Ielpo
Alessandro Anselmo • Edoardo Rosso
Editors

Minimally Invasive Pancreatoduodenectomy in Cancer

Springer

Editors
Benedetto Ielpo
Hepato-Biliary and Pancreatic Surgery Unit, Department of Surgery, Hospital del Mar
Pompeu Fabra University
Barcelona, Spain

Alessandro Anselmo
HPB Surgery and Transplants Unit
Policlinico Tor Vergata, Surg. Dept.
Rome, Italy

Edoardo Rosso
Centre de Chirurgie Digestive – Pole Santé Sud
Le Mans, France

This work contains media enhancements, which are displayed with a "play" icon. Material in the print book can be viewed on a mobile device by downloading the Springer Nature "More Media" app available in the major app stores. The media enhancements in the online version of the work can be accessed directly by authorized users.

ISBN 978-3-031-99694-8 ISBN 978-3-031-99695-5 (eBook)
https://doi.org/10.1007/978-3-031-99695-5

This Springer imprint is published by the registered company Springer Nature Switzerland AG
The registered company address is: Gewerbestrasse 11, 6330 Cham, Switzerland

In Loving Memory of Professor Cristiano Huscher

This book is dedicated to the late Professor Cristiano Huscher, a true pioneer and visionary in the field of minimally invasive surgery. His innovative spirit and relentless pursuit of excellence have profoundly shaped the evolution of surgical techniques, particularly in minimally invasive pancreatoduodenectomy. Professor Huscher not only revolutionized surgical practices but also left a lasting legacy as a mentor to numerous students and surgeons worldwide. His passion for teaching and his commitment to advancing the field have inspired a new generation of surgeons to carry forward his groundbreaking work.

Even in the final years of his life, Professor Huscher continued to innovate, pursuing new research with the same enthusiasm and curiosity that had defined his career. His legacy as a pioneer, educator, and researcher remains an enduring source of inspiration for all who had the privilege of learning from him.

To honor his enduring legacy, we have asked his daughter, Dr. Alessandra Huscher, to share her personal memories and reflections of her remarkable father.

With deep affection and highest respect, dear Cristiano, this book is dedicated to you.

Benedetto Ielpo
Alessandro Anselmo
Edoardo Rosso

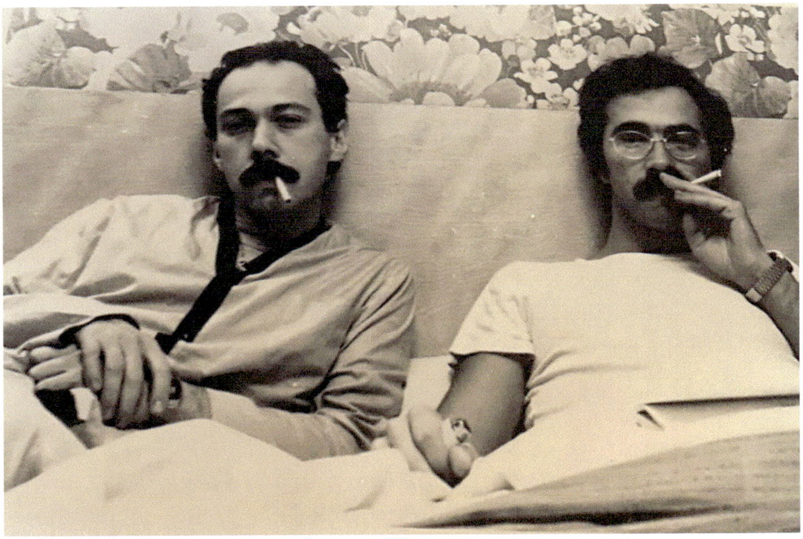

It all started in a hotel in the Marais... in 1983.
More friendship than money in your pocket…
A general surgeon and a gynecologist from a provincial town, in a village hospital.
Curiosity, the ability to recognize the value of large centers of reference brought them, together, into the international reality of Paris…
They were Dad and Luca Minelli.
Luca a few years later presented that strange thing that was laparoscopy at the time. The sentence was, as expected, without appeal: "… in general surgery it will never make sense" …
Knowing him, it could only end like that...
Then came the years of Vallecamonica, of my thesis on laparoscopic hemicolectomy… and from there a preferential relationship with technologies, both for one and the other, up to robotics, my latest traveling companion.
And amidst great successes and very difficult moments, the best that remains of you are the bonds from that time, which are still there, and the desire to look at the world and life as a great gift.
I like to think of you together again and I am sure it will please many who knew you.
Dr. Alessandra HUSCHER in memory of Professor Cristiano HUSCHER

Contents

Part I

Overview

Update and Current Indications of Minimally Invasive Pancreatoduodenectomy

1

Greta Donisi, Giovanni Capretti, Cristina Ridolfi, and Alessandro Zerbi

1.1 Minimally Invasive Pancreatic Surgery

Minimally invasive surgery has become nowadays the standard of care for many general surgery procedures. The process of development of minimally invasive pancreatic surgery (MIPS) have encountered some initial difficulties due to the intrinsic complexity of this surgical field, that, even when performed with an open approach, is still associated to notable morbidity and mortality. Nowadays the role of minimally invasive distal pancreatectomy is well established with international guidelines recommending performing minimally invasive approach when not strictly contraindicated [1, 5]. The role of minimally invasive pancreaticoduodenectomy (PD) is still under investigation [46] as PD remains the most complex pancreatic operation, involving not only a challenging resection phase due to the intricate anatomy of the pancreatic head but also a complex reconstruction phase entailing a high risk of severe complications and mortality, with rates of approximating 40% and 5% [31], respectively, even in high-volume centers. Nevertheless, more and more centers around the world have in place processes of MIPD implementation.

The first report of laparoscopic PD (LPD) traces back to the 1992 when Gagner performed the first successful LPD [20]. He concluded that, despite being feasible, it appeared not to provide advantages relatively to open approach. The technical complexity of laparoscopic approach related to a diminished dexterity, reduced tactile feedback, and constrained movement of laparoscopic instruments caused an initial setback in implementation of LPD. Trying to overcome these limits, Giulianotti [23] in 2001 performed the first robotic PD, taking advantages of the benefits provided by the robotic platform such as tremor filtration, enhanced dexterity, greater freedom of movement facilitated by the EndoWrist system, and superior visualization of the operative field through 3D imaging. Recent technological advances, improving the laparoscopic instruments, along with the implementation of robotic platforms, favored an escalation of reports on MIPD worldwide.

G. Donisi (✉) · G. Capretti · A. Zerbi
Department of Biomedical Sciences, Humanitas University, Milan, Italy

Pancreatic Surgery Unit, IRCCS Humanitas Research Hospital, Milan, Italy
e-mail: greta.donisi@humanitas.it; giovanni.capretti@hunimed.eu; alessandro.zerbi@hunimed.eu

C. Ridolfi
Pancreatic Surgery Unit, IRCCS Humanitas Research Hospital, Milan, Italy
e-mail: cristina.ridolfi@humanitas.it

B. Ielpo et al. (eds.), *Minimally Invasive Pancreatoduodenectomy in Cancer*,
https://doi.org/10.1007/978-3-031-99695-5_1

1.2 Minimally Invasive Pancreaticoduodenectomy: Feasibility and Safety

Despite the diffusion, starting from the late 2000s, of reports on MIPD worldwide, the general surgeons' opinion on MIPD remains skeptical. Initial presented results on LPD were quite heterogenous. On one hand reports from high-volume referral centers supported the safety of the procedure not observing an increase in morbidity and mortality and even proposing some benefits provided by minimally invasive approach such as reduced intraoperative blood loss and length of stay at the expense of a longer operative time [6, 11, 14, 17, 24, 25, 32, 50]. On the other hand, distinct results were reported in the case of low-volume centers and not dedicated pancreatic surgeons. A real-world US portrait was presented by Adam et al. [2] in a nation-wide analysis which included 7061 pancreaticoduodenectomies, of which 52% performed in low-volume centers showing that the rate of PD performed with a minimally invasive approach attested at 14% with an associated increase in postoperative mortality and lack of observed advantages. More authors in monocentric series reported suboptimal results such as higher rate of severe morbidity, grade C-POPF, post-pancreatectomy hemorrhage, and reoperation rate in case of LPD [12, 16]. Trying to provide high-quality evidence on safety and feasibility of LPD, a collective effort was put in producing randomized clinical trials comparing LPD to OPD. The first two monocentric Indian [39] and Spanish [40] RCTs supported the diffusion of LPD, showing comparable morbidity and mortality rate relatively to open and an advantage in terms of reduced length of stay. Moreover, the PLOT study [39] reported a reduced estimated blood loss and rate of surgical site infections, while the PADULAP trial [40] reported a decrease major morbidity rate and reintervention rate in the case of LPD. Unfortunately, the multicentric LEOPARD 2 trial [47] from Netherlands depicted a different picture, the trial was interrupted early due to safety concerns with a reported mortality of 10% in the LPD group. Reportedly, operating surgeons had a personal experience of more than 20 LPDs before trial initiation. This experience raised some relevant concerns on the real number of procedures necessary to master the technique and on the patients' safety during this initial phase of the learning curve. The largest and most recent trial focusing on LPD by Wang et al. [49], reassured to some extent the scientific community showing how in experienced and trained hands LPD can be implemented safely without endangering the patient, nevertheless failed to demonstrate a substantial benefit of this technique over the open approach.

With a more widespread availability of robotic platform and a decrease in cost, we are observing in recent years a net shift toward RPD, with more and more surgeons worldwide approaching MIPS through robotic platform. A recently published monocentric RCT, the EUROPA trial [30], compared 29 RPD to 33 OPD showing comparable results in terms of postoperative morbidity and mortality, with no mortality events observed in the robotic group. Therefore, relatively to the primary endpoint of the study, cumulative postoperative morbidity within 90 days, RPD appeared comparable to OPD. Nevertheless, it reported an increase in incidence of grade B/C pancreas-specific complication in addition to increased operative time and higher cost. Concretely, the only complication that occurred more frequently in the robotic arm was grade B/C DGE, with as proposed explanation the use of different techniques used for reconstruction, notably manual anastomosis in open and mechanical anastomosis in robotic arm; moreover, 72% of patients in the robotic arm underwent a pylorus-resecting PD versus only 39% in the open arm.

Moreover, it needs to be noted that in the robotic arm 17% of patients required a venous resection, 14% an additional organ resection, and 20% of cases required conversion, and for both RPD and OPD, reported operative time and estimated blood loss were greater than those of the reported in analogous RCTs suggesting the complexity of enrolled cases. These results underly the importance of patients' selection in case of MIPS and how, despite its safety in experienced hand, it may still be overperformed by open surgery in case of intrinsically challenging cases. The latest published Chinese RCT by Liu [35] presented encouraging results, showing not only a similar morbidity and mortality across the two approaches but also a decreased operative time, estimated blood loss, and postoperative length of stay in case of a robotic approach.

Currently, high-level evidence demonstrating the superiority of one minimally invasive approach over the other is lacking but registries and surveys are reporting a growing preference toward RPD [4, 19, 21, 26, 27, 36, 38]. A recent snapshot of Italian clinical practice from the Italian Group of Minimally Invasive Pancreatic Surgery showed how more than 60% of MIPD in the Italian territory are performed robotically [7], while an International Survey on MIPS practice reported how from 2016 to 2022 the percentage of LPD decreased from 51% to 36.8% and the proportion of RPD increased from 23% to 47.9% [48].

Confirming these findings, the preliminary results of the DIPLOMA-2 trial [15, 18], presented in May 2024 at the IHPBA Meeting in Cape Town, comparing OPD to MIPD reported how around 90% of included MIPD were carried out robotically. Moreover, it is worth reporting how, in this large trial enrolling 288 patients from 14 centers across 6 European countries, the short-term outcomes leaned in favor of MIPD with a comparable CCI and mortality rate among groups, and a significantly decrease in CR-POPF rate (23% vs. 36%), surgical site infection rate (13% vs. 23%), length of stay (9 vs. 11 days), and time to functional recovery (7 vs. 8 days) in case of MIPD. These results, most likely, reflected the strict criteria for center inclusion, with surgeon previous experience of >60 MIPD, reporting the outcomes of few excellent centers.

Results of Minimally Invasive versus Open Pancreaticoduodenectomy published Randomized Clinical Trials are summarized in Table 1.1.

Table 1.1 Minimally invasive versus open pancreaticoduodenectomy published randomized clinical trials

RCTs	*N*	OT, min	EBL, ml	CR-POPF, %	Severe morbidity (CD ≥ 3), %	LOS, days	90-day mortality, %
Palanivelu 2017 (PLOT) Lps vs. Open	32 vs. 32	**359 vs. 320**	**250 vs. 401**	6 vs. 12	9 vs. 12	**7 vs. 13**	3 vs. 3
Poves 2018 (PADULAP) Lps vs. Open	34 vs. 32	**486 vs. 365**	–	13 vs. 28	**16 vs. 38**	**13.5 vs. 17**	0 vs. 2
Van Hilst 2019 (LEOPARD 2) Lps vs. Open	50 vs. 59	**410 vs. 274**	300 vs. 450	28 vs. 24	50 vs. 39	11 vs. 10	10 vs. 2
Wang 2021 Lps vs. Open	297 vs. 297	**325 vs. 300**	**200 vs. 300**	10 vs. 11	29 vs. 23	**15 vs. 16**	2 vs. 2
Klotz 2024 (EUROPA) Robotic vs. Open	29 vs. 33	**431 vs. 367**	742 vs. 814	38 vs. 21	–	17 vs. 13	0 vs. 9
Liu 2024 Robotic vs. Open	81 vs. 80	**245 vs. 298**	**245 vs. 298**	14 vs. 13	22 vs. 24	**11 vs. 13.5**	1 vs. 1

CD Clavien-Dindo, *OT* operative time, *EBL* estimated blood loss, *CR-POPF* clinically relevant postoperative pancreatic fistula, *LOS* length of stay, *Lps* laparoscopic, **Bold** $p < 0.05$

1.3 Minimally Invasive Pancreaticoduodenectomy for Pancreatic Ductal Adenocarcinoma

Despite the growing body of evidence, it remains difficult to draw definitive conclusion on the role of MIPD for cancer. On one hand, resection for cancer entails a more radical and therefore challenging surgical procedure; on the other hand, it is the field in which patients may get the most advantage, firstly, the robotic platform may allow an easier and more extended dissection thanks to the magnified vision and flexible instrumentation, and secondly, a faster recovery from surgery may lead to an easier access to adjuvant therapy. The majority of available comparative studies do not focus exclusively on pancreatic resection for cancer, concentrating on safety of MIPD. Nevertheless, stratifying the data for oncological head resections, the majority of the available literature, including retrospective and prospective studies, reports a similar rate of R0 resections and number of harvested lymph nodes among the two techniques with a few reports even proposing a superiority of robotic approach [9, 13, 22, 29, 32, 34, 37, 41, 42, 45, 52]. A recent metanalysis by Kamarajah et al. [28] focused on long-term oncological outcomes after pancreatic resections and reported similar 5-year overall survival (OS) after OPD and MIPD performed for pancreatic cancer. Similarly, Sun et al. [43] reported a similar OS in OPD and MIPS and a better DFS in case of MIPD, and Chen et al. [10] observed a higher 3-, 4-, and 5-year survival in case of MIPD. When analyzing these results, it is imperative to take into account the selection bias factor, because in absence of randomization or patients' matching, fitter patients with smaller lesions will be more frequently selected for minimally invasive approach and the open approach will be only reserved for more advanced lesions and unfit patients, who may be unfit to aggressive chemotherapy regimens as well. Overcoming these biases, all the available RCTs comparing OPD and MIPD have reported a comparable R0 resection rate and number of harvested lymph nodes, providing a good estimate of the oncological appropriateness of a minimally invasive resection. Nevertheless, whether these findings translate in a long-term survival benefit remains unclear. A 2022 monocentric study from Leuven [44], in which patients were matched using propensity score models reported a better median disease free and overall survival in the case of minimally invasive pancreatic resection. Nevertheless, high-level evidence will only be provided by RCTs providing patients' long-term oncological outcomes. In the current era of neoadjuvant therapy and increasing treatment opportunities for borderline resectable and locally advanced patients, the role of MIPD in cases of tumor vascular involvement cannot be overlooked. Few reports are available in the literature regarding its feasibility. Nevertheless, despite acceptable morbidity and mortality reported by a few dedicated, experienced centers, the majority of the surgical community still considers vascular involvement a contraindication to a minimally invasive approach [3, 8, 33, 51].

1.4 Evidence-Based Guidelines

Currently, scientific community has produced two international evidence-based guidelines papers on MIPS, The Miami guidelines [5] published in 2020 after a worldwide consensus meeting and the European Brescia Guidelines [1] published in 2024. Despite conspicuous number of scientific reports published between the two consensus meetings, both provide similar statements relatively to MIPD: LPD and RPD appear to be acceptable alternative to OPD for both benign/premalignant lesions and periampullary and pancreatic cancers when performed by experienced surgeons in the context of high-volume centers. In accordance with available literature, as showed earlier, the evidence remains low and the recommendation weak. The Miami guidelines conclude relatively to PD that there is insufficient data to recommend MIPD over OPD and that a strict outcome monitoring is recommended through inclusion to registries (GRADE 2A). Nevertheless, they add how both approaches, MIPD and OPD, are valid for selected patients with adenocarcinoma, with a lower degree of evidence (GRADE 2B). Regarding the always contemporary comparison among RPD and LPD, in light of the absence of evidence of a clear superiority of one approach of the other, the guidelines conclude how surgeon training, experience, and available resources currently guide which approach to utilize (GRADE 2C). The most recent Brescia Guidelines divide the recommendations based on the indications and the type of minimally invasive technique utilized. Regarding the role of both LPD and RPD in the management of benign and premalignant lesions of pancreatic head, the statement recites that both MI approaches can be considered as an alternative approach OPD, when performed by experienced surgeons in high-volume centers with a low-evidence level and a weak form of recommendation (GRADE 2C). Moving to malignant lesions, for pancreatic head PDAC, both RPD and LPD represent acceptable alternative. For LPD, the evidence level was high with weak recommendation (GRADE 2A) and that for RPD was low with weak recommendation (GRADE 2C), reflecting the absence of published RCTs on RPD at the time when the consensus meeting was held, in September 2022. Even in this case, the limitation to experienced surgeons and high-volume centers setting is underlined and the authors added how these MIPD cases need to be included in registries and prospectively maintained database to follow outcomes. Superimposable conclusions were drawn in the setting of resectable non pancreatic periampullary adenocarcinomas (GRADE 2C).

Despite this lack of definitive evidence, the process of MIPD implementation is unstoppable, with more and more surgeons worldwide starting their learning curve. In this evolving panorama, it is crucial the need to ensure patients safety through a structured and recognized training program and through outcomes monitoring via inclusion of cases in national and international registries.

References

1. Abu Hilal M, Van Ramshorst TME, Boggi U, et al. The Brescia internationally validated European guidelines on minimally invasive pancreatic surgery (EGUMIPS). Ann Surg. 2024;279:45–57.
2. Adam MA, Choudhury K, Goffredo P, et al. Minimally invasive distal pancreatectomy for cancer: short-term oncologic outcomes in 1733 patients. World J Surg. 2015;39:2564–72. https://doi.org/10.1007/s00268-015-3138-x.
3. Addeo P. Minimally invasive pancreaticoduodenectomy with venous resection: results of a systematic review. Mini-invasive Surg. 2020;4:64.
4. Valle V, Pakataridis P, Marchese T, et al. Comparative analysis of open, laparoscopic, and robotic pancreaticoduodenectomy: a systematic review of randomized controlled trials. Medicina (Kaunas). 2025;61(7):1121. https://doi.org/10.3390/medicina61071121. PMID: 40731751; PMCID: PMC12298437.
5. Asbun HJ, Moekotte AL, Vissers FL, et al. The Miami international evidence-based guidelines on minimally invasive pancreas resection. Ann Surg. 2020; https://doi.org/10.1097/SLA.0000000000003590.
6. Asbun HJ, Stauffer JA. Laparoscopic vs open pancreaticoduodenectomy: overall outcomes and severity of complications using the accordion severity grading system. J Am Coll Surg. 2012;215:810.
7. Boggi U, Donisi G, Napoli N, et al. Prospective minimally invasive pancreatic resections from the IGOMIPS registry: a snapshot of daily practice in Italy on 1191 between 2019 and 2022. Updat Surg. 2023;75:1439–56. https://doi.org/10.1007/s13304-023-01592-7.
8. Boggi U, Napoli N, Costa F, et al. Robotic-assisted pancreatic resections. World J Surg. 2016;40:1. https://doi.org/10.1007/s00268-016-3565-3.
9. Chapman BC, Gajdos C, Hosokawa P, et al. Comparison of laparoscopic to open pancreaticoduodenectomy in elderly patients with pancreatic adenocarcinoma. Surg Endosc. 2018;32:2239–48. https://doi.org/10.1007/s00464-017-5915-0.
10. Chen K, Zhou Y, Jin W, et al. Laparoscopic pancreaticoduodenectomy versus open pancreaticoduodenectomy for pancreatic ductal adenocarcinoma: oncologic outcomes and long-term survival. Surg Endosc. 2020;34:1948–58. https://doi.org/10.1007/s00464-019-06968-8.
11. Chen XM, Sun DL, Zhang Y. Laparoscopic versus open pancreaticoduodenectomy combined with uncinated process approach: a comparative study evaluating perioperative outcomes (retrospective cohort study). Int J Surg. 2018;51:170–3. https://doi.org/10.1016/j.ijsu.2018.01.038.

12. Chopinet S, Fuks D, Rinaudo M, et al. Postoperative bleeding after laparoscopic pancreaticoduodenectomy: the Achilles' heel? World J Surg. 2018;42:1. https://doi.org/10.1007/s00268-017-4269-z.
13. Croome KP, Farnell MB, Que FG, et al. Total laparoscopic pancreaticoduodenectomy for pancreatic ductal adenocarcinoma: oncologic advantages over open approaches? Ann Surg. 2014;260:633.
14. Dang C, Wang M, Zhu F, et al. Comparison of laparoscopic and open pancreaticoduodenectomy for the treatment of nonpancreatic periampullary adenocarcinomas: a propensity score matching analysis. Am J Surg. 2021;222:377–82. https://doi.org/10.1016/j.amjsurg.2020.12.023.
15. de Graaf N, Emmen AMLH, Ramera M, et al. Minimally invasive versus open pancreatoduodenectomy for pancreatic and peri-ampullary neoplasm (DIPLOMA-2): study protocol for an international multicenter patient-blinded randomized controlled trial. Trials. 2023;24. https://doi.org/10.1186/s13063-023-07657-7.
16. Dokmak S, Ftériche FS, Aussilhou B, et al. Laparoscopic pancreaticoduodenectomy should not be routine for resection of periampullary tumors. J Am Coll Surg. 2015;220:831–8. https://doi.org/10.1016/j.jamcollsurg.2014.12.052.
17. El Nakeeb A, Attia M, El Sorogy M, et al. Laparoscopic pancreaticodudenectomy for periampullary tumor: should it be a routine? A propensity score–matched study. Surg Laparosc Endosc Percutan Tech. 2020;30:7.
18. Emmen AMLH, de Graaf N, Ramera M, et al. Minimally invasive versus open pancreatoduodenectomy for pancreatic and periampullary neoplasm (DIPLOMA-2): an international patient-blinded randomized trial. HPB. 2024a;26:S42–3. https://doi.org/10.1016/j.hpb.2024.03.072.
19. Emmen AMLH, Zwart MJW, Khatkov IE, et al. Robot-assisted versus laparoscopic pancreatoduodenectomy: a pan-European multicenter propensity-matched study. Surgery (United States). 2024b;175:1587–94. https://doi.org/10.1016/j.surg.2024.02.015.
20. Gagner M, Pomp A. Laparoscopic pylorus-preserving pancreatoduodenectomy. Surg Endosc. 1994;8(5):408–10.
21. Gavriilidis P, Lim C, Menahem B, et al. Robotic versus laparoscopic distal pancreatectomy—the first meta-analysis. HPB. 2016;18:567–74. https://doi.org/10.1016/j.hpb.2016.04.008.
22. Girgis MD, Zenati MS, King JC, et al. Oncologic outcomes after robotic pancreatic resections are not inferior to open surgery. Ann Surg. 2021;274:e262.
23. Giulianotti PC, Coratti A, Angelini M, et al. Robotics in general surgery personal experience in a large community hospital. Arch Surg. 2003;138(7):777–84.
24. Han SH, Kang CM, Hwang HK, et al. The Yonsei experience of 104 laparoscopic pancreaticoduodenectomies: a propensity score-matched analysis with open pancreaticoduodenectomy. Surg Endosc. 2020;34:1658–64. https://doi.org/10.1007/s00464-019-06942-4.
25. Ielpo B, Caruso R, Duran H, et al. Robotic versus standard open pancreatectomy: a propensity score-matched analysis comparison. Updat Surg. 2019;71:137–44. https://doi.org/10.1007/s13304-018-0529-1.
26. Jiang DJ, Hogg ME. Robotic pancreaticoduodenectomy versus laparoscopic pancreaticoduodenectomy. Laparosc Surg. 2021:1–7. https://doi.org/10.21037/ls-20-53.
27. Kamarajah SK, Bundred J, Saint MO, et al. Robotic versus conventional laparoscopic pancreaticoduodenectomy a systematic review and meta-analysis. Eur J Surg Oncol. 2020;46:6–14.
28. Kamarajah SK, Gujjuri R, Bundred JR, et al. Long-term survival after minimally invasive resection versus open pancreaticoduodenectomy for periampullary cancers: a systematic review, meta-analysis and meta-regression. HPB. 2021;23:197–205.
29. Kantor O, Talamonti MS, Sharpe S, et al. Laparoscopic pancreaticoduodenectomy for adenocarcinoma provides short-term oncologic outcomes and long-term overall survival rates similar to those for open pancreaticoduodenectomy. Am J Surg. 2017;213:512–5. https://doi.org/10.1016/j.amjsurg.2016.10.030.
30. Klotz R, Mihaljevic AL, Kulu Y, et al. Robotic versus open partial pancreatoduodenectomy (EUROPA): a randomised controlled stage 2b trial. 2024; https://doi.org/10.1016/j.lanepe.2024.100900.
31. Krautz C, Nimptsch U, Weber GF, et al. Effect of hospital volume on in-hospital morbidity and mortality following pancreatic surgery in Germany. Ann Surg. 2018;267:411–7. https://doi.org/10.1097/SLA.0000000000002248.
32. Kuesters S, Chikhladze S, Makowiec F, et al. Oncological outcome of laparoscopically assisted pancreatoduodenectomy for ductal adenocarcinoma in a retrospective cohort study. Int J Surg. 2018;55:162–6. https://doi.org/10.1016/j.ijsu.2018.05.026.
33. Kung JWC, Parks RW. Vascular resections in minimally invasive surgery for pancreatic cancer. Laparosc Endosc Robot Surg. 2022;5:3–9.
34. Kwon J, Song KB, Park SY, et al. Comparison of minimally invasive versus open pancreatoduodenectomy for pancreatic ductal adenocarcinoma: a propensity score matching analysis. Cancers (Basel). 2020;12. https://doi.org/10.3390/cancers12040982.
35. Liu Q, Li M, Gao Y, et al. Effect of robotic versus open pancreaticoduodenectomy on postoperative length of hospital stay and complications for pancreatic head or periampullary tumours: a multicentre, open-label randomised controlled trial. Lancet Gastroenterol Hepatol. 2024; https://doi.org/10.1016/s2468-1253(24)00005-0.
36. Lof S, Vissers FL, Klompmaker S, et al. Risk of conversion to open surgery during robotic and laparoscopic pancreatoduodenectomy and effect on outcomes: international propensity score-matched

comparison study. Br J Surg. 2021;108:80–7. https://doi.org/10.1093/bjs/znaa026.
37. Nussbaum DP, Adam MA, Youngwirth LM, et al. Minimally invasive pancreaticoduodenectomy does not improve use or time to initiation of adjuvant chemotherapy for patients with pancreatic adenocarcinoma. Ann Surg Oncol. 2016;23:1026–33. https://doi.org/10.1245/s10434-015-4937-x.
38. Ouyang L, Zhang J, Feng Q, et al. Robotic versus laparoscopic pancreaticoduodenectomy: an up-to-date system review and meta-analysis search strategy and study selection. Front Oncol. 2022;12:1–10. https://doi.org/10.3389/fonc.2022.834382.
39. Palanivelu C, Senthilnathan P, Sabnis SC, et al. Randomized clinical trial of laparoscopic versus open pancreatoduodenectomy for periampullary tumours. Br J Surg. 2017;104(11):1443–50. https://doi.org/10.1002/bjs.10662.
40. Poves I, Burdío F, Morató O, et al. Comparison of perioperative outcomes between laparoscopic and open approach for pancreatoduodenectomy: the Padulap randomized controlled trial. In: Annals of surgery. Lippincott Williams and Wilkins; 2018. p. 731–9.
41. Sharpe SM, Talamonti MS, Wang CE, et al. Early National experience with laparoscopic pancreaticoduodenectomy for ductal adenocarcinoma: a comparison of laparoscopic pancreaticoduodenectomy and open pancreaticoduodenectomy from the National Cancer Data Base. J Am Coll Surg. 2015;221:175.
42. Stauffer JA, Coppola A, Villacreses D, et al. Laparoscopic versus open pancreaticoduodenectomy for pancreatic adenocarcinoma: long-term results at a single institution. Surg Endosc. 2017;31:2233–41. https://doi.org/10.1007/s00464-016-5222-1.
43. Sun R, Yu J, Zhang Y, et al. Perioperative and oncological outcomes following minimally invasive versus open pancreaticoduodenectomy for pancreatic duct adenocarcinoma. Surg Endosc. 2021;35:2273–85. https://doi.org/10.1007/s00464-020-07641-1.
44. Topal H, Aerts R, Laenen A, et al. Survival after minimally invasive vs open surgery for pancreatic adenocarcinoma. JAMA Netw Open. 2022;5:E2248147. https://doi.org/10.1001/jamanetworkopen.2022.48147.
45. Uijterwijk BA, Wei K, Kasai M, et al. Minimally invasive versus open pancreatoduodenectomy for pancreatic ductal adenocarcinoma: individual patient data meta-analysis of randomized trials. Eur J Surg Oncol. 2023;49:1351–61. https://doi.org/10.1016/j.ejso.2023.03.227.
46. Underwood PW, Gerber MH, Hughes SJ. Pitfalls of minimally invasive pancreatoduodenectomy. Ann Pancreat Cancer. 2019;2:2. https://doi.org/10.21037/apc.2018.12.02.
47. van Hilst J, De Rooij T, Bosscha K, et al. Laparoscopic versus open pancreatoduodenectomy for pancreatic or periampullary tumours (LEOPARD-2): a multicentre, patient-blinded, randomised controlled phase 2/3 trial. Lancet Gastroenterol Hepatol. 2019;4:199–207. https://doi.org/10.1016/S2468-1253(19)30004-4.
48. van Ramshorst TME, van Hilst J, Bannone E, et al. International survey on opinions and use of robot-assisted and laparoscopic minimally invasive pancreatic surgery: 5-year follow up. HPB. 2024;26:63–72. https://doi.org/10.1016/j.hpb.2023.09.004.
49. Wang M, Li D, Chen R, et al. Laparoscopic versus open pancreatoduodenectomy for pancreatic or periampullary tumours: a multicentre, open-label, randomised controlled trial. Lancet Gastroenterol Hepatol. 2021;6:438–47. https://doi.org/10.1016/S2468-1253(21)00054-6.
50. Yan Y, Hua Y, Chang C, et al. Laparoscopic versus open pancreaticoduodenectomy for pancreatic and periampullary tumor: a meta-analysis of randomized controlled trials and non-randomized comparative studies. Front Oncol. 2023;12:1093395.
51. Yang E, Chong Y, Wang Z, et al. Minimally-invasive versus open pancreatoduodenectomies with vascular resection: a 1:1 propensity-matched comparison study. J Minim Access Surg. 2022;18:420–5. https://doi.org/10.4103/jmas.jmas_201_21.
52. Zhou W, Jin W, Wang D, et al. Laparoscopic versus open pancreaticoduodenectomy for pancreatic ductal adenocarcinoma: a propensity score matching analysis. Cancer Commun. 2019;39. https://doi.org/10.1186/s40880-019-0410-8.

Benchmarking in Pancreatoduodenectomy

2

María Martín Ramos and Patricia Sánchez-Velázquez

2.1 Benchmarking in Healthcare

2.1.1 Definition

Originally, benchmarking was conceived as a tool in industry and economics to evaluate and promote quality. The aim was to establish a comparison among the best-performing results, identify how these organizations operated, and adopt the best ideas to improve one's outcomes. In healthcare, benchmarking has been defined as a process of comparative evaluation and identification of the underlying causes leading to high levels of performance [1]. The goal of benchmarking is to identify areas for improvement by comparing with realistic outcomes rather than merely the average ones, as often happens in routine practice, thereby pushing clinicians to perform at their highest possible level [2, 3]. By identifying potential improvements, this process encourages clinicians to pursue excellence.

Benchmarking serves as a robust methodology to facilitate constructive comparisons and also foster discussions among different cohort groups such as types of patients, centers, geographical areas, or even countries [4]. This practice promotes the sharing of methods and results, leading to effective communication and the potential for visits to other institutions to learn about their practices. As benchmarking helps identify potential differences among practitioners and indicates which practices lead to the best results, it promotes homogenization in healthcare performance [3]. However, it is not a static snapshot; it is designed as a tool for continuous quality improvement. The essence of benchmarking is to share, analyze, and implement changes constantly. This ongoing flow of information can offer new options and perspectives on the subject, contributing to the enhancement of healthcare, training, and surgical techniques [5].

2.1.2 Steps for Implementing Benchmarking in Surgery

Staiger et al. (2019), in their paper in *Annals of Surgery*, suggest several steps that can be followed to identify and apply benchmarking in surgical procedures [2]:

1. *Define the event of interest*: Focus on complex events with a high risk of poor outcomes, as these have greater potential for improvement. For example, pancreaticoduodenectomy, which is among the general surgery procedures with the highest complication rates, can particularly benefit from benchmarking assessments.
2. *Select the group of patients*: For the selection of patients and hospitals in benchmarking, it

M. M. Ramos · P. Sánchez-Velázquez (✉)
HPB Unit, Hospital del Mar, Barcelona, Spain
e-mail: maria.martin.ramos@psmar.cat; psanchezvelazquez@psmar.cat

B. Ielpo et al. (eds.), *Minimally Invasive Pancreatoduodenectomy in Cancer*,
https://doi.org/10.1007/978-3-031-99695-5_2

is important to establish clear selection criteria and clearly define the exclusion criteria.

3. *Determine endpoints*: It is crucial for benchmarking to target clinically relevant endpoints. The parameters studied need to be objective, anonymous, universally applicable, simple to interpret, up to date, have clear exclusion criteria, and be uniform.
4. *Choose the number of centers needed*: The greater the differences in results, the more centers are required.
5. *Find collaborating centers*: Collect the necessary data, with leader-to-leader communication being the most efficient method.
6. *Calculate benchmark values*: Determine benchmark cutoffs for each endpoint. Although several methodologies have been proposed, there is no standardized procedure for establishing benchmarking values. Weissman et al. (1999) proposed the Achievable Benchmark of Care (ABC), which uses an unselected cohort and benchmarks the tenth percentile of the median value across all centers. This approach includes real-life surgical patients rather than only low-risk ones, setting it apart from the "best patient in the best center" (BPBC) method [6]. In the BPBC method, the cutoff point for a benchmarking indicator is set above the 75th percentile of the median value for each indicator across organizations, but only for low-risk patients in high-volume units. This percentile represents the threshold for the best possible achievable outcome for a given parameter.

   The Expert Delphi Consensus in 2022 endorsed the best patient in best center (BPBC) methodology as the preferred approach [7]. However, Van Horst et al. (2022) proposed a method that balances both ABC and BPBC, establishing different benchmarks for different risk groups using ABC benchmarks to evaluate individual surgeons and BPBC to compare departments or hospitals [8].
7. *Analyse the gap*: Assess the gap within the established benchmark values.
8. *Perform modifications*: Implement necessary changes to drive improvement.

Upon reaching the final step, the benchmarking process should restart with new topics of interest identified during the previous cycle, as it is designed to be a tool for continuous improvement and support for change.

2.1.3 Application of Benchmarking in Pancreatoduodenectomy

Benchmarking is particularly crucial in high-complexity procedures, as it allows for comparisons among the limited number of centers that perform these techniques. Pancreatoduodenectomy, a procedure with significant impact on patient outcomes due to its high morbidity and mortality rates, serves as a prime example. Postoperative complications from this surgery affect health, quality of life, and healthcare costs. The purpose of benchmarking in this context is to reduce morbidity by comparing outcomes with the optimal and achievable standards [2].

Moreover, in the era of minimally invasive surgery, it is crucial to have realistic comparison tools that allow for meaningful evaluations of new techniques such as laparoscopic and robotic PD.

In pancreatic surgery, there have been attempts to establish outcome comparisons using average performance from various cohort studies as a cut-off value. However, these studies often lack a structured methodology that enables reliable comparisons and therefore the extrapolation of outcomes to other populations or patient groups. In recent years, several publications in the field of pancreatic surgery have focused on establishing benchmark outcomes, primarily using the BPBC methodology. Among these, two studies stand out when discussing pancreaticoduodenectomy:

In 2019, Sánchez-Velázquez et al. [4] conducted a multicentric study involving 23 international renowned expert centers in pancreatic surgery, analyzing a total of 6186 PDs. These high-volume centers for pancreatic surgery (performing ≥50 complex pancreatic interventions per year, with relevant publications in the field and a maintained prospective database) from Europe, Asia, and America compiled the "best center" definition and focused on a target population without significant comorbidities (i.e., "benchmark cases").The rationale behind this selection is to pursue excellence and, therefore, to emulate the best performance in patients where optimal outcomes are expected.

The data were analyzed to establish 20 clinically relevant outcome benchmarks for pancreaticoduodenectomy (PD), derived from the 75th percentile of the medians for each outcome indicator across centers, based on a cohort of low-risk patients. Only patients with a minimum follow-up of 1 year were included, with outcomes evaluated at discharge and periodically at 3, 6, and 12 months. The 6-month period was chosen as the cutoff because overall median cumulative patient morbidity, as measured by the Comprehensive Complication Index (CCI), is known to increase up to 2.4 times from the initial hospital discharge (20.9 vs. 8.6) (Table 2.1). Beyond this point, CCI did not increase significantly. Therefore, reliable outcome reports should cover at least the first six postoperative months.

This study was the first to establish key benchmark parameters for pancreatic surgery, including a clinically relevant pancreatic fistula (CR-POPF) rate of less than 19%, indicating that all surgeons should aim for this target, along with a desired mortality rate of under 1.6%. Additionally, it provided benchmarks for oncological indicators, such as 1-year disease-free survival and the minimum number of desired harvested lymph nodes. The study also revealed significant variation in the proportion of benchmark cases relative to the total number of pancreaticoduodenectomy (PD) cases across centers. Interestingly, centers with a higher proportion of "low-risk patients" experienced higher rates of index complications, such as pancreatic fistula. One possible explanation is that handling a higher proportion of complex cases enhances surgeons' skills and improves the effectiveness of the multidisciplinary team, leading to a reduction in failure-to-rescue rates, which the paper suggests should be kept under 9%.

Table 2.1 The 20 outcome measurements established for low-risk cases from the 23 international high-volume centers

	Median across the 23 centers (range)	Benchmark cutoff
Operating duration	6.1 h (3.4–8.6)	≤ 7.5 h
Blood transfusions	13% (2–36.4)	≤ 23%
Hospital stay	12 d (6–31)	≤ 15 d
Postoperative 6-mo morbidity		
Patients with at least 1 complication (graded as Clavien-Dindo)	65.3% (43.5–89.6)	≤ 73%
Patients with complication grades I–III	53% (30.6–86.5)	≤ 62%
Patients with complication grades ≥ III	19% (4.4–52.3)	≤ 30%
Patients with complication grade IV	2% (0–14)	≤ 5%
CCI®[a]	20.9 (0–33.5)	≤ 20.9
Pancreatic fistula rate (ISGPF classification B–C)	10% (0–35.4)	≤ 19%
Grade B	8% (0–35.4)	≤ 15%
Grade C	2% (0–12)	≤ 5%
Biochemical leak	8% (1.3–22.7)	≤ 13%
Severe postoperative bleeding (≥III)	4% (0–14)	≤ 7%
In-hospital mortality	0% (0–4)	≤ 1.6%
Failure-to-rescue rate	0% (0–25)	≤ 9%
Readmission rate	16% (1.6–29.1)	≤ 21%
Oncological outcomes in patients with PADC (*n* = 1091)		
R1 rate	27% (2.3–67)	≤ 39%
Number of lymph nodes resected	19 (14–43)	≥ 16%
1-year DFS survival (actual)	42% (22.6–100)	≥ 53%
3-year DFS survival (actuarial)	0% (0–15.4)	≥ 9%

From Sánchez-Velázquez et al. [4]
[a]CCI® ranges from 0 (no complication) to 100 (death)

To illustrate a practical application of the benchmark tool, the authors selected three different cohorts of minimally invasive pancreatoduodenectomy (MIPD) performed in three high-volume centers (see Table 2.2). The comparison revealed some discrepancies in surgical outcomes. As expected, there were differences in surgical time across the centers, with minimally invasive approaches generally taking longer. However, the analysis also uncovered higher rates of clinically relevant postoperative pancreatic fistula (CR-POPF) and increased mortality in one of the centers whereas this fact was not the same in the others. This variation underscores the importance of applying benchmark values to assess and improve the quality of surgical care, highlighting that even among high-volume centers, outcomes can vary significantly. This comparison, while based on a small cohort of patients and acknowledging its limitations, sug-

Table 2.2 Comparison of benchmarks in four different cohorts: one cohort with a poorer preoperative physical status (ASA ≥ 3) and three single-center MIS cohorts

	ASA class ≥3 (*n* = 931)	Center MIS 1 (*n* = 8)	Center MIS 2 (*n* = 8)	Center MIS 3 (*n* = 62)	Benchmark cutoff (75th percentile of medians from 23 centers)
% Benchmark cases		8/37 (22%)	8/51 (16%)	62/100 (62%)	–
Operating duration	6 h	**7.6 h**	n.a.	**8.3 h**[b]	≤7.5 h
Blood transfusions	14.7%	12.5%	n.a.	4.8%	≤23%
Hospital stay	10d	4.5d	6.5d	16d	≤ 16d
Postoperative 6-mo morbidity					
Patients with at least 1 complication (graded as Clavien-Dindo)	60%	38%	63%	68%	≤73%
Patients with complication grades I–III	50%	38%	12.5%	62%	≤62%
Patients with complication grades ≥ III	19%	13%	**50%**[b]	13%	≤30%
Patients with a complication grade IV	4%	0%	0%	0	≤5%
CCI®[a]	20.9	4	17.5	20.9	≤20.9
Pancreatic fistula rate (ISGPF classification B–C)	10%	13%	0%	**23%**[b]	≤19%
Grade B	7%	13%	0%	**21%**[b]	≤15%
Grade C	3%	0%	0%	2%	≤5%
Biochemical leak	5%	13%	0%	8%	≤13%
Severe postoperative bleeding (≥III)	3%	0%	0%	**10%**[b]	≤7%
In-hospital mortality	**3%**[b]	0%	0%	**3%**[b]	≤1.6%
Failure-to-rescue rate	**16%**[b]	0%	0%	**25%**[b]	≤9%
Readmission rate	20%	**25%**[b]	**50%**[b]	7%	≤21%
Oncological outcomes in patients with PADC (*n* = 1091)					
R1 rate	21%	0	n.a	n.a.	≤38%
Number of lymph nodes resected	22	32	**13**[b]	35	≥16
1-year DFS survival (actual)	**41%**[b]	n.a.	n.a.	n.a.	≥53%
3-year DFS survival (actuarial)	**2.5%**[b]	n.a.	n.a.	n.a.	≥9%

From Sánchez-Velázquez et al. [4]

[a] CCI ranges from 0 (no complication) to 100 (death)

[b]Values are outside of the benchmark

gests that some groups performing MIPD achieved outcomes comparable to those seen with the open approach. Despite variations in surgical time and higher rates of certain complications in specific centers, the overall data indicate that MIPD, when performed by experienced teams in high-volume centers, can yield results on par with traditional open PD. This finding supports the potential for minimally invasive techniques to be a viable alternative to open surgery in selected cases.

In 2020, the same research group published a follow-up study that established 19 benchmarks for pancreaticoduodenectomy (PD) with porto-mesenteric venous resection (PVR) [9]. Using a similar methodology, they conducted a multi-center study involving nearly the same 23 international expert centers in pancreatic surgery, analyzing 1462 patients undergoing PD with PVR. The benchmark values were again defined as the 75th percentile for outcome parameters where higher values are associated with worse outcomes (e.g., mortality and morbidity) and the 25th percentile for variables where lower values indicate worse outcomes (e.g., R0 resection or 1-year survival rates).

The study revealed higher cut-offs for in-hospital mortality rates (4% vs. 1.6%) and overall complication rates compared to PD alone, which was expected given the added morbidity from vascular resection. However, procedure-associated complications were similar between PD with PVR and PD alone. Significant differences among centers were observed in the 90-day CCI, major complications (Clavien-Dindo ≥3a), and in-hospital mortality rates. Notably, there was no correlation between the volume of procedures performed at a center and postoperative morbidity, which the authors attributed to the inclusion of only high-volume centers. Regarding different PVR techniques, only splenic vein ligation was associated with a slight increase in morbidity. No significant differences in morbidity were found among other types of PVR or reconstruction techniques (Table 2.3).

Table 2.3 Outcome benchmarks for PD with PVR in 840 low-risk cases

Benchmark cutoffs				
Operation duration	<8 h			
Intraoperative blood transfusion rate	≤27%			
Intensive therapy unit stay	≤1 day			
Hospital stay	≤14 day			
Postoperative morbidity	**At discharge**	**At 90 d**	**At 6 mo**	
Any complication	≤79%	≤83%	≤83%	
Clavien-Dindo grade ≥ 3a	≤28%	≤34%	≤36%	
Comprehensive complications index (CCI)	<21	≤23%	≤26%	
Pancreatic leak rate (all grades) (ISGPF)	≤19%			
Clinically relevant POPF (grades B or C)	≤14%			
Severe postoperative bleeding grade ≥ 3a	≤7%			
In-hospital mortality	≤4%			
1-year hospital readmission rate	≤32%			
Portal vein thrombosis rate	≤14%			
Occlusive only rate	≤4%			
Oncological outcomes (PDAC only, *n* = 679)	**R0 rate**	**R1 rate**	**R2 rate**	
Resection margins status	≥35%	≤63%	≤2%	
Portal vein positive resection margin rate	≤3%			
Total number or lymph nodes resected	≥16			
Survival (PDAC only, *n* = 589)	**1-year**	**2-year**	**3-year**	**5-year**
Overall survival rate	≥68%	≥37%	≥21%	≥9%
Disease-free survival rate	≥22%	≥9%	≥2%	≥0%

From Raptis et al. [9]

2.2 Conclusion

Benchmarking is a tool recently adopted in medical analysis to promote continuous quality improvement. It involves comparing achievable results in surgical procedures and fosters comparison and collaboration among centers to enhance individual outcomes. The essence of benchmarking lies in the ongoing sharing, analysis, and implementation of improvements.

This approach is particularly useful in high-complexity surgical procedures, such as pancreatoduodenectomy, which is known for its high morbidity and mortality rates. In this context, benchmarking proves invaluable. With the advent of minimally invasive surgery, having these reference values is essential, as it allows for the comparison of the safety and efficacy of new techniques. This comparison not only ensures that innovations meet established standards but also serves as a practical tool to foster meaningful comparisons and guide improvements in surgical practice.

Two landmark international multicenter studies have established benchmark values for open pancreatoduodenectomy, focusing on clinically relevant outcomes. These studies, analyzed in this book chapter, are the first to set such cutoffs. The benchmarks provide valuable insights into expected morbidity and mortality rates, as well as oncological indicators, serving as important thresholds for comparing surgical performance in pancreatic surgery.

References

1. Ellis J. All inclusive benchmarking. J Nurs Manag. 2006;14(5):377–83.
2. Staiger RD, Schwandt H, Puhan MA, Clavien PA. Improving surgical outcomes through benchmarking. Br J Surg. 2019;106(1):59–64.
3. Ettorchi-Tardy A, Levif M, Michel P. Benchmarking: a method for continuous quality improvement in health. Healthc Policy [Internet]. mayo de 2012 [citado 10 de marzo de 2018];7(4):e101–19. Disponible en: http://www.ncbi.nlm.nih.gov/pubmed/23634166.
4. Sánchez-Velázquez P, Muller X, Malleo G, Park JS, Hwang HK, Napoli N, et al. Benchmarks in pancreatic surgery: a novel tool for unbiased outcome comparisons. Ann Surg. 2019;270(2):211–8.
5. Muller X, Marcon F, Sapisochin G, Marquez M, Dondero F, Rayar M, et al. Defining benchmarks in liver transplantation: a multicenter outcome analysis determining best achievable results. Ann Surg [Internet]. septiembre de 2018 [citado 11 de marzo de 2018];267(3):419–25. Disponible en: http://www.ncbi.nlm.nih.gov/pubmed/28885508.
6. Weissman NW, Allison JJ, Kiefe CI, Farmer RM, Weaver MT, Williams OD, et al. Achievable benchmarks of care: the ABCs of benchmarking. J Eval Clin Pract. 1999;5(3):269–81.
7. Gero D, Muller X, Staiger RD, Gutschow CA, Vonlanthen R, Bueter M, et al. How to establish benchmarks for surgical outcomes?: a checklist based on an international expert Delphi consensus. Ann Surg. 2022;275:115–20.
8. van Ramshorst TME, Giani A, Mazzola M, Dokmak S, Ftériche FS, Esposito A, et al. Benchmarking of robotic and laparoscopic spleen-preserving distal pancreatectomy by using two different methods. Br J Surg [Internet]. 2022;110(1):76–83. Disponible en: 10.1093/bjs/znac352.
9. Raptis DA, Sánchez-Velázquez P, Machairas N, Sauvanet A, Rueda de Leon A, Oba A, et al. Defining benchmark outcomes for Pancreatoduodenectomy with Portomesenteric venous resection. Ann Surg. 2020;272(5):731–7.

3 Vascular Variant of Hepatic Artery

Antonio Iannelli and Edoardo Rosso

3.1 Introduction

There is considerable variation in the arterial supply to the liver as shown by several studies conducted on liver donors and individuals undergoing hepatic, biliary, or pancreatic surgery. The arterial vascular supply to the liver consisting of the common hepatic artery arising from the celiac trunk, becoming the proper hepatic artery (PHA) after the origin of the gastroduodenal artery (GDA) and giving rise to a right (RHA) and a left hepatic artery (LHA), is only found in the 55–75% of the individuals [1–4] as several anatomical variants exist. Knowing the exact anatomy of arterial supply to the liver during liver and pancreatic surgery is of critical importance to avoid injuries that may affect postoperative outcomes.

Pancreatoduodenectomy (PD) is a well-established surgical procedure, mainly done in the setting elective surgery for pancreatic head cancer. Currently, this procedure is more and more done through minimally invasive (MI) approaches, including laparoscopy and robotics which may challenge the identification of vascular arterial variants and may lead to a vascular injury [5, 6]. Thus, it is of mainstay importance when planning a PD to carefully evaluate the identification of the anatomy of the arterial supply to the liver, which is typically evaluated by computed tomography with contrast, that ensures high sensitivity and specificity [7]. This information can also be useful to assess the feasibility of radical tumor resection with negative margins.

The presence of an aberrant hepatic artery (AHA) may be a concern in the setting of MI approach, and special attention should be paid to clarify the arterial anatomy when scheduling a MIPD in order to avoid an inadvertent division of an AHA which has not been carefully identified preoperatively and/or not identified at the time of surgery.

This chapter focuses on the possible management of AHAs, their impact before and during MIPD, and outlines the most important factors that should influence the surgical strategy facing AHAs in this setting.

A. Iannelli
University of Côte d'Azur, Nice, France

Department of Digestive Surgery, Hopital Archet 2, University Hospital of Nice, Nice, France

Hepatic Complications in Obesity, Nice, France

Adipocible Research Study Group (University of Nice Côte d'Azur and Idex), Nice, France
e-mail: IANNELLI.A@chu-nice.fr

E. Rosso (✉)
Centre de Chirurgie Digestive – Pole Santé Sud, Le Mans, France
e-mail: edoardo_rosso@hotmail.com

B. Ielpo et al. (eds.), *Minimally Invasive Pancreatoduodenectomy in Cancer*,
https://doi.org/10.1007/978-3-031-99695-5_3

Table 3.1 Elements of arterial vascular supply to the liver that are to be taken into account when planning a DP

1	Accessory or replaced RHA
2	RHA from SMA, CT, GDA, or aorta
3	Presence of an accessory or replaced LHA
4	Diameter of the aberrant artery
5	Diameter of an eventual proper RHA
6	Tumor encasement of the artery
7	Distance of the tumor from the aberrant artery

RHA right hepatic artery, *LHA* left hepatic artery, *SMA* superior mesentery artery, *GDA* gastroduodenal, *LGA* left gastric artery

3.2 Aberrant Arterial Anatomy Relevant to a MIDP (Table 3.1)

The AHAs that must systematically be considered when planning a MIPD are those that arise from the superior mesenteric artery (SMA) or less commonly directly from the aorta, which can be either an accessory right hepatic artery (aRHA) (supplying the right liver or a portion of it along with another artery, generally a RHA coming from the proper HA) or a replaced right hepatic artery (rRHA) (supplying the right liver of part of it solely). The other variants that should be identified before DP are as follows: the trifurcation of the CHA into the RHA, LHA, and gastroduodenal artery (GDA), which implies the absence of PHA; the vascular supply to the left liver including an accessory or replaced LHA generally from the left gastric artery; and the CHA coming from SMA that occurs in around 2% of individuals [8].

3.3 Elements of Vascular Physiology Relevant to the Vascular Supply to the Liver

There is evidence from the literature on bile duct injuries sustained during laparoscopic cholecystectomy that the occlusion of the RHA without a concomitant biliary or portal vein injury rarely results in clinically significant ischemia to the liver or bile ducts [9]. This is due to the complex arterial vascular supply of the bile ducts that relies on three systems, afferent vessels, marginal arteries, and an epicholedochal plexus that can effectively provide backup in the form of continuing arterial inflow to the bile ducts when some supplying vessels are disrupted. The transverse hilar marginal artery can function as an arterial shunt between the two sides of the liver. Besides the evidence obtained from anatomical studies on cadavers through injection of fluid resins into this complex arterial network confirming the opacification of the right liver after occlusion of the RHA, arteriographic studies have confirmed reflow after occlusion of the right or left hepatic artery occurs from the unaffected side through the hilar marginal artery and hilar plexus, which function as a preformed collateral arterial route [10–12]. The use of preoperative angiography may, thus, allow to test the effectiveness of the reflow of an aberrant RHA. While vascular anatomy for a safer MIPD is mainly assessed through contrast-enhanced triphasic CT-scan, which is easily accessible and has few contraindications, its most evident drawback is represented by the fact that it does not provides dynamic static imaging of the arterial vascular supply it produces. On the other hand, angiography allows to confirm the presence of vascular aberrancies through direct contrast injection followed by active image records. Moreover, the dynamic visualization of the arterial flow gives additional information concerning which is the preferential pathway for the right hepatic lobe vascular supply. Furthermore, selective catheterization with temporary vascular occlusion or injection of the contrast agent under variable degrees of pressure can simulate what would happen in case of aberrant RHA ligation with the eventual identification of arterial shunts through the hilar plate. However, it must be considered that the effectiveness of the arterial shunts during arteriography may be influenced by the injection pressure that may contribute to force the reflow. This is why some authors privilege an interval of few days or weeks after the embolization of an aRHA. Ishikawa et al. [13], Cloyd et al. [14], and El Amrani et al. [15] reported the successful embolization of a rRHA originating from the SMA in a total of five patients. The aim of this procedure was to stimulate arterial shunt formation in order to perform PD with aberrant RHA ligation without compromising liver arterial supply. Shunts' opening was confirmed by preoperative CT-scan 3 weeks after angioembolization with no evidence of liver ischemia in any of the included patients. In inly one study, right liver lobe revascularization through arterial shunts was confirmed only with an immediate post-embolization angiography. No embolization- and postoperative-related ischemia complications were reported. While this strategy may be interesting especially when an adjuvant chemotherapy is planned, it may be at the origin of an inflammatory reaction around the artery and complicate the surgical dissection. The value of embolization in favoring the reflow and its effectiveness in potentiating the vascular supply to the contralateral hemi-liver remains a debated issue.

3.4 Elements of the Aberrant Hepatic Artery to Consider Before MIPD

Aberrant RHAs are the most common variants and their precise identification and radiological characterization is mandatory before planning the MIDP to avoid any injury to arterial supply to the liver. While the ligation of an aRHA has no serious consequences, the ligation of a rRHA may lead to ischemia-related complications after MIPD. The most dreadful consequences of an acute partial ischemia of liver parenchyma consist of liver abscesses and biliary ischemic post-PD complications. This mainly occur when the arterial supply to the right liver coming through the opening of the arterial shunts at liver hilum is inadequate. This may occur due to injury to the epicholedochal plexus or to the transverse hilar marginal during dissection if this is pushed too high in the liver hilum or due to inadvertent coagulation.

In addition, injury to hepatic arteries during surgery may be responsible for thrombosis or pseudoaneurysm formation that can lead to postoperative hemorrhage, especially in the setting of a postoperative pancreatic fistula. This is why the arteries should be manipulated carefully avoiding direct grasping during robotic dissection. To this scope, robotic surgeons encircle the vessels with a soft vessel loop and avoid direct manipulation of the arteries.

An aberrant RHA can have many different characteristics depending on its origin, its path toward the liver, and its eventual contact or invasion by the tumor. As said above, all these characteristics should be defined before surgery with the aid of CT scan and in selected cases of arteriography. Extreme cases include a large rRHA or a CHA coming from SMA that needs to be preserved or reimplanted if it's infiltrated or too close to the tumor. While infiltration by the tumor implies the division of the artery with or without reimplantation, the close proximity may not contraindicate a safe dissection especially after neoadjuvant chemotherapy. The more the distance between them is reduced, the more increases the risk of a marginal oncological status in case of a conservative approach with the only study published on this topic setting the cutoff at 10 mm [16]. On the other hand, the eventual encasement of the aberrant artery by the tumor can induce the progressive formation of arterial shunts and make its ligation without reconstruction safe. Finally, the use of vascular divestment technique may allow to dissect free the aberrant artery in MIDP [17].

3.5 Intraoperative Approach

Once the preoperative work-up definition of vascular anatomy has been appropriately defined and discussed, in the case of an aberrant RHA, the first step is to decide whether to do a preoperative embolization and its timing. In the case of an aRHA, this is rarely needed as it can be safely ligated during surgery especially when the caliber of the aRHA is small. A rare exception may be represented by an aRHA presenting a caliber comparable to that of the RHA coming from the PHA when the tumor is in proximity of the RHA or an inflammatory liver pedicle (due to endoscopic stenting) may be anticipated or in the setting of bile duct cancer that needs a more extensive dissection of the liver pedicle high in the hilum. In this case, the aRHA may be kept until the completion of the dissection. If a rRHA with a large caliber far away from the tumor is identified, the plan is generally to spare it during surgery (*see below*) as it is the case for a CHA coming from the SMA. It may happen that a large rRHA is infiltrated, and in this case, a preoperative functional angiographic study with temporary occlusion of this vessel may allow to safely embolize the aberrant HA or ligate it during surgery. If a doubt persists, it has to be reimplanted contraindication the MI approach. However, we believe that this is an exceedingly rare clinical situation.

If a trifurcation of the CHA without PHA is shown, then the exact anatomy of the trifurcation should be identified especially when the RHA stems from the GDA.

In the case of an aberrant RHA that has to be spared, the initial intraoperative approach should be focused on the identification and isolation of this artery. Most of the descriptions of MIPD in presence of this anatomical peculiarity delineate a posterior approach with rapid identification of the SMA as the most suitable strategy in this situation [18]. After a full Kocher maneuver with exposure of the inferior vena cava, the left renal vein is isolated and the SMA is carefully dissected at its origin from the aorta. This, in turn, allows to recognize the aberrant artery arising from the SMA avoiding its inadvertent injury during dissection. Once the origin of the aberrant RHA is isolated, the next step is to identify it distally in the hepatic pedicle. The access to the aberrant RHA in the liver hilum is gained isolating and dividing the common bile duct, usually after removing the gallbladder. The artery is then encircled in the liver pedicle and then fully mobilized avoiding any manipulation and excessive traction that can lead to subsequent thrombosis. PD can be then completed with the division of the stomach and the first jejunal loop, pancreatic body division above the superior mesenteric vein, and pancreatoduodenal bloc resection. The preemptive identification of the variant RHA helps reducing possible unintentional lesions and leaves the possibility to take the best choice in terms of surgical strategy with regard to the artery.

Nguyen et al. [19] were the first to publish their experience of MIPD in the presence of an aberrant RHA. In a cohort of 30 patients with vascular anomalies undergoing robotic PD, 15 were found to have a rRHA from the SMA. A conservative approach toward the aberrant RHA was applied in all cases, and no differences in postoperative and oncological outcomes were identified comparing patients with and without vascular anomalies. The same results were reported by Wang et al. [20] in 58 patients with an aRHA or rRHA undergoing a laparoscopic PD with preservation of the aberrant artery. No difference in terms of conversion rate, intraoperative outcomes such as operative time and estimated blood loss, post-PD complications, number of harvested lymph nodes, and R0 resection margins was also highlighted by Kim et al. [21] when comparing patients with aberrant RHA to patients with normal vascular anatomy undergoing robotic PD. In this cohort, 11 patients underwent successful rRHA conservative management while 2 out of 4 with an aRHA needed aberrant RHA ligation and division; one of them experimented an initial postoperative increase in liver enzymes that rapidly normalized with no other complications.

Considering oncological outcomes in the setting of MIPD in patients with vascular anomalies, Giani et al. [22] identified a significant increased median number of harvested lymph nodes in the aberrant vascular group compared to the modal vascular anatomy group. They analyzed nine patients with a rRHA and one with an aRHA from the SMA undergoing laparoscopic PD but did not report how the aberrant arteries had been managed. Lastly, Zhang et al. [23], in their comparative study including 22 patients with aberrant RHA (12 aRHA and 10 rRHA), found a significant increased operative time for these patients compared to those with a modal anatomy. The increased operative time was related to the time spent to spare the RHA arising from the SMA.

Focusing on the necessity to resect or conserve the aberrant RHA, although the most frequently described behavior is conservative, the anatomy of the tumor deeply affects the choice. In a cohort of 25 patients with a rRHA undergoing laparotomic PD, Okada et al. [14] report a significantly different rate of R0/R1 margins depending on the distance between the tumor and the aberrant RHA with an increased incidence of R1 margins for tumors with ≤10 mm interspace between the tumor and the rRHA.

In the case of a trifurcation, the dissection of the arterial supply to the liver can be done proximally and distally to the trifurcation isolating the CHA and then its branches distally in the liver pedicle to identify the GDA as the last step. Once the vascular anatomy corresponds to the preoperative cartography, vascular division can be achieved.

When an aberrant artery has to be divided, it can be reimplanted on the origin of the divided GDA when its caliber is small (and in this case its reimplantation should be justified as any anastomotic thrombosis may lead to the occlusion of the whole vascular supply to the liver) or to the splenic artery that is in most of the cases of large caliber and can be easily turned toward the liver. This complex vascular reconstruction is best done by open surgery.

The anatomical aberrancies involving the left hepatic artery (LHA) are also frequently reported, and the coexistence of an anatomical variation of both RHA and LHA can be found in 4–8% of patients [4]. This eventuality may represent a pitfall as a double aberrancy logically increases the risk to determine a severe liver ischemic damage in case of injury or necessity to perform resection of one or both of liver arteries; a second anatomical aberrancy adds another element whose management must be considered not to compromise the radicality and to guarantee the best oncological results to the patient. On the other hand, an accessory LHA generally provides for arterial supply compensation in case of aberrant RHA ligation without reconstruction also when the former is a rRHA.

3.6 Conclusions

The presence of a trained minimally invasive surgeon in the setting of a tertiary center and a careful selection of patients are the most important factors that affect the outcomes of this demanding procedure [24–26]. The first step is distinguishing between an aRHA and a rRHA; the existence of a modal RHA leaves the possibility to the pancreatic surgeon to perform the aRHA ligation without reconstruction with almost no risk to develop postoperative ischemia-related complications. This reduces the complexity and operative time of the surgical procedure, the risk of a R1 resection margin if in case of a tumor in contact with the aberrant artery, and any risk linked to the formation of a pseudoaneurysm of the latter. Contrast-enhanced CT scan is the key imaging technique to identify vascular anomalies of the liver arterial supply, discriminate between an aRHA and a rRHA, and precisely define other anatomical features, such as the proximity of the tumor to the aberrant artery and the path and diameter of the latter, that can influence the preoperative and intraoperative strategy. It should also be considered that, although aRHA and rRHA most commonly originates from the SMA, aberrant RHAs originating from other vessels such as the gastroduodenal artery, the celiac trunk, or the aorta are also documented.

If arterial reconstruction is needed in case of a large caliber RHA arising from the SMA to avoid an unduly ischemic injury, laparotomic conversion to perform the anastomosis is suggested.

Finally, one more factor that must be considered when conducting a MIPD is the tumor anatomy. The necessity to perform a ligation and division of a previously identified aberrant RHA often depends on its relationship with the tumor.

References

1. Varotti G, Gondolesi GE, Goldman J, et al. Anatomic variations in right liver living donors. J Am Coll Surg. 2004;198(4):577–82. https://doi.org/10.1016/j.jamcollsurg.2003.11.014.
2. Hiatt JR, Gabbay J, Busuttil RW. Surgical anatomy of the hepatic arteries in 1000 cases. Published online. 1994:50–2.
3. Gruttadauria S, Foglieni CS, Doria C, Luca A, Lauro A, Marino IR. The hepatic artery in liver transplantation and surgery: vascular anomalies in 701 cases. Clin Transpl. 2001;15(5):359–63.
4. Suzuki T, Nakayasu A, Kawabe K, Takeda H, Honjo I. Surgical significance of anatomic variations of the hepatic artery. Am J Surg. 1971;122(4):505–12.
5. Nickel F, Haney CM, Kowalewski KF, et al. Laparoscopic versus open pancreaticoduodenectomy: a systematic review and meta-analysis of randomized controlled trials. Ann Surg. 2020;271(1):54–66.
6. García-Picazo A, Sánchez-Velázquez P, Burdio F, et al. Anatomical variations of the hepatic artery in duodenopancreatectomy: tips and tricks in the minimally invasive surgical approach. Updates Surg. 2025. https://doi.org/10.1007/s13304-025-02307-w. PMID: 40593390.
7. Sahani D, Saini S, Pena C, et al. Using multidetector CT for preoperative vascular evaluation of liver neoplasms: technique and results. Am J Roentgenol. 2002;179(1):53–9.
8. Michels NA. Blood supply and anatomy of the upper abdominal organs with a descriptive atlas. Philadelphia/Montreal: JB Lippincot Co.; 1955. p. 3–137.
9. Strasberg SM, Helton WS. An analytical review of vasculobiliary injury in laparoscopic and open cholecystectomy. HPB (Oxford). 2011;13(1):1–14. https://doi.org/10.1111/j.1477-2574.2010.00225.x. Epub 2010 Nov 15. PMID: 21159098; PMCID: PMC3019536.
10. Redman HC, Reuter SR. Arterial collaterals in the liver hilus. Radiology. 1970;94:575–9.
11. Bengmark S, Rosengren K. Angiographic study of the collateral circulation to the liver after ligation of the hepatic artery in man. Am J Surg. 1970;119:620–4.
12. Mays ER, Wheeler CS. Demonstration of collateral arterial flow after interruption of hepatic arteries in man. N Engl J Med. 1974;290:993–6.
13. Ishikawa M, Yamagami T, Kakizawa H, et al. Preoperative coil embolization in patients with a replaced hepatic artery scheduled for pancreatectomy with splanchnic artery resection helps to prevent ischemic organ injury. J Comput Assist Tomogr. 2016;40(1):172–6.
14. Okada K-I, Kawai M, Hirono S, et al. A replaced right hepatic artery adjacent to pancreatic carcinoma should be divided to obtain R0 resection in pancreaticoduodenectomy. Langenbecks Arch Surg. 2015;400(1):57–65.
15. Cloyd JM, Chandra V, Louie JD, Rao S, Visser BC. Preoperative embolization of replaced right hepatic artery prior to pancreaticoduodenectomy. J Surg Oncol. 2012;106(4):509–12.
16. El Amrani M, Leteurtre E, Sergent G, et al. Pancreatic head carcinoma and right hepatic artery: embolization management – a case report. J Gastrointest Oncol. 2014;5(4):E80–3.
17. Rosso E, Petrucciani N, El Zibawi M, Iannelli A. Pancreaticoduodenectomy with vascular divestment for locally advanced pancreatic neuroendocrine tumour. ANZ J Surg. 2021;91(7–8):E551–3. https://doi.org/10.1111/ans.16569. Epub 2021 Jan 8.
18. Ogiso S, Conrad C, Araki K, Basso V, Gayet B. Posterior approach for laparoscopic pancreaticoduodenectomy to prevent replaced hepatic artery injury. Ann Surg Oncol. 2013;20(9):3120. https://doi.org/10.1245/s10434-013-3058-7.
19. Nguyen TK, Zenati MS, Boone BA, et al. Robotic pancreaticoduodenectomy in the presence of aberrant or anomalous hepatic arterial anatomy: safety and oncologic outcomes. HPB. 2015;17(7):594–9.
20. Wang S, Chen Q, Liu S, Zhang W, Ji B, Liu Y. The impact of aberrant hepatic artery on resection margin and outcomes of laparoscopic pancreatoduodenectomy: a single-center report. World J Surg. 2021;45(10):3183–90.
21. Kim JH, Gonzalez-Heredia R, Daskalaki D, Rashdan M, Masrur M, Giulianotti PC. Totally replaced right hepatic artery in pancreaticoduodenectomy: is this anatomical condition a contraindication to minimally invasive surgery? HPB. 2016;18(7):580–5. https://doi.org/10.1016/j.hpb.2016.04.009.
22. Giani A, Mazzola M, Morini L, et al. Hepatic vascular anomalies during totally laparoscopic pancreaticoduodenectomy: challenging the challenge. Updat Surg. 2021:0123456789. https://doi.org/10.1007/s13304-021-01152-x.
23. Zhang W, Wang K, Liu S, et al. A single-center clinical study of hepatic artery variations in laparoscopic pancreaticoduodenectomy. Medicine (Baltimore). 2020;99(21):e20403. https://doi.org/10.1097/md.0000000000020403.
24. Dokmak S, Aussilhou B, Ftériche FS, Dembinski J, Romdhani C, Sauvanet A. The outcome of laparoscopic pancreatoduodenectomy is improved with patient selection and the learning curve. Surg Endosc. 2021:0123456789.
25. Coppola A, Stauffer JA, Asbun HJ. Laparoscopic pancreatoduodenectomy: current status and future directions. Updat Surg. 2016;68(3):217–24.
26. Ielpo B, Anselmo A, Koh Y, et al. Minimally invasive pancreatic anastomosis after pancreaticoduodenectomy: multi-institutional step by step video description of the technique. Updates Surg. 2023;75(1):255–59. https://doi.org/10.1007/s13304-022-01389-0. Epub 2022 Nov 12. PMID: 36371550.

4 The Role and Anatomy of the Mesopancreas in Pancreatoduodenectomy

Leandro Siragusa, Luigi Eduardo Conte, Silvio Caringi, Renato De Martino, and Alessandro Anselmo

Precise anatomical understanding and meticulous technique in surgical management of pancreatic cancer, particularly during a pancreatoduodenectomy, is fundamental. A crucial aspect of this procedure is mesopancreas handling, a controversial and complex anatomical structure that plays a significant role in both surgical and oncological outcomes [1–3].

4.1 The Mesopancreas: A Contested Anatomical Structure

The term "mesopancreas" refers to retropancreatic tissue, microscopically consisting of areolar and adipose tissue, peripheral nerves and plexuses, blood and lymphatic vessels or capillaries, and lymph nodes [3]. However, despite its frequent use in surgical literature, there is no consensus regarding the precise anatomy and terminology of this plate-like structure. Over the years, numerous terms and definitions have been proposed without reaching a definitive agreement.

The first definition of the "mesopancreas" was introduced by Gockel et al., who described it as a firm and well-vascularized structure extending from the posterior surface of the pancreatic head to the area behind the superior mesenteric vessels, including the superior mesenteric vein (SMV) and the superior mesenteric artery (SMA). According to Gockel et al., the boundaries of the mesopancreas are correlated with its developmental embryology: extending to the descending duodenum on the right, behind the spleen on the left, and caudally beyond the mesenteric vessels [2].

Anatomically, the term "mesentery" is defined as a fold of peritoneum that attaches an organ to the posterior wall of the abdomen and contains all its blood vessels and draining lymphatics and lymph nodes [4]. By this definition, a "true" mesopancreas would need to encompass all the arterial supply and draining veins of the pancreatic head. However, it is well-known that the head of the pancreas is supplied by the inferior pancreaticoduodenal artery (a branch of the superior mesenteric artery or the first jejunal artery) and the superior pancreaticoduodenal artery (a branch of the gastroduodenal artery). The pancreaticoduodenal veins, located near these

L. Siragusa (✉)
IRCCS Humanitas Research Hospital, Milan, Italy
e-mail: leandros93@hotmail.it

L. E. Conte · S. Caringi · A. Anselmo
Department of Surgical Science, University of Rome "Tor Vergata", Rome, Italy
e-mail: conteluigieduardo@gmail.com; silviocaringi.ptv@gmail.com; alessandroanselmo.ptv@gmail.com

R. De Martino
IRCCS Humanitas Research Hospital, Milan, Italy

Department of Biomedical Science, Humanitas University, Milan, Italy
e-mail: renatodimartino.ptv@gmail.com

B. Ielpo et al. (eds.), *Minimally Invasive Pancreatoduodenectomy in Cancer*,
https://doi.org/10.1007/978-3-031-99695-5_4

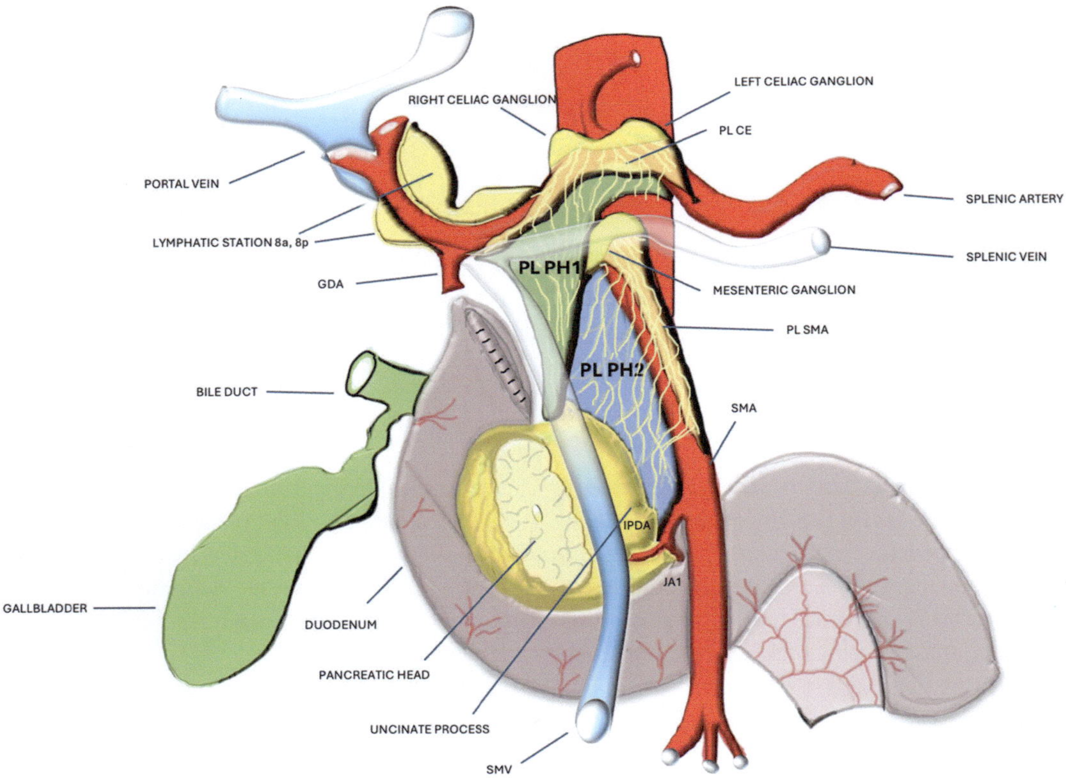

Fig. 4.1 Anatomic definition of mesopancreas according to the Japan Pancreas Society [21]. GDA gastro-duodenal artery, IPDA inferior pancreaticoduodenal artery, JA1 first jejunal artery, PL CE celiac plexus, PL PH1 pancreatic head plexus 1, PL PH2 pancreatic head plexus 2, PL SMA superior mesenteric artery plexus, SMA superior mesenteric artery, SMV superior mesenteric vein

arteries, drain into the superior mesenteric or portal veins. Since the mesopancreas contains only the inferior pancreaticoduodenal artery, this challenges the concept of a "true" mesopancreas [1] (Fig. 4.1).

4.2 Embryological Perspective

Understanding the embryology of the pancreas is crucial to grasp the concept of the mesopancreas. The pancreas develops from two buds: the ventral bud, located in the ventral mesogastrium, and the dorsal bud, in the dorsal mesogastrium, adjacent to the lateral aspect of the duodenum. These buds receive their blood supply from the gastroduodenal artery, inferior pancreaticoduodenal artery, and splenic artery. As development progresses, the ventral bud rotates and fuses with the dorsal bud to form the pancreas. The proximal part of the duct of Wirsung originates from the ventral pancreatic duct, while the distal part comes from the dorsal pancreatic duct. The duct of Santorini, on the other hand, is derived from the duct of the dorsal bud [5].

4.3 Nomenclature Debate

Over the years, several alternative names and concepts have been proposed to describe the mesopancreas. For instance, in 2013, Bouassida et al. introduced the term "retro-portal lamina" to describe the loose areolar tissue extending between the head, neck, and uncinate process of the pancreas to the aortocaval groove. This tissue contains nerve plexuses, lymphatics, and capillaries [6].

In 2016, Sharma and Isaji suggested that the term "mesopancreas" is a misnomer, proposing instead the name "Pancreatic Head Plexus II" based on the classification by the Japan Pancreas Society (JPS). The JPS clearly distinguishes between the pancreatic head plexus I (PLphI) and pancreatic head plexus II (PLphII), with the latter being the region primarily involved in nerve tissue distribution to the uncinate process from the SMA plexus, including the inferior pancreaticoduodenal artery. Sharma and Isaji argue that the tissue surrounding PLphII has been incorrectly identified as the mesopancreas and should be correctly named [7].

In the same year, Kawabata et al. introduced the term "mesopancreatoduodenum" to describe a common mesentery located behind the SMA, including the mesentery of the third and fourth portions of the duodenum and proximal jejunum. This structure, supplied by the inferior pancreaticoduodenal artery and the first jejunal artery, encompasses the lymph nodes on the left side of the SMA, extending beyond the traditional limits of the mesopancreas [8].

In 2020, Yi et al. analyzed the relationships between the mesopancreas and the pancreatic head plexus from a morphological and clinical perspective, suggesting the use of the term "mesopancreatoduodenum" instead of "mesopancreas" due to the complex interplay between the duodenum, pancreas, and SMA [9].

Most recently, in 2021, Muro et al. proposed the term "pancreas–major arteries ligament" (P–A ligament) to describe the structure connecting the pancreas to the major arteries, including the aorta, celiac trunk, and SMA. The P–A ligament comprises three components: the ventral part, the dorsal part, and the IPDA part, each with distinct locations and fibrous bundle directions [10].

4.4 Surgical Technique and the Mesopancreas

During pancreatoduodenectomy, the jejunum is typically divided using a linear stapler approximately 15–20 cm distal to the Treitz ligament [8, 11–13]. This division allows a careful separation of the mesentery at its entry point into the proximal jejunal loop. The loop, along with the fourth portion of the duodenum, is then passed posterior to the mesenteric vessels, clearing the operative field on the right side. This maneuver facilitates the separation of the head and uncinate process of the pancreas from the superior mesenteric vessels. The mesopancreas, a key structure in this dissection, is divided along the superior mesenteric artery (SMA) using ligatures, bipolar cautery, clips, or advanced energy-based devices such as Thunderbeat™ or Harmonic™ shears. Given the delicate nature of this procedure, stapling the entire resection surface is not recommended due to the high risk of injuring nearby vessels. Careful dissection is essential when exposing the anterolateral aspect of the SMA, as it is fundamental to avoid injury to this vital vessel. Ensuring that all soft tissues along the superior mesenteric vessels are adequately harvested is of particular importance, as the medial and posterior margins are common sites of R1 resections, which are associated with residual tumor cells and a poorer prognosis [14, 15].

Three different levels of mesopancreasectomy are described and differentiated based on grade of malignancy of the tumors, both in open and in robotic surgery [16, 17]. Level 1 is used for benign or low-grade tumors, where full mesopancreas dissection is not always necessary. The dissection starts by identifying variations in the inferior pancreaticoduodenal vein (IPDV) and superior mesenteric vein (SMV). The mesopancreas is partially divided, preserving key arteries like the first jejunal artery, without proceeding to full resection. Level 2 is applied to malignant tumors where complete mesopancreas removal is essential for oncological resection. In this case, the dissection includes ligating and dividing the inferior pancreaticoduodenal artery (IPDA) and the first jejunal artery while preserving the neurovascular bundle around the superior mesenteric artery (SMA). The mesopancreas and mesojejunum are removed en bloc. Level 3 is reserved for aggressive or borderline tumors with potential tissue infiltration. In this extended dissection, the mesopancreas and surrounding tissue near the SMA are fully extirpated using an "anterior approach," known as the "triangular operation," which clears tissue between the SMV, SMA, and hepatic artery. This method is also used when venous resection is required (for further detail see Chaps. 8 and 18).

4.5 Oncological Considerations

The oncological importance of the mesopancreas lies in its potential role as a route for cancer spread, particularly via its rich network of lymphatic and neural structures [15, 18–20]. As such, thorough resection of the mesopancreas during pancreatoduodenectomy is crucial to achieving clear surgical margins and reducing the likelihood of R1 resections [15].

However, the variability in how surgeons define and approach the mesopancreas can lead to inconsistencies in surgical outcomes and complicate the interpretation of clinical studies.

4.6 Need for Consensus

Despite the ongoing debate and lack of a universally accepted definition, understanding the mesopancreas is essential for surgeons specializing in hepato-pancreato-biliary surgery. The structure's potential oncological relevance, coupled with the complexity of its anatomical relationships, underscores the need for a clear and consistent definition. Convening a consensus conference that brings together anatomists, pathologists, radiologists, oncologists, and surgeons is necessary to establish the definitive definition, anatomy, and boundaries of the mesopancreas.

In conclusion, while the mesopancreas remains a somewhat nebulous concept in surgical anatomy, its importance in pancreatic surgery cannot be overstated. As research continues to evolve, so too must our understanding and approach to this critical structure in the pursuit of improved surgical outcomes and patient care.

References

1. Agrawal MK, et al. Mesopancreas: myth or reality? J Pancreas. 2010;11(3):230–3.
2. Gockel I, Domeyer M, Wolloscheck T, et al. Resection of the mesopancreas (RMP): a new surgical classification of a known anatomical space. World J Surg Onc. 2007;5:44.
3. Boggi U, Lombardo C, Napoli N. Robotic pancreatoduodenectomy for pancreatic cancer with superior mesenteric/portal vein resection and reconstruction. In: Boggi U, editor. Minimally invasive surgery of the pancreas. Updates in surgery. Milano: Springer; 2018.
4. Morgado PJ. Total mesorectal excision: a misnomer for a sound surgical approach. Dis Colon Rectum. 1998;41:120–1.
5. Borghi F, Gattolin A, Garbossa D, Bogliatto F, Garavoglia M, Levi AC. Embryologic bases of extended radical resection in pancreatic cancer. Arch Surg. 1998;133(3):297–301.
6. Bouassida M, Mighri MM, Chtourou MF, Sassi S, Touinsi H, Hajji H, et al. Retroportal lamina or mesopancreas? Lessons learned by anatomical and histological study of thirty three cadaveric dissections. Int J Surg. 2013;11:834–6.
7. Sharma D, Isaji S. Mesopancreas is a misnomer: time to correct the nomenclature. J Hepatobiliary Pancreat Sci. 2016;23(12):745–9.
8. Kawabata Y, Tanaka T, Ishikawa N, Hayashi H, Tajima Y. Modified total meso-pancreatoduodenum excision with pancreaticoduodenectomy as a mesopancreatic plane surgery in borderline resectable pancreatic cancer. Eur J Surg Oncol. 2016;42:698–705.
9. Yi SQ, Nagakawa Y, Ren K, Dai YD, Zhang M, Chen JF, et al. The mesopancreas and pancreatic head plexus: morphological, developmental, and clinical perspectives. Surg Radiol Anat. 2020;42:1501–8.
10. Muro S, et al. What comprises the plate-like structure between the pancreatic head and the celiac trunk and superior mesenteric artery? A proposal for the term "P-A ligament" based on anatomical findings. Anat Sci Int. 2021;96(3):370–7.
11. Mihaljevic AL, Hackert T, Loos M, Hinz U, Schneider M, Mehrabi A, Hoffmann K, Berchtold C, Müller-Stich BP, Diener M, Strobel O, Büchler MW. Not all Whipple procedures are equal: proposal for a classification of pancreatoduodenectomies. Surgery. 2021;169(6):1456–62.
12. Kawabata Y, Hayashi H, Ishikawa N, Tajima Y. Total mesopancreatoduodenum excision with pancreaticoduodenectomy in lower biliary tract cancer. Langenbeck's Arch Surg. 2016;401:463–9.
13. Diener MK, Mihaljevic AL, Strobel O, Loos M, Schmidt T, Schneider M, Berchtold C, Mehrabi A, Müller-Stich BP, Jiang K, Neoptolemos JP, Hackert T, Miao Y, Büchler MW. Periarterial divestment in pancreatic cancer surgery. Surgery. 2021;169(5):1019–25.

14. García-Picazo A, Sánchez-Velázquez P, Burdio F, Ielpo B. Anatomical variations of the hepatic artery in duodenopancreatectomy: tips and tricks in the minimally invasive surgical approach. Updates Surg. 2025.
15. Peparini N, Chirletti P. Mesopancreas: a boundless structure, namely R1 risk in pancreatico- duodenectomy for pancreatic head carcinoma. Eur J Surg Oncol. 2013;39(12):1303–8.
16. Inoue Y, Saiura A, Yoshioka R, Ono Y, Takahashi M, Arita J, Takahashi Y, Koga R. Pancreatoduodenectomy with systematic mesopancreas dissection using a supracolic anterior artery-first approach. Ann Surg. 2015;262(6):1092–101.
17. Ielpo B, d'Addetta MV, Anselmo A, Rosso E, de Blasi V, Sanchez-Velazquez P, Vellalta G, Podda M, Burdio F. Levels of robotic mesopancreas dissection according to malignancy and vascular anatomy: what surgeons need to know. Ann Surg Oncol. 2024;31(3):1916–8.
18. Kitagawa H, Ohta T, Makino I, Tani T, Tajima H, Nakagawara H, et al. Carcinomas of the ventral and dorsal pancreas exhibit different patterns of lymphatic spread. Front Biosci. 2008;13:2728–35.
19. Makino I, Kitagawa H, Ohta T, Nakagawara H, Tajima H, Ohnishi I, et al. Nerve plexus invasion in pancreatic cancer: spread patterns on histopathologic and embryological analyses. Pancreas. 2008;37:358–65.
20. Ielpo B, Anselmo A, Masuda Y, et al. Superior mesenteric artery first approach for minimally invasive pancreaticoduodenectomy: a step-by-step surgical technique video. Ann Surg Oncol. 2023;30(3):1500–03.
21. Japan Pancreas Society. Classification of pancreatic carcinoma. 4th ed. Tokyo: Kanehara & Co., Ltd.; 2017.

Part II

Minimally Invasive Approach

Standard Laparoscopic Pancreatoduodenectomy

5

Levan Tsamalaidze, Filipe Kunzler, Domenech Asbun, and Horacio Asbun

5.1 Introduction

Since the first laparoscopic pancreaticoduodenectomy (LPD) was performed 20 years ago, advancements in medical technology and surgeon's experience have enabled the widespread adoption of the minimally invasive technique for treating lesions in the head of the pancreas. Pancreaticoduodenectomy (PD) demands advanced skills and a precise understanding of the surgical steps involved in this highly complex abdominal procedure. Numerous studies and guidelines appear to indicate that laparoscopic and robotic pancreatic resections are equally effective and, in some cases, potentially superior to open surgery [1–8].

Complex procedures can be standardized by dividing them into well-delineated steps. This allows for simplification of the procedure and better reproducibility. Standardization of multiple different surgical procedures have been reported over time by different groups of experts worldwide [9–14].

Numerous studies have detailed standardized surgical techniques for minimally invasive pancreaticoduodenectomy (MIPD), including both laparoscopic and robotic-assisted PD [15–17]. This chapter describes the authors technique for MIPD based on the review of about 80 operative reports and surgical videos to identify the most commonly used sequence of surgical steps and describe them in detail, along with practical tips and tricks.

5.2 Standardized Surgical Technique (Video)

The patient is placed supine, in split–leg position, and secured to the operating table in a standard, safe fashion. Review of the imaging preoperatively for mapping and planning the surgery is

Supplementary Information The online version contains supplementary material available at https://doi.org/10.1007/978-3-031-99695-5_5. The videos can be accessed individually by clicking the DOI link in the accompanying figure caption or by scanning this link with the SN More Media App.

L. Tsamalaidze
Division of Hepatobiliary and Pancreas Surgery, Miami Cancer Institute, Miami, FL, USA

New Vision University, Tbilisi, Georgia
e-mail: tsamalaidze.l@gmail.com

F. Kunzler · D. Asbun
Division of Hepatobiliary and Pancreas Surgery, Miami Cancer Institute, Miami, FL, USA
e-mail: kunzler.filipe@gmail.com; Domenech.asbun@baptisthealth.net

H. Asbun (✉)
Division of Hepatobiliary and Pancreas Surgery, Miami Cancer Institute, Miami, FL, USA

Herbert Wertheim College of Medicine, Florida International University, Miami, FL, USA
e-mail: horacioA@baptisthealth.net

B. Ielpo et al. (eds.), *Minimally Invasive Pancreatoduodenectomy in Cancer*,
https://doi.org/10.1007/978-3-031-99695-5_5

done routinely immediately prior to starting the surgery. This allows for mental preparedness of what the surgical team will encounter during the dissection. Important aspects to attend to are the vascular anatomy and its anatomic variations, angle of the PV-SMV junction, areas of proximity of the lesion to the vascular structures, and location of the pancreatic duct within the pancreatic parenchyma, which is better seen on a sagittal view of a pancreas protocol MRI.

5.2.1 Enter the Abdomen

A 5-mm skin incision in the mid left abdomen is used, and the abdomen is entered with a 5-mm optical insufflating port using a 0° scope. This entry site is usually 8 cm to the left of the midline and about 16 cm of the xyphoid. A total of two 5-mm ports and four 12-mm ports are inserted under direct visualization as shown in the Fig. 5.1. Usually, the midline port ends located about 16 cm from the xyphoid with the abdomen insufflated. Two 12-mm ports are located at each side about 8 cm to the left (the initial entry site that has been converted to 12 mm) and right, respectively. A 5-mm port is located in the subxiphoid area, and the other 5-mm port is placed as lateral and superior as feasible on the right upper quadrant. Once in the abdominal cavity, visual laparoscopic exploration is done of the abdominal organs and peritoneum to rule out distant metastatic disease.

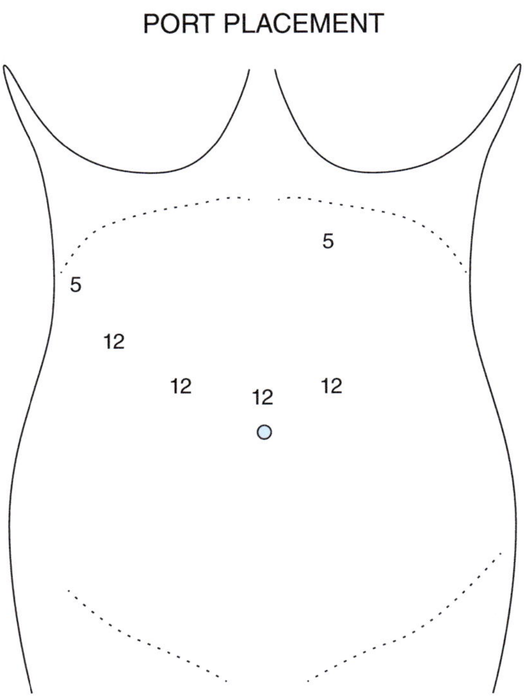

Fig. 5.1 Trocar placement. (Figure reproduced with the permission of Horacio J. Asbun)

5.2.2 Omentum and the Lesser Sac

The surgery is started by splitting the greater omentum up to the transverse colon creating two omental flaps. This facilitates access to the area of the ligament of Treitz and decreases any potential tension on the future antecolic gastrointestinal anastomoses. The omentum is therefore divided at the anticipated place were the future duodenojejunostomy will be positioned in an antecolic manner (usually aligned at about half point of a normal size left lateral liver lobe), as shown in the video. The gastrocolic ligament is then widely opened along the greater curve of the stomach entering into the lesser sac, preserving the gastroepiploic arcade (Fig. 5.2). Dissection is continued towards the hepatic flexure of the colon from left to right towards the gastroepiploic pedicle (Trunk of Henle) which will be transected later. Mobilizing the right colon and taken down adhesions to the area of the gallbladder early facilitates the exposure of the trunk of Henle.

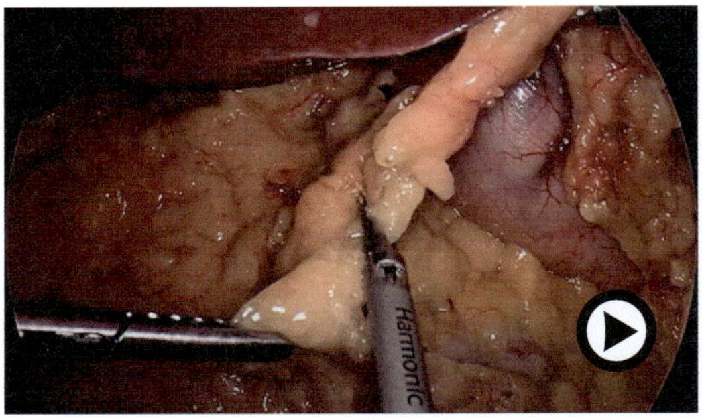

Fig. 5.2 Wide opening of the lesser sac (Standardized surgical technique (▶ https://doi.org/10.1007/000-hej))

5.2.3 Hepatic Flexure of the Colon

The patient is placed in reverse Trendelenburg with the left side down. The proximal transverse colon, hepatic flexure of the colon, distal ascending colon, and mesocolon are dissected off the retroperitoneum and Gerota's fascia along the avascular plane and retracted inferomedially (Fig. 5.3). This maneuver gives wide exposure of the head of the pancreas, the first, second, and third portion of the duodenum. The wide mobilization and spontaneous caudad retraction of the colon by gravity will help in exposing the gastroepiploic pedicle in the lesser sac as the posterior aspect of the stomach is retracted superiorly.

5.2.4 Cholecystectomy

The cystic duct and artery are identified, a critical view of safety is obtained, and both structures are ligated and divided in the usual fashion. The cholecystectomy is completed, or in some patients, the gallbladder maybe left attached to the liver if it facilitates its retraction, depending on the patient's body habitus.

5.2.5 Gastroepiploic Vessels

The gastroepiploic pedicle is then isolated in the prepyloric area as it begins its course inferiorly away from the greater curve. The veins in this pedicle join with colic veins to form the trunk of Henle. The vascular pedicle and its surrounding adipose tissue are encircled with the help of an esophageal finger retractor and divided with a stapler using a vascular load with closed height of 0.75–1.0 mm (transecting vessels close to the pylorus/duodenal wall helps avoid injury to the superior right colic vein). The first portion of the duodenum is better mobilized after this step, especially at its inferior edge.

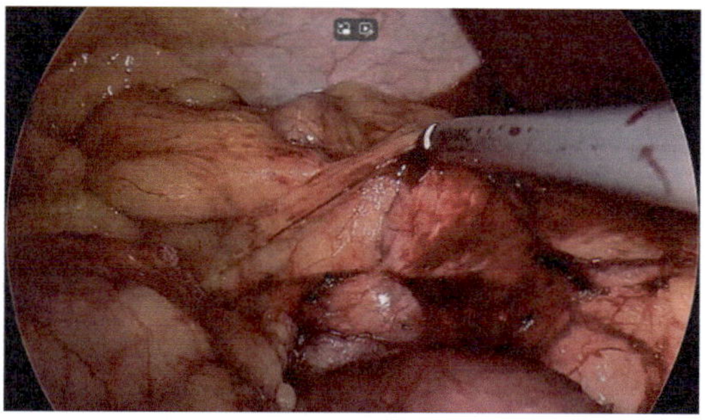

Fig. 5.3 Mobilization of the hepatic flexure of the colon

5.2.6 Duodenum

The first portion of the duodenum is approached posteriorly within the lesser sac and carefully dissected circumferentially, especially at its superior edge. Care is taken to avoid injury to the gastroduodenal artery (GDA) and common hepatic artery (CHA). The first portion of the duodenum is divided with a stapler in about 2–3 cm from the pylorus (closed height of 1.2–1.5 mm). Care is taken to transect the duodenum in the correct angle, which will serve for construction of the duodenojejunostomy later. The stomach is retracted to the patient's left which allows wide exposure of the retrogastric and peripancreatic area. Right gastric artery is usually encountered at this point and divided.

When significant adhesions are present along the area of the duodenum, and anterior dissection is done along the superior border at the level of the pylorus and duodenal bulb. In that case, the right gastric artery may be divided prior to the transection of the duodenum.

5.2.7 Lymph Node 8a

The area of the celiac trunk tributaries is inspected, and the CHA lymph node (8a) is identified. This is usually the gateway to the common hepatic artery below, and sometimes, the portal vein is visible deeper as well. The lymph node is meticulously dissected (Fig. 5.4) and excised exposing CHA. Dissection is continued along the CHA towards the origin of the GDA. A frozen examination of the CHA lymph node may be performed to assess the extent of the disease but by itself, a positive result would not affect the decision to continue proceeding with the resection.

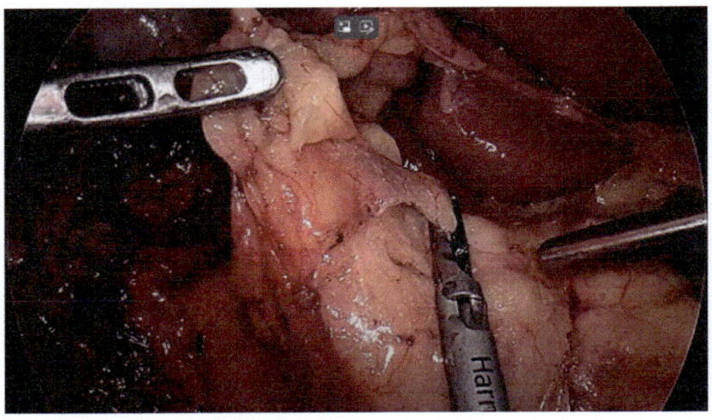

Fig. 5.4 8a lymph node dissection

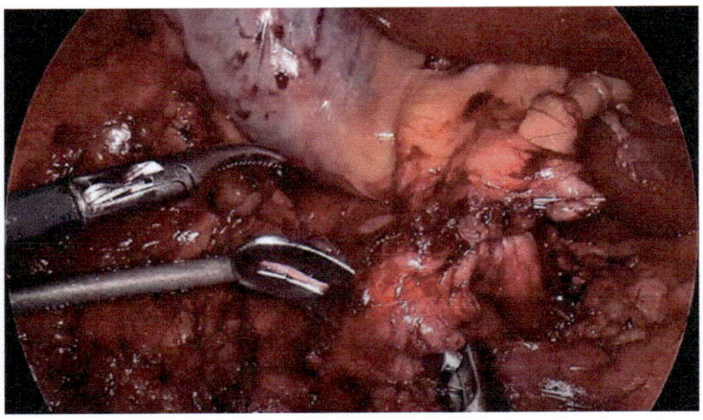

Fig. 5.5 Encircling the common bile duct

5.2.8 Gastroduodenal Artery

The GDA is identified as it takes off from the CHA and crosses towards the head of the pancreas. Intraoperative Doppler ultrasound may be utilized to follow the course of the hepatic artery and confirm hepatic flow while temporarily clamping the GDA, but this is not routinely needed. The GDA is carefully encircled at the origin avoiding injury to the suprapancreatic portal vein (located dorsally) and divided with a stapler using a vascular load (closed height of 0.75–1.0 mm). A 5-mm stump is usually left, which allows endovascular embolization in case the patient develops postpancreatectomy hemorrhage from the GDA stump. Careful dissection behind the GDA stump is carried out, and the suprapancreatic portal vein is exposed. Dividing the GDA early facilitates better access to the hepatoduodenal ligament and its structures.

5.2.9 Common Bile Duct

The dissection of the hepatoduodenal ligament is carried out next. Attention is turned to identifying the common bile duct (CBD) in the lateral aspect of the hepatoduodenal ligament. The peritoneum anterior to the hepatoduodenal ligament is opened, and CBD is dissected circumferentially (Fig. 5.5). Much care is taken to avoid injury to the portal vein (PV), which is located dorsomedially to the CBD. The CBD transection line is chosen taking into consideration the location of the tumor and its biology. The goal is clear margins while preserving as much bile duct length as possible. As such, if feasible, the CBD may be divided even below the insertion of the cystic duct. The bile duct is encircled, clamped with an endoscopic bulldog (Fig. 5.6), and divided with scissors, keeping the posterior wall 2–3 mm longer than the anterior. This will facilitate creation of the hepaticojejunostomy in the reconstruction phase. If there is a preoperatively placed biliary stent, cultures are taken, and the stent is either removed or pushed into the duodenum to be removed with the specimen. Bile duct margin may be sent to frozen pathology if there is suspicion of tumor involvement. The transected CBD at the specimen side is closed by clipping or suturing. ICG infusion is started after clamping the CBD at a 0.4 mg/min infusion rate if the patient is not allergic to iodine.

5.2.10 Retropancreatic Tunnel

Inferior edge of the pancreas is widely exposed at the proposed location of the superior mesenteric vein (SMV). Intraoperative ultrasound may help to identify the SMV. A window between the SMV-PV trunk and the neck of the pancreas is created. This retropancreatic tunnel is developed cephalad along the avascular plane by gently lifting the neck of the pancreas anteriorly. A wide opening at the inferior aspect of the pancreas facilitates the creation of the plane and the identification of the different structures. A finger retractor is carefully introduced in the retropancreatic space and advanced towards the previously exposed suprapancreatic PV, and the tip is exposed at this level (Fig. 5.7). Care should be

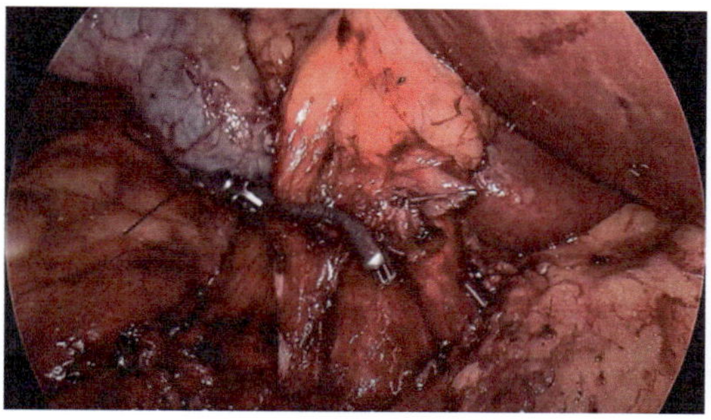

Fig. 5.6 Clamping the common bile duct

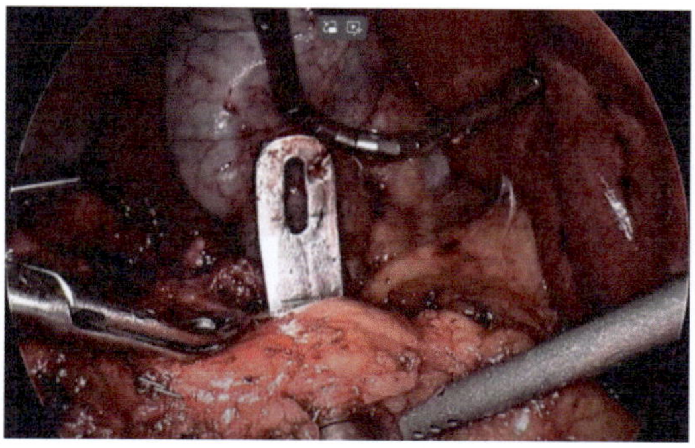

Fig. 5.7 Retropancreatic tunnel

taken to avoid injuring the vascular structures including the CHA when dissecting with the finger retractor. A Penrose drain is inserted into the finger retractor fenestration and passed around the neck of the pancreas for retraction in a hanging maneuver.

5.2.11 Groove

The exposure of the mesenteric–uncinate groove may be achieved by retracting the neck of the pancreas with the Penrose drain anteriorly. This anterior traction allows for better exposure of tributaries to the SMV near the pancreas that should be either protected or ligated, such as the right gastroepiploic vein and anterior superior pancreatoduodenal vein. Gently dissecting the colon mesentery off the uncinate process will facilitate uncinate process dissection at later stages. Care should be taken to avoid injury to the right superior colic vein during this step.

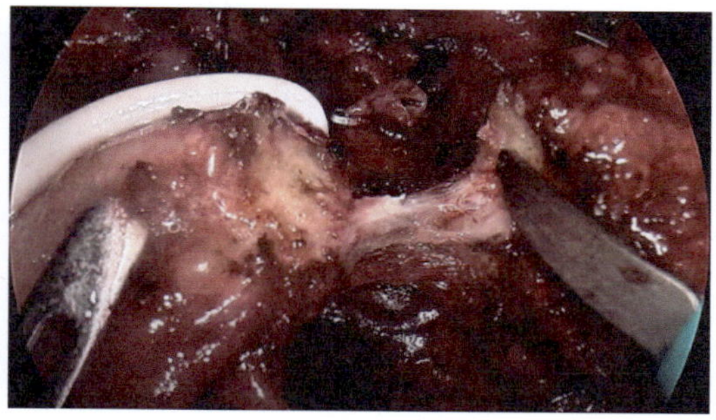

Fig. 5.8 Division of the pancreas

5.2.12 Pancreas

Division of the pancreatic parenchyma is started with ultrasonic shears by using the lower active blade by itself taking advantage of the ultrasonic dissection. When dissection nears the main pancreatic duct, care is taken to avoid thermal injury to the duct. Ultrasonic evaluation and oscillating movements of the ultrasonic active blade will help identify the main pancreatic duct (MPD) and safely dissect it circumferentially (Fig. 5.8). The MPD is divided with scissors, creating a 2–3-mm stump to be used for anastomosis later.

5.2.13 Kocher Maneuver

A complete Kocher maneuver is performed. For this part, the camera is moved to the right-sided port. The second and third portions of the duodenum are widely mobilized by dissecting it off the other retroperitoneal structures (Fig. 5.9). An assistant long limb bowel grasper is placed through the subxiphoid port to retract the earlier mobilized right colon medially and caudally towards the left, while the divided duodenal stump is retracted cephalad. Kocherization is considered sufficient when IVC and the base of the left renal vein are exposed, and ideally the lateral edge of the aorta as well. In the event of a posterior tumor further exposure of the aortocaval groove can be readily done if an extended lymphadenectomy in this area is desired. Dissection is carried out towards the third and fourth portion of the duodenum behind superior

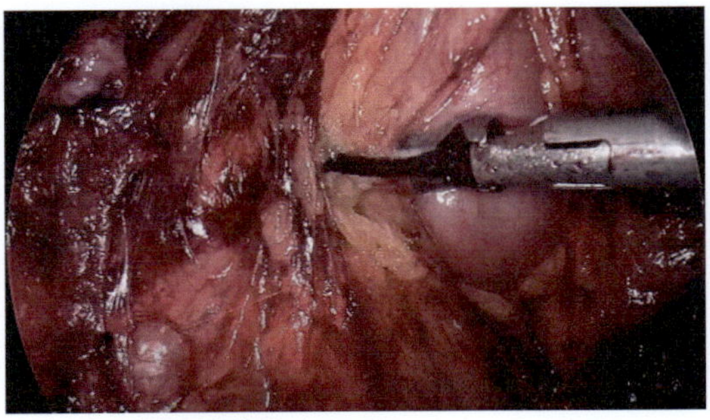

Fig. 5.9 Extensive Kocher Maneuver

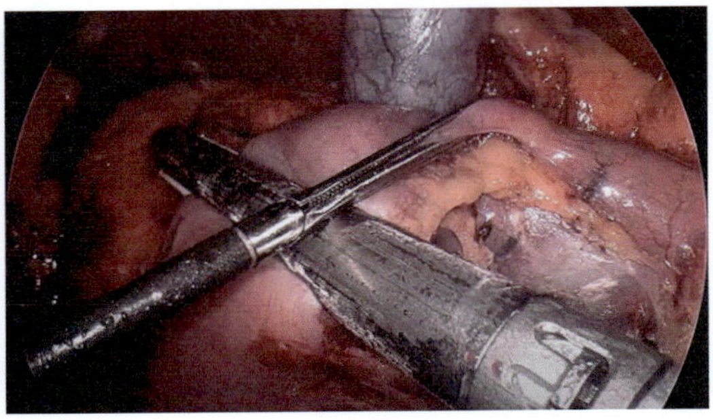

Fig. 5.10 Division of the small bowel

mesenteric vessels. The ligament of Treitz is accessed and opened from the right side. Once a wide window has been created opening the ligament of Treitz, the jejunum is not immediately pulled, the fourth portion of duodenum is first dissected free from its attachments up to its junction with the jejunum. Rarely, supramesocolic takedown of the ligament of Treitz from the right cannot be achieved, and an inframesocolic approach must be taken from the left side under the transverse colon mesentery. Proximal jejunum is gently pulled and passed behind the superior mesenteric vessels, bringing it to the right upper quadrant. The dissection in this stage includes the retropancreatic lymph node groups keeping them in block with the specimen.

5.2.14 Bowel

After bringing the proximal jejunum to the right upper quadrant, a site is chosen for its division. A window is created in the mesentery of the jejunum and the mesenteric vessels are ligated with an advanced bipolar device. The mesentery is cut near the bowel, and excessive mesenteric cutting is avoided, as bleeding from these vessels can occur postoperatively. The jejunum is divided with a stapler (Fig. 5.10), usually about 5 cm beyond the fourth portion of the duodenum (closed staple height of 0.75–1.0 mm) or at a site that would allow the pancreaticojejunal limb to reach without tension for the anastomoses.

5.2.15 Uncinate Process

Dissection of the uncinate process is done from caudate to cephalad. The wide exposure of this area can be attained by retracting the specimen towards the right, by means of a large bowel grasper straddling the pancreas with its opened limbs. The assistant role is crucial in retracting the mesenteric vessels towards the left with the aid of an endokittner and a suction device. ICG infusion may help to delineate pancreatic parenchyma and facilitate this challenging part of the surgery, but its benefit varies according to the degree of fibrosis of the pancreatic parenchyma (Fig. 5.11). Meticulous dissection between uncinate process and SMA and the SMV-PV trunk is performed under direct visualization. Small vessels are ligated with an advance bipolar device, larger veins, usually a caudad, and a more cephalad branch, as well as the inferior pancreatoduodenal artery, originating from SMA, are identified, isolated, clipped, and divided. In case of a replaced RHA, care should be taken to identify and secure this vessel from injury.

5.2.16 Specimen

The specimen is placed in an endoscopic bag with the jejunal end oriented within the edge of the endobag. This facilitates the orientation and extraction of the specimen through a smaller incision, usually 4 cm. It is removed either by enlarging one of the lateral port sites up to 4–5 cm or less frequently through a Pfannenstiel incision.

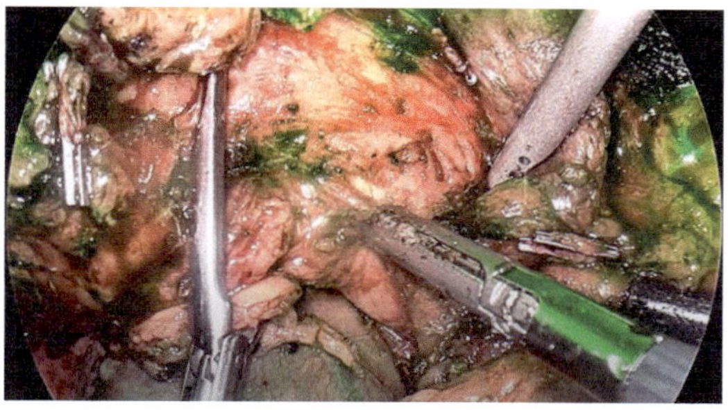

Fig. 5.11 Dissection of the uncinate process

The wound is closed, and pneumoperitoneum reestablished. Cholecystectomy is completed if not done so already while the resection margins are checked by a pathologist.

5.2.17 Margins

Specimen margins are evaluated according to NCCN protocol by a pathologist in coordination with a surgeon, to make sure R0 resection is achieved.

5.2.18 Hepaticojejunostomy

The reconstruction is started by the bilioenteric anastomosis. The authors feel that doing it first gives better access to this anastomosis since the loop of jejunum is free and also helps anchoring the jejunum for the subsequent pancreatic anastomoses.

The jejunum that was left in the right upper quadrant is further advanced and accommodated for the hepaticojejunostomy. It is important to preserve adequate length of the afferent limb proximally (15–20 cm) to allow for construction of the subsequent pancreaticojejunostomy. The patient is rotated left-side down, and the surgeon stands at the patient's right side. The camera is moved to the most lateral 12-mm port. The previously placed bulldog on the bile duct is usually placed cephalad enough that allows for the performance of the anastomosis, and it is not removed until the anastomosis is completed. An enterotomy slightly smaller than the diameter of the CBD is made. A running posterior layer of size 4–0 absorbable barbed suture is started from medial to lateral. The first stitch is placed from inside the bowel out and brought from outside the duct into the lumen at the most medial aspect of the anastomoses. The knot or barbed loop end inside the anastomoses in the posterior layer. The presence of a longer posterior CBD wall facilitates placement of the stitches during the construction of this layer. The anterior wall is then started at the most medial aspect in close proximity to the first stitch of the posterior wall but this time from outside-in maintaining the knot/loop outside. This layer is sutured in similar fashion from medial to lateral. Both sutures are tied at the most lateral corner of the anastomosis. A posterior15-Fr Blake drain is placed at this stage, prior to the construction of the pancreaticojejunostomy to avoid manipulation of this anastomosis once constructed. The drain is positioned behind but not in direct contact with the hepaticojejunostomy and advanced to the posterior aspect of the future pancreaticojejunostomy site.

5.2.19 Pancreaticojejunostomy

A two-layer duct-to-mucosa pancreaticojejunostomy is performed with the surgeon standing between the patient's legs. Reverse Trendelenburg position is added to an extent depending on the patient's body habitus. It is broken in five consecutive steps:

1. Posterior outer pancreatojejunal layer (dorsal pancreatic parenchyma to seromuscular jejunal layer)
2. Enterotomy
3. Posterior inner pancreaticojejunal (duct-to-mucosa) layer
4. Anterior inner pancreaticojejunal (duct-to-mucosa) layer
5. Anterior outer pancreatojejunal (ventral pancreatic parenchyma to seromuscular jejunal) layer

1. Posterior outer pancreatojejunal layer (dorsal pancreatic parenchyma to seromuscular jejunal layer)

A running absorbable barbed 4–0 suture is started at the superior edge of the pancreas including the dorsal portion of the pancreas and a seromuscular layer of the jejunum close to the mesentery. This will be the posterior outer layer of the anastomosis. The suture runs in cranio-caudal direction and finishes at the inferior border of the pancreas. The lower end of this running sutures to be tied with the anterior-outer pancreatojejunal suture later. The stitches in the pancreas side are placed well in the posterior aspect of the pancreas but not the cut edge. Those in the jejunal side are placed in the same place of the seromuscular layer to create a "ledge" of small bowel that opposes the pancreatic capsule posteriorly and ends covering the posterior aspect of the inner duct-to-mucosa anastomoses. Furthermore, it everts the cut edge of the pancreas upwards, better exposing the pancreatic duct.

2. Enterotomy

An enterotomy is created using the ultrasonic shears, slightly larger in diameter than the pancreatic duct. We usually place a 3.5 or 5 Fr pediatric feeding tube into the pancreatic duct to facilitate construction of anastomosis but pulled out prior to completion of the anastomosis.

3. Posterior inner pancreaticojejunal layer (duct-to-mucosa)

The posterior inner layer of the anastomosis is fashioned with interrupted 5–0 absorbable polyglactin suture mounted on an RB2 or, if available, a TF needle. Usually, alternating suture colors are used (using a surgical marker) to avoid confusion during placement. The first stitch of this duct-to-mucosa anastomosis is placed at the 6 o'clock (most posterior) position. The needle is passed inside-out the duct and outside-in the jejunum. This assumes that 12 o'clock is the most anterior aspect. This suture is left untied and together with the pancreatic stent can be gently used to help open the lumen of the duct for subsequent suture placement. Care is taken to avoid excessive manipulation of the suture/stent to prevent damage to the pancreatic duct. The amount of posterior layer interrupted sutures will depend on duct size but is usually at least two more, one at approximately 8 o'clock and one at 4 o'clock. The posterior stitches are tied as they are placed except for the first 6 o'clock stitch which is tied last.

4. Anterior inner pancreaticojejunal layer (duct-to-mucosa)

A 12 o'clock stitch is placed on the anterior layer of the pancreatic duct only to help gently manipulate and expose the duct during anastomosis. Further interrupted (outside-in the duct and inside-out the jejunum) stitches are placed on the ventral aspect of the pancreatic duct and left untied. Care is taken not to cross the stitches, and the tails are aligned. Placing the stitches from caudad to cephalad is helpful. Ideally, at least 3–4 anterior stitches are used for the anterior layer. The 12 o'clock stitch, which was initially placed through the pancreas to help expose the duct, is the last stitch to be completed by being passed through the jejunum. All anterior stitches are tied.

5. Anterior outer pancreatojejunal layer (ventral pancreatic parenchyma to seromuscular jejunal layer)

The suture from the posterior outer layer is now advanced further by coming around the inferior edge of the pancreas and ending at the lower portion to join the future anterior layer. This anterior outer layer is constructed with a running craniocaudal absorbable 4–0 barbed suture in a similar fashion to the posterior outer layer. This includes the ventral portion of the pancreatic parenchyma (trying to avoid the cut edge) and anterior seromuscular layer of the jejunum, creating an anterior "ledge" of bowel. This suture is tied to the suture from the dorsal pancreatojejunal layer, and this concludes the pancreaticojejunostomy.

5.2.20 Duodenojejunostomy

For the construction of end-to-side duodenojejunostomy, the same pancreatobiliary jejunal loop is used at about 30–50 cm beyond the previous Treitz ligament or were the loop reaches the divided post-pyloric duodenum without tension. The jejunal loop is brought in antecolic fashion at the site where the greater omentum was previously split. A two-layer duodenojejunostomy is started with a running posterior seromuscular layer using 3–0 absorbable barbed suture. Small bites are taken and the staple-line at the duodenal stump is incorporated in this posterior outer layer. After finishing the posterior layer, openings in the duodenum and jejunum are created using ultrasonic shears. The opening in the duodenum is done close to the staple line. The pylorus is gently dilated. The inner running posterior layer incorporates the small rim of duodenum that it is between the staple and the opening by placing the stitches passed the staple line internally. Then, the anterior layer is created in the usual fashion for a bowel anastomosis. Once the outer posterior and anterior layers are completed, they are tied to each other.

In high-risk patients, we place a second 15-Fr Blake drain which is placed anteriorly to the pancreaticojejunostomy and duodenojejunostomy from the left superior port site.

5.3 Discussion

MIPD is a complex operation. We present our operative technique developed with over two decades of experience in a standardized format that may make learning and teaching the procedure simpler. The technical steps can be adapted to a laparoscopic or robotic approach. Other well-established surgeons have also proposed similarly deconstructed explanations of this complex procedure [7, 16].

Deviation from the standardized technique in each individual patient is uncommon and the authors agree with the literature, artery-first approach with its different variations is used [18–20]. In a similar manner, vascular resections are performed routinely and proximal and distal control as well as reconstruction for type II–IV resections require modifications of the described technique.

In conclusion, as more patients are offered a minimally invasive option for PD, standardized and reproducible teaching methods for MIPD will be of continued importance.

References

1. Gagner M, Pomp A. Laparoscopic pylorus-preserving pancreatoduodenectomy. Surg Endosc. 1994;8(5):408–10.
2. Asbun HJ, Stauffer JA. Laparoscopic vs open pancreaticoduodenectomy: overall outcomes and severity of complications using the accordion severity grading system. J Am Coll Surg. 2012 Dec;215(6):810–9.
3. Mantzavinou A, Uppara M, Chan J, Patel B. Robotic versus open pancreaticoduodenectomy, comparing therapeutic indexes; a systematic review. Int J Surg Lond Engl. 2022;101:106633.
4. Cai J, Ramanathan R, Zenati MS, Al Abbas A, Hogg ME, Zeh HJ, et al. Robotic pancreaticoduodenectomy is associated with decreased clinically relevant pancreatic fistulas: a propensity-matched analysis. J Gastrointest Surg. 2020;24(5):1111–8.
5. Asbun HJ, Moekotte AL, Vissers FL, Kunzler F, Cipriani F, Alseidi A, et al. The Miami International Evidence-based Guidelines on minimally invasive pancreas resection. Ann Surg. 2020;271(1):1–14.
6. Abu Hilal M, van Ramshorst TME, Boggi U, Dokmak S, Edwin B, Keck T, et al. The Brescia Internationally Validated European Guidelines on Minimally Invasive Pancreatic Surgery (EGUMIPS). Ann Surg. 2024;279(1):45–57.
7. Palanivelu C, Senthilnathan P, Sabnis SC, Babu NS, Srivatsan Gurumurthy S, Anand Vijai N, et al. Randomized clinical trial of laparoscopic versus open pancreatoduodenectomy for periampullary tumours. Br J Surg. 2017;104(11):1443–50.
8. Croome KP, Farnell MB, Que FG, Km R-L, Truty MJ, Nagorney DM, et al. Total laparoscopic pancreaticoduodenectomy for pancreatic ductal adenocarcinoma: oncologic advantages over open approaches? Ann Surg. 2014;260(4):633–40.
9. Conticchio M, Delvecchio A, Ferraro V, Stasi M, Casella A, Filippo R, et al. Standardization of robotic right liver mobilization. Int J Med Robot Comput Assist Surg MRCAS. 2023;19(6):e2551.
10. Miskovic D, Ahmed J, Bissett-Amess R, Gómez Ruiz M, Luca F, Jayne D, et al. European consensus on the standardization of robotic total mesorectal excision for rectal cancer. Colorectal Dis Off J Assoc Coloproctology G B Irel. 2019;21(3):270–6.

11. Villeneuve LM, Evans AR, Bowen I, Gernsback J, Balsara K, Jea A, et al. A systematic review of the power of standardization in pediatric neurosurgery. Neurosurg Rev. 2023;46(1):325.
12. Yoshimura K, Okubo K, Matsui Y, Nishiyama H, Ogawa O. Laparoendoscopic single-site surgery for left adrenalectomy: standardization of technique. J Endourol. 2011;25(6):1031–5.
13. Asbun HJ, Stauffer JA. Laparoscopic approach to distal and subtotal pancreatectomy: a clockwise technique. Surg Endosc. 2011;25(8):2643–9.
14. Asbun HJ, Van Hilst J, Tsamalaidze L, Kawaguchi Y, Sanford D, Pereira L, et al. Technique and audited outcomes of laparoscopic distal pancreatectomy combining the clockwise approach, progressive stepwise compression technique, and staple line reinforcement. Surg Endosc. 2020;34(1):231–9.
15. Asbun HJ, Harada E, Stauffer JA. Tips for laparoscopic pancreaticoduodenectomy. J Hepato-Biliary-Pancreat Sci [Internet]. 2016 [cited 2024 Apr 9];23(3). Available from: https://onlinelibrary.wiley.com/doi/10.1002/jhbp.325.
16. Kendrick ML, Cusati D. Total laparoscopic pancreaticoduodenectomy. Arch Surg. 2010;145:1.
17. How i do it: robotic pancreaticoduodenectomy – PubMed [Internet]. [cited 2024 Apr 10]. Available from: https://pubmed.ncbi.nlm.nih.gov/31152344/.
18. Sanjay P, Takaori K, Govil S, Shrikhande SV, Windsor JA. "Artery-first" approaches to pancreatoduodenectomy. Br J Surg. 2012;99(8):1027–35.
19. Kurosaki I, Minagawa M, Takano K, Takizawa K, Hatakeyama K. Left posterior approach to the superior mesenteric vascular pedicle in pancreaticoduodenectomy for cancer of the pancreatic head. J Pancreas. 2011;12(3):220–9.
20. Cai Y, Gao P, Li Y, Wang X, Peng B. Laparoscopic pancreaticoduodenectomy with major venous resection and reconstruction: anterior superior mesenteric artery first approach. Surg Endosc. 2018;32(10):4209–15.

Robotic Pancreato Duodenectomy

6

Benedetto Ielpo, Greta Donisi, Patricia Sanchez-Velazquez, Alberto Garcia-Picazo, and Fernando Burdio

6.1 Main Indications and Contraindications

Since the pioneering report of the first robotic PD by Giulianotti et al. in 2003 [1], numerous studies have demonstrated the feasibility and safety of robotic PD in treating malignancies of the pancreatic head.

Based on the current body of literature reviewed, mainly being retrospective non-randomized studies, robotic PD is as safe and effective as the open approach for both benign and malignant disease [2–7]. The recently published EUROPA trial [8] and the Chinese trial by Liu et al. [9], the first RCTs comparing open versus robotic PD, have confirmed these results, reporting comparable postoperative short-term outcomes for a variety of pancreatic head diseases and periampullary tumors.

Supplementary Information The online version contains supplementary material available at https://doi.org/10.1007/978-3-031-99695-5_6. The videos can be accessed individually by clicking the DOI link in the accompanying figure caption or by scanning this link with the SN More Media App.

B. Ielpo (✉) · G. Donisi · P. Sanchez-Velazquez · A. Garcia-Picazo · F. Burdio
HPB Unit, Hospital del Mar, Pompeu Fabra University, Barcelona, Spain
e-mail: ielpo.b@gmail.com; greta.donisi@icloud.com; psanchezvelazquez@hmar.cat; alberto.gpicazo@gmail.com; fburdio@hmar.cat

Invasion of major vessels is a relative contraindication for minimally invasive approach and only expert surgeons in high-volume centers should perform such procedure.

It is worth underlining that mastering the techniques involved in this procedure requires extensive training due to its complexity.

6.2 Surgical Technique (Video)

- *Patient Position*
  As shown in the Fig. 6.1, the patient is positioned supine in a 20-degree reverse Trendelenburg, slight left side tilt, with arms adducted and legs apart. We suggest a slight left side rotation in order to get a better visualization during the Kocher maneuver.
- *Trocar placement*
  Trocar placement is illustrated in Fig. 6.2. We suggest adapting its placement according to the conformation of the patient's abdominal wall. To determine the optimal trocar placement area, it is important to identify the subcostal arch, superior anterior iliac spine, and the midline and transverse line through the umbilicus. In this way, surgeons get a better picture of abdominal wall landmarks to better orientate trocars placement.

  Based on our experience, we prefer aligning the trocars with the umbilicus. Robotic trocars 2 and 3 are positioned approximately

B. Ielpo et al. (eds.), *Minimally Invasive Pancreatoduodenectomy in Cancer*,
https://doi.org/10.1007/978-3-031-99695-5_6

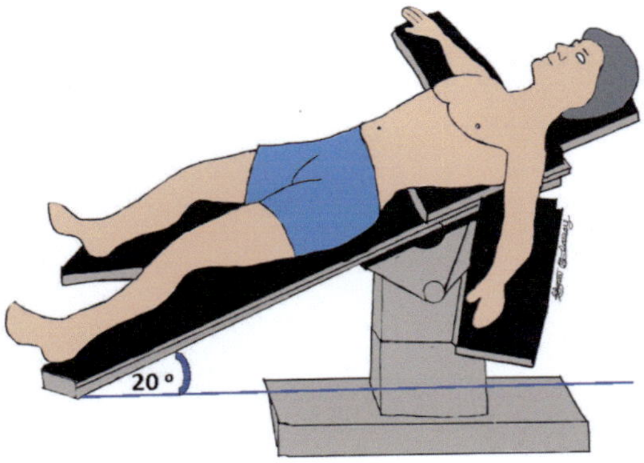

Fig. 6.1 Patient position

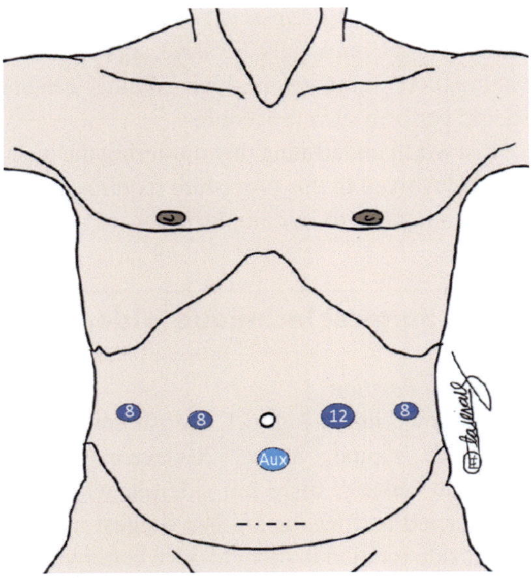

Fig. 6.2 Robotic trocars placement

10–12 cm apart, with the assistant's 12-mm trocar placed in between, 1–2 cm below, as depicted. This placement allows for ample space between these two robotic arms, facilitating assistant's access and range of motion.

Trocars 1 and 4 are situated roughly 5 cm apart from trocars 2 and 3, respectively, approximately 1 cm above the transverse umbilical line. Induction of pneumoperitoneum is achieved through a Verres needle enabling refining of trocars placement after abdominal distension. We then directly insert the robotic trocars, starting with number 2, which primarily serves as the optic trocar throughout the surgery. Following its insertion, we sequentially place trocars 4, 3, and finally the arm 1. The assistant trocar is inserted only at the end of this process.

The robot is positioned on the patient's right side, and docking begins at this point. Through the initial surgical steps, robotic instruments are placed as follows: the endoscope is positioned in trocar 2, the fenestrated bipolar in trocar 1, the vessel sealer in trocar 3, and the tip-up in trocar 4.

- *Exploration and Mobilization*

  As for any oncological procedure, exploration of the abdominal and pelvic cavities precedes surgery.

  If there is no radiological suspicion of vascular invasion, our current practice, as depicted in the video, involves an artery first approach. The Treitz ligament and the mesentery of the first jejunal loop are initially sectioned, dissecting as far as possible up to the superior mesenteric artery (SMA) (Fig. 6.3). Sectioning the jejunal mesentery, as shown in the video, facilitate this step. This is known as the left approach, or Treitz ligament approach, among the SMA first approaches [10], which is contraindicated if the tumor is deemed potentially not resectable after the exploration. In this approach, after dividing the ligament of Treitz, the proximal jejunum is pulled to the left to expose the first and second jejunal arteries, which are then divided at their origin from the SMA, as shown in the video. Further traction on the proximal jejunum facilitates a counterclockwise rotation of the superior mesenteric artery, aiding in the identification and division of the inferior pancreaticoduodenal artery. Additionally, traction of the proximal jejunum clears the posterior and right aspects of the superior mesenteric artery. Subsequently, the jejunum is divided, and the duodenum is moved to the right to expose and divide the remaining connective tissue attached to the superior mesenteric pedicle.

  We propose using this approach for tumors located along the uncinate and ventral pan-

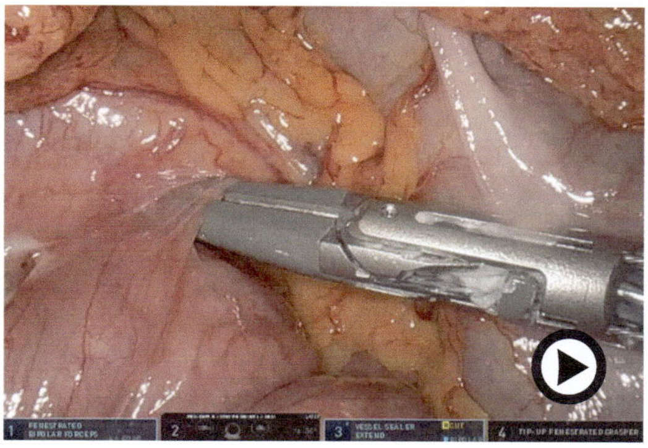

Fig. 6.3 Treitz section (Surgical technique (▶ https://doi.org/10.1007/000-hek))

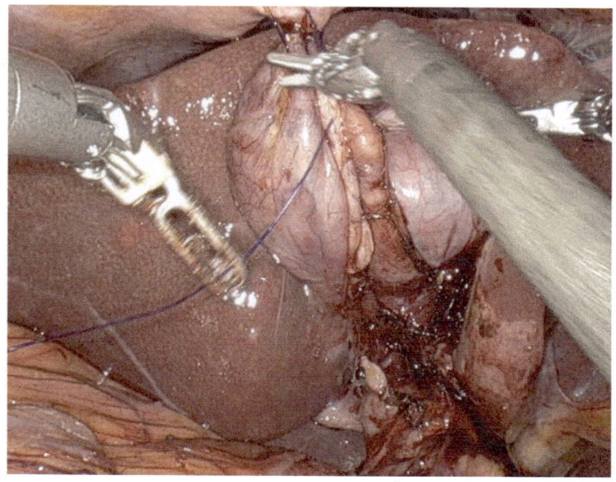

Fig. 6.4 Gallbladder lifting up

creas. Nevertheless, it may be challenging in patients with fatty mesentery. In such case, indocyanine green fluorescence imaging can assist in localizing the superior mesenteric artery, thereby enhancing procedural ease.

Alternatively, when tumor is located far from the uncinate process or in challenging cases with fatty mesentery, we suggest a partial left approach, involving only Treitz ligament section, jejunum mobilization, and section. The dissection of the SMA will be further detailed posteriorly, as described below. This is not an obligatory step which may be skipped according to surgeon preferences. But, in our experience, this maneuver facilitates the completion of the following Kocher maneuver, allowing a full first jejunal loop mobilization.

6.2.1 Surgical Field Exposure

A fundamental initial step is achieving wide exposure of the surgical field. We recommend lifting the liver by passing a stitch through the falciform ligament at its origin, a straight needle is used which is passed transabdominally and knotted externally, as shown in the video. In case of a particularly large hemiliver, especially in cases of fatty liver, which may obstruct the surgical field, we suggest placing an additional transhepatic stitch for further elevation. In certain cases, an additional suture to the left liver lobe is also required to further expose the surgical field for a better dissection.

Subsequently, the gallbladder is freed by dissecting and sectioning the cystic artery and duct with a partial cholecystectomy technique (Fig. 6.4). Finally, the gallbladder fundus is secured to the abdominal wall using a barbed suture. This approach ensures a broad surgical field exposure, facilitating safe dissection, as it is shown in the video.

6.2.2 Kocher Maneuver and SMA Dissection

Right hepatic flexure is taken down partially starting with the separation of the duodenum from the transverse colon.

Surgery continues with mobilization of the duodenum. This maneuver should be performed as extensively as possible, as part of the "posterior approach to the SMA," to ensure correct dissection of the SMA [10].

The posterior approach begins with wide Kocherization to expose the vena cava and left renal vein, as demonstrated in the video. An important suggestion is to move the tip-up instrument of the fourth robotic arm retracting the duodenum and subsequently adjusting the traction to allow further mobilization of the duodenum, as shown in the video.

The origin of the SMA is exposed where it passes above the left renal vein (Fig. 6.5). This approach offers advantages in early identification of SMA, and it also aids in an early identification of a replaced right hepatic artery from the superior mesenteric artery and, additionally, allows for aorto-caval node sampling. As shown in the video, this step allows for an initial mesopancreas dissection from the SMA and, whenever possible, to divide the superior pancreaticoduodenal artery (Fig. 6.6).

A useful trick is to use a gauze to protect the duodenum when manipulated by the Tip-up grasper. To prevent any nerve plexus injury, dissection of the SMA is performed only on its superior border, which is considered a margin of the mesopancreas [11]. While this approach may be challenging in patients with peripancreatic inflammation around the pancreatic head, we recommend it for posteromedial tumors in the pancreatic head and neck, as well as periampullary tumors extending from the pancreatic body to the head. We believe that combining the left and posterior approaches to the SMA allows for a safer and oncologically radical mesopancreas dissection [10].

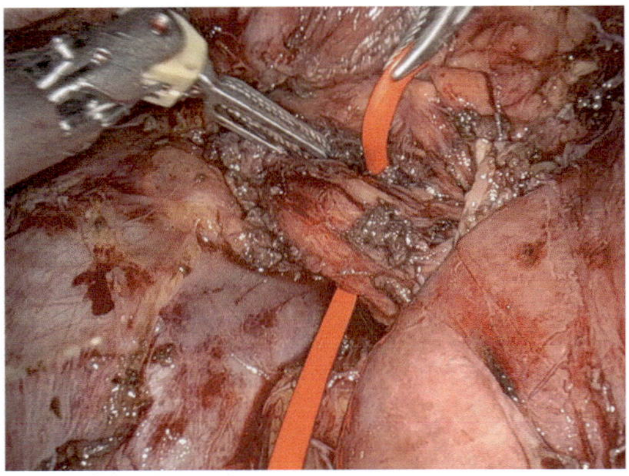

Fig. 6.5 Superior mesenteric artery identification

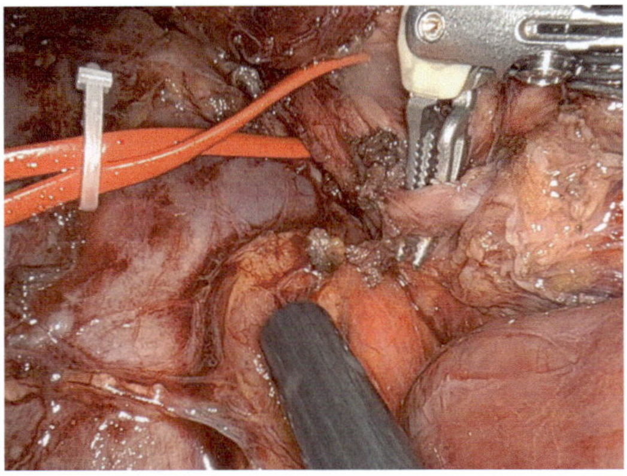

Fig. 6.6 Early-stage inferior pancreatoduodenal artery section

Robotic surgery may facilitate this approach thanks to increased maneuverability, precise dissection, and a shorter learning curve, as demonstrated in the video.

6.2.3 Hilar Dissection

Dissection progresses to the liver hilum, where the common hepatic artery, proper hepatic artery, gastroduodenal artery, and main biliary duct are identified. It is crucial to perform at least a standard lymphadenectomy of the specified stations as shown in the video.

This dissection can be conducted using various robotic instruments interchangeably, depending on the surgeon's experience and the procedural stage. The hook instrument is particularly useful to open the fat tissues around the arteries, while the vessel sealer is effective for node dissection. Once the gastroduodenal artery (GDA) is identified, we recommend, before its section, to check for proper liver vascularization from the hepatic artery by clamping GDA with a bulldog as demonstrated in the video with or without indocyanine green (ICG) fluorescence imaging. Subsequently, the GDA can be sectioned using Hem-o-Lock or ligation, according to the surgeon's preference. We suggest to leave a relatively long GDA stump in order to be radiologically embolized in case of post operative bleeding.

After the GDA is sectioned, dissection continues until the portal vein is identified, followed by sectioning the fine lamina between the vein and the superior margin of the neck of the pancreas. This maneuver facilitates the subsequent dissection of the tunnel between the pancreatic neck and the superior mesenteric vein (SMV).

Before proceeding to the next step, the stomach is transected using a stapler.

6.2.4 Pancreatic Transection

At this stage, the mesocolon is gently lifted downward using the tip-up forceps, and a careful dissection of the inferior pancreatic border is performed using either the hook or the vessel sealer. This dissection is carried out carefully until the SMV is identified. Once identified, a tunnel between the vein and the pancreatic neck is created. The vessel sealer, with its smooth tip, is particularly useful for this maneuver. If the passage cannot be completed up to the superior border of the pancreas, we recommend using an alternative device through the assistant port, such as a gold finger, as demonstrated in the video. A loop can be placed to lift the pancreatic neck.

Transection at this step can be accomplished using robotic scissors, avoiding electrocautery when very close to the pancreatic duct. Hemorrhage from the pancreatic stump can be controlled by the bipolar fenestrated forceps placed in the robotic arm number 1 and the hook placed in the number 3.

Following completion of the transection, in case of small ducts, we suggest placing a temporary plastic stent in the pancreatic stump to maintain patency of the pancreatic duct.

6.2.5 Mesopancreas Dissection

In the video demonstration, the initial phase entails traction and transection of the proximal portion of the first jejunal loop, previously dissected up to the Treitz ligament, using a mechanical stapler.

The second phase involves separating the uncinate process from the mesentery of the first jejunal loop, proceeding between the uncinate process and the terminal branch of the SMV. A vessel-free space allows direct dissection with scissors. The first jejunal branch of the SMV is dissected and sacrificed to facilitate exposure of the SMA. Subsequently, the uncinate process is dissected off the SMA with a caudal to cranial approach.

During superficial dissection of the mesopancreas, the inferior pancreaticoduodenal vein (IPDV) is encountered first. Section is performed using LigaSure or, in case of a larger IPDV, a ligature is applied. The robotic platform offers significant advantages when ligatures are required.

If the previous posterior SMA approach mesopancreas dissection was not done, deep dissection of the mesopancreas involves identifying and transecting the inferior pancreaticoduodenal arteries (IPDA). Robotic Vessel Sealer and, if necessary, any assistant radiofrequency devices, are employed to control bleeding at this stage.

As shown in the video and in Fig. 6.7, the previous dissection of SMA performed at an early stage allows for a safer identification, decreasing the risk of damaging it and increasing the chance for a more complete mesopancreas dissection.

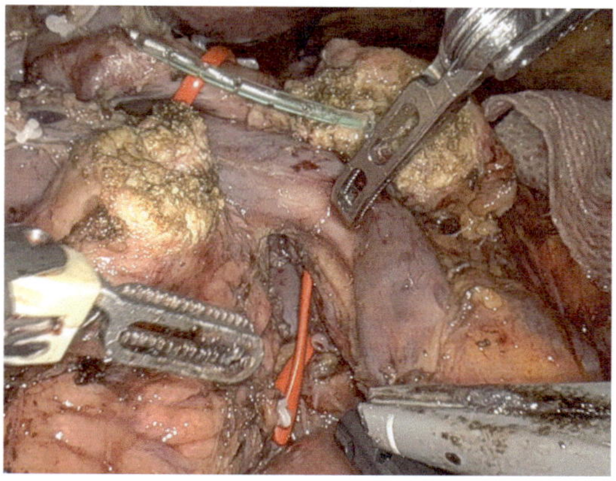

Fig. 6.7 SMA identification during mesopancreas dissection

6.2.6 Specimen Extraction

An endobag is inserted through a Pfannenstiel incision, once the demolition phase is completed, to extract the surgical specimen, as demonstrated in the video. Subsequently, the incision is closed. This step is typically performed by fellows or training residents and may take approximately 30 min. We strongly recommend that the surgeon take a break during this step to rest, eat, and drink.

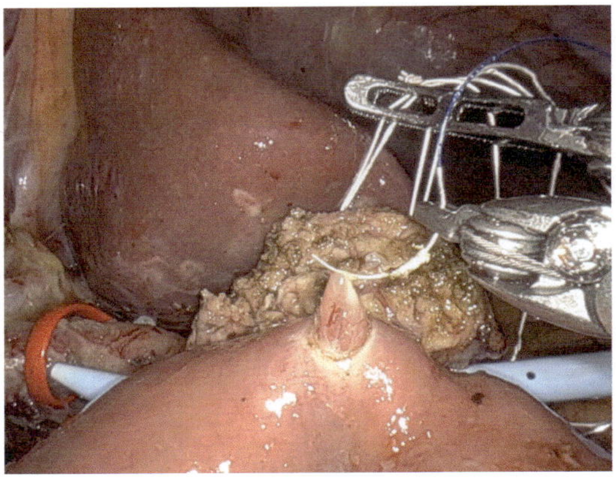

Fig. 6.8 Jejunum orifice

6.2.7 Reconstruction

A single-loop reconstruction is performed according to the Child technique.

6.2.7.1 Pancreatic Anastomosis

In the video, we demonstrate a modified Blumgart anastomosis.

Before starting the anastomosis, a pigtail drainage is inserted. In our opinion, this is an important tip as it allows for a safe and effective drainage placement posteriorly to the anastomosis.

A double-needle 3/0 Gore-Tex stitch is utilized, the needle is modified in order to have a straight angle. To manage the length, we recommend cutting the suture and knotting it in the middle, resulting in a 15 cm overall length.

This suture is passed through the jejunal loop and the entire stump thickness, starting from the upper part, creating two trans-pancreatic stitches—one on each side of the pancreatic duct. These stitches are grasped by the tip-up robotic forceps with slight traction, allowing the jejunal loop to lie behind the posterior face of the pancreas.

Another 3/0 single-needle Gore-Tex suture is placed just posterior to the main pancreatic duct, between the pancreas and the jejunal loop.

The orifice for the duct-to-mucosa is created just in front of the pancreatic duct using the needle of a 5/0 polyglactin suture, which is passed through the jejunal loop wall and coagulated with the hook, resulting in a smaller and precise orifice opening (Fig. 6.8).

In our opinion, a smaller opening might decrease potential pancreatic leaks.

The duct-to-mucosa anastomosis is performed using interrupted 5/0 polyglactin sutures, usually 3–4 posteriorly and 5–7 anteriorly. Once the sutures are passed the two extremities are included in a Hem-o-lok, which can be easily released later, to avoid confusion among the different sutures. The posterior sutures are tied, except for the lateral ones, to avoid tension.

Typically, a stent is inserted into the pancreatic duct after completing the posterior wall of the duct-to-mucosa anastomosis, removing the previous one, if placed. Currently, we are using a biodegradable stent, Q3 Medical, Dublin, Ireland, as shown in the video.

Once the anastomosis is finished, the two sutures grasped by the tip-up forceps are freed, and the jejunum is sutured again, enclosing the neck of the pancreas within the jejunal loop. Subsequently, two single-needle Gore-Tex sutures are placed in the corner to further invaginate both sides.

6.2.7.2 Biliary Anastomosis

This anastomosis is performed following the same jejunal loop of the previous anastomosis.

An end-to-side hepatic-jejunum anastomosis is performed, with a posterior double semicon-

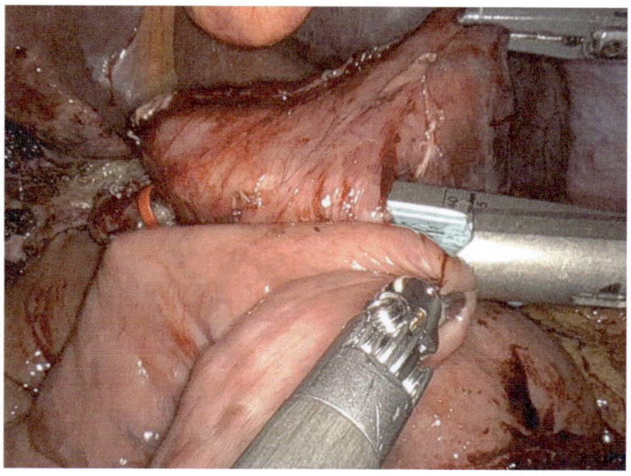

Fig. 6.9 Gastroenteric anastomosis

tinuous and single layer anteriorly. A 5/0 polyglactin sutures are used. As for any anastomosis, it is important to avoid any tension in order to decrease fistulas. Contrary to common opinion, this is considered a difficult anastomosis, as well. Robotic approach clearly facilitates this step allowing for a backwards suture, which, otherwise, by laparoscopy is very difficult.

6.2.7.3 Gastric Anastomosis

Using the same jejunal loop as of the previous pancreatic and hepatic anastomosis, we perform a side-to-side anastomosis with the posterior gastric wall, as shown in Fig. 6.9. After the opening of both jejunum and stomach with scissors or hook, a stapler is introduced and fired. Finally, the wall discontinuation is closed with a single-layer barbed suture 3/0. If a robotic stapler is used for this anastomosis, we suggest introduce through the third robotic arm trocar. Sometime, even this procedure can be difficult, especially in thin patients where there is not enough space to correctly maneuver the robotic stapler. An alternative option can be the use of a laparoscopic standard stapler through the auxiliary laparoscopic trocar.

6.3 Special Tricks and Tips and Personal Suggestions

We suggest always to study preoperatively the vascular anatomy of the patient, looking at any vascular variant that might complicate the procedure. The 3D vascular reconstruction can be visualized in the robotic screen.

Some laparoscopic extra energy devices used through the assistant trocar may provide advantages in some surgical steps. On one hand, they may speed up the surgery; on the other hand, if the Synchroseal is not available, a fine-tip laparoscopic energy device may help in achieving finer dissection.

Whenever possible, we also suggest to wrap the GDA with the round ligament, as shown in the video. This maneuver might decrease the risk of potential GDA bleeding in case of pancreatic fistula.

As no evidence exist on the best anastomosis, pancreatic anastomosis should be performed according to surgeons and institution practice [12].

Additionally, this is a very complex surgery, and we strongly suggest that surgeons who are approaching this procedure for the first time adhere to the “See One, Do One, Teach One Approach” whereby they spend time in an external lab reviewing the full procedures either remotely or in person until they are comfortable, invite a certified proctor to advise them on the initial cases, and get comfortable with the equipment and procedure well enough that you feel comfortable teaching your colleagues what you have learned. Surgeons should be humble and not overly proud, always seeking help and guidance [2].

In our opinion, at least in the current era, it is important that surgeons approaching this procedure already get enough experience with open procedures.

At the initial stage of the learning curve, surgeons should avoid being too dogmatic. A hybrid procedure, with some anastomoses or steps performed using an open approach, can serve as a bridge to help overcome the initial learning curve. This flexibility is also a key point for success along with continued review of videotaped procedures or viewing live procedures where you can focus in on the steps you find more challenging.

A fundamental key point to the success of such a complex surgery is also the collaboration among all members of the team so it is important that the team participates in the "See 1, Do 1, Teach 1," strategy for the greatest chance of success. Since the very beginning of our series we have been sharing the different steps of the procedure among colleagues, resulting in a less stressful procedure, better knowledge transfer, and a more rapid adoption of the robotic procedure.

In our opinion, this procedure should not be performed by a single surgeon. Through collaboration, it is also possible to accelerate the learning curve. Like many other procedures, this is not a one-surgeon operation.

Main Key Points

- Proper patient positioning and trocar placement are critical for optimal access and visualization during surgery.
- Wide exposure of the surgical field, achieved through liver lifting and securing the gallbladder, is useful to keep robotic arms free.
- Extensive mobilization of the duodenum and meticulous dissection of the superior mesenteric artery (SMA) are essential steps to ensure safety in case of intraoperative accidents.
- Careful dissection of the mesopancreas and hepatic hilum is neoessary, ensuring lymphadenectomy and proper vascular control.
- Successful outcomes depend on team collaboration and initial proctoring by experienced surgeons for those new to the procedure.

Acknowledgments The authors thanks Miss Flavia Ielpo Fuentes and Chiara Ielpo Fuentes for their contributions with the drawing of the pictures.

References

1. Giulianotti PC, et al. Robotics in general surgery personal experience in a large community hospital. Arch Surg. 2003;138(7):777–84.
2. Uijterwijk BA, Wei K, Kasai M, Ielpo B, Hilst JV, Chinnusamy P, Lemmers DHL, Burdio F, Senthilnathan P, Besselink MG, Abu Hilal M, Qin R. Minimally invasive versus open pancreatoduodenectomy for pancreatic ductal adenocarcinoma: individual patient data meta-analysis of randomized trials. Eur J Surg Oncol. 2023;49(8):1351–61. https://doi.org/10.1016/j.ejso.2023.03.227. Epub 2023 Apr 7.
3. Lof S, et al. Outcomes of elective and emergency conversion in minimally invasive distal pancreatectomy for pancreatic ductal adenocarcinoma: an international multicenter propensity score-matched study. Ann Surg. 2021;274:e1001–7.
4. Gavriilidis P, et al. Robotic versus laparoscopic distal pancreatectomy—the first meta-analysis. HPB. 2016;18:567–74.
5. Ouyang L, Zhang J, Feng Q, Zhang Z, Ma H. Robotic versus laparoscopic pancreaticoduodenectomy: an up-to-date system review and meta-analysis search strategy and study selection. Front Oncol. 2022;12:1–10.
6. Jiang DJ, Hogg ME. Robotic pancreaticoduodenectomy versus laparoscopic pancreaticoduodenectomy. Laparosc Surg. 2021;5:1–7. https://doi.org/10.21037/ls-20-53.
7. Aiolfi A, Lombardo F, Bonitta G, Danelli P, Bona D. Systematic review and updated network meta – analysis comparing open, laparoscopic, and robotic pancreaticoduodenectomy. Updat Surg. 2021;73:909–22.
8. Klotz R, et al. Robotic versus open partial pancreatoduodenectomy (EUROPA): a randomised controlled stage 2b trial. Lancet Reg Health Eur. 2024;39:100864. https://doi.org/10.1016/j.lanepe.2024.100864.
9. Liu Q, et al. Effect of robotic versus open pancreaticoduodenectomy on postoperative length of hospital stay and complications for pancreatic head or periampullary tumours: a multicentre, open-label randomised controlled trial. Lancet Gastroenterol Hepatol. 2024; https://doi.org/10.1016/s2468-1253(24)00005-0.
10. Ielpo B, Anselmo A, Masuda Y, Xuan MYH, Burdio F, De Blasi V, Sanchez-Velazquez P, Giuliani A, Azagra JS, Viola GM, Podda M, Pellino G, Rosso E. Superior mesenteric artery first approach for minimally invasive pancreaticoduodenectomy: a step-by-step surgical technique video. Ann Surg Oncol. 2023;30(3):1500–3. https://doi.org/10.1245/s10434-022-12743-2. Epub 2022 Nov 5.
11. Ielpo B, d'Addetta MV, Anselmo A, Rosso E, de Blasi V, Sanchez-Velazquez P, Vellalta G, Podda M, Burdio F. Levels of robotic mesopancreas dissection according to malignancy and vascular anatomy:

what surgeons need to know. Ann Surg Oncol. 2024;31(3):1916–8. https://doi.org/10.1245/s10434-023-14686-8. Epub 2023 Dec 10. PMID: 38071705; PMCID: PMC10838235.

12. Ielpo B, Anselmo A, Koh Y, Burdio F, De Blasi V, Sanchez-Velazquez P, Azagra JS, Huscher C, Giuliani A, Pellino G, Rosso E. Minimally invasive pancreatic anastomosis after pancreaticoduodenectomy: multi-institutional step by step video description of the technique. Updat Surg. 2023;75(1):255–9. https://doi.org/10.1007/s13304-022-01389-0. Epub 2022 Nov 12.

Artery-First Approaches

7

Benedetto Ielpo, Yoshio Masuda,
Patricia Sanchez-Velazquez, and Fernando Burdio

7.1 Introduction

With the rapid propagation of minimally invasive pancreatic surgery among the international surgical community, it is important to reinforce key oncological steps established in the traditional open approach. The primary objective of this chapter is to examine one of the most important oncological steps in minimally invasive pancreaticoduodenectomy (MIPD).

Understanding and mastering the various approaches to superior mesenteric artery (SMA) dissection for MIPD is crucial to achieve negative margins, more complete lymphadenectomy, and a safer mesopancreatic dissection [1]. Moreover, these techniques enable early visualisation of a replaced right hepatic artery (RHA) and any vascular variant or recognition of non-resectability before irreversible steps are taken. They are also successful in reducing intraoperative bleeding due to the early identification of SMA and superior mesenteric vein (SMV) branches and tributaries [2]. Each approach offers unique advantages depending on the patient's anatomy and the specifics of the tumour's location. There are six different approaches in SMA dissection for MIPD, which will be explored in this chapter (Fig. 7.1).

The right approach offers direct access to the uncinate process, allowing for excellent exposure of the SMA, retroperitoneal, and para-aortic tissues, and facilitating tumour dissection in this challenging area [3]. The right posterior approach is advantageous for tumours that extend into the retroperitoneum, while the left posterior approach is better suited for accessing the infracolic retroperitoneum lateral to the duodenojejunal flexure [4]. The anterior and superior approaches each have their distinct benefits for tumours situated in different anatomical regions, allowing for more comprehensive and tailored surgical strategies [3].

Each approach is accompanied with its risks and technical demands; thus, being proficient in all approaches provides the performing surgeon with the flexibility to adapt mid-operation if unexpected anatomical or pathological challenges arise. This is crucial in complex surgeries such as MIPD, where precision and adaptability

---

Supplementary Information The online version contains supplementary material available at https://doi.org/10.1007/978-3-031-99695-5_7. The videos can be accessed individually by clicking the DOI link in the accompanying figure caption or by scanning this link with the SN More Media App.

B. Ielpo (✉) · P. Sanchez-Velazquez · F. Burdio
HPB Unit, Hospital del Mar, Pompeu Fabra University, Barcelona, Spain
e-mail: ielpo.b@gmail.com; psanchezvelazquez@psmar.cat; fburdio@hotmail.com

Y. Masuda
Ministry of Health Singapore, Singapore, Singapore

Yong Loo Lin School of Medicine, National University of Singapore, Singapore, Singapore
e-mail: ymasuda3398@gmail.com

B. Ielpo et al. (eds.), *Minimally Invasive Pancreatoduodenectomy in Cancer*,
https://doi.org/10.1007/978-3-031-99695-5_7

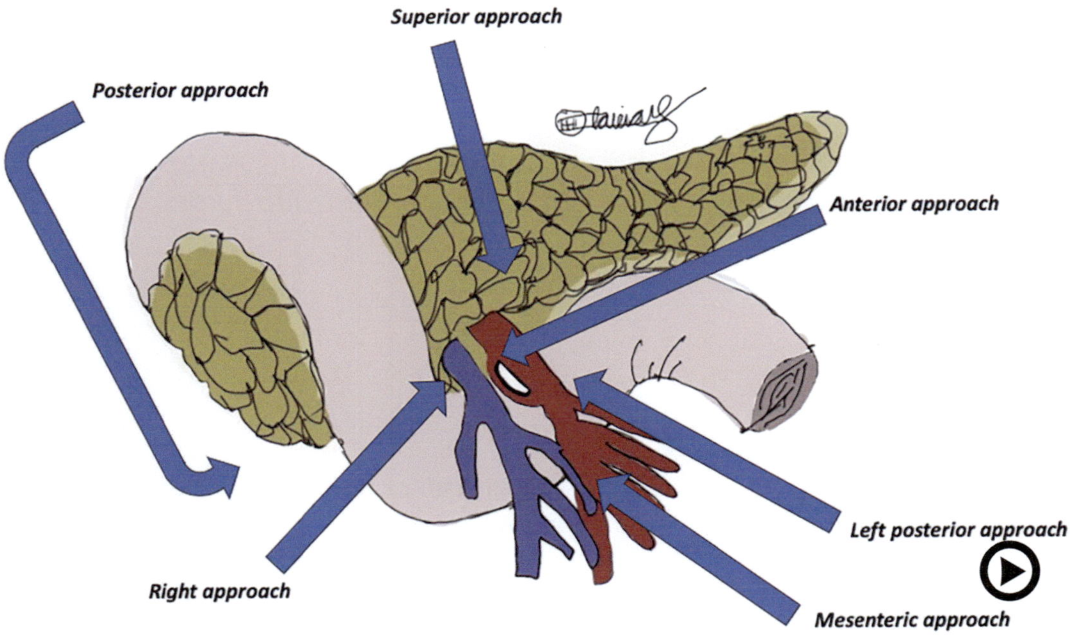

Fig. 7.1 The six different approaches in superior mesenteric artery dissection for minimally invasive pancreaticoduodenectomy (Artery first approaches (▶ https://doi.org/10.1007/000-hem))

enable surgeons to tailor individualised treatment plans which can lead to significant impact in patient outcomes. Such patient outcomes include clearer margins of resection, decreased rates of postoperative complications, and shorter recovery times [5]. Surgeons will be able to leverage these benefits more effectively, promoting enhanced recovery protocols and better prognosis. Moreover, achieving negative margins is particularly important in surgical oncology, as the preservation of healthy tissue is paramount for both oncological control and quality of life post-surgery [6, 7].

As the field of minimally invasive surgery rapidly advances, it is important to keep abreast of these novel MIPD techniques. This not only improves local clinical outcomes, but also contributes to the broader adoption of these techniques globally. Accordingly, international surgical standards will assuredly progress, and patient outcomes will continue to improve. In this chapter, we will explore five different SMA dissection approaches for MIPD in greater depth for the remainder of this chapter.

7.2 Right Approach (Uncinate-First Approach)

In the included video, a dissection of the SMV from the uncinate process was first performed. A landing zone was subsequently created through a cranial dissection of the uncinate process. The next step involves the identification and exposure of the SMA, which was achieved through the dissection of the first jejunal branch of the SMV. Subsequently, the uncinate process was dissected off the SMA using a caudal to cranial approach. As shown in the video, this exposed the pancreaticoduodenal artery, which can be dissected using various approaches (Fig. 7.2).

The right/medial uncinate approach is frequently performed in both open and MIPD due to the excellent exposure and easier identification of the SMA, retroperitoneal, and para-aortic tissues. Furthermore, most surgeons find dissections to be safer and more accurate when started distally, as the pancreatic uncinate process lacks precise anatomical and surgical landmarks [8]. However, surgeons should be aware of the risk of injury of the SMV, as early dissection of the SMV is necessary for this approach. Its relationship with the superior mesenteric vessels poses a challenge to resection, leading to it being one of the most common sites of margin positivity [9].

The right/medial uncinate approach should be primarily utilised for malignant tumours of the uncinate process, as well as for bulky tumours arising in the superior aspect of the pancreatic head [10].

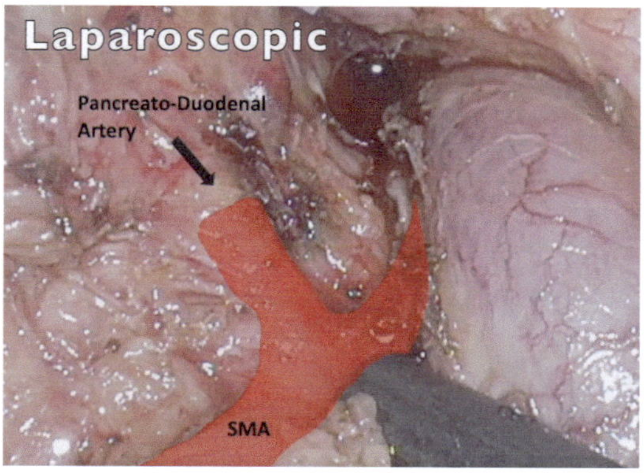

Fig. 7.2 Right/uncinate first approach: identification of the pancreaticoduodenal artery after dissection of the uncinate process from the superior mesenteric artery

7.3 Posterior Approach (Left Renal Vein Approach)

This approach begins with a wide Kocherization to expose the vena cava and left renal vein, as demonstrated in the video. The origin of the SMA will then be exposed at its origin, where it passes above the left renal vein. The right posterior approach is advantageous as it allows for early identification of the SMA and SMV, thus facilitating en bloc resection.

This approach is especially useful for early identification of a replaced RHA originating from the SMA and for aorto-caval node sampling (Fig. 7.3) [3]. Moreover, it enables an earlier dissection of the mesopancreas from the SMA, which decreases the complexity of such dissections in later steps, as shown in Fig. 7.4, where common hepatic artery arises from the SMA. Proper mesopancreas dissection is crucial as local recurrence of pancreatic cancer is often thought to be due to insufficient dissection in this area [2].

However, this approach is known to be difficult in patients with peripancreatic inflammation around the pancreatic head [11]. There is also a risk of inferior vena cava injury, which can be mitigated with a wide Kocher manoeuvre and by

Fig. 7.3 Posterior/left renal vein approach: early identification of a replaced right hepatic artery originating from the superior mesenteric artery

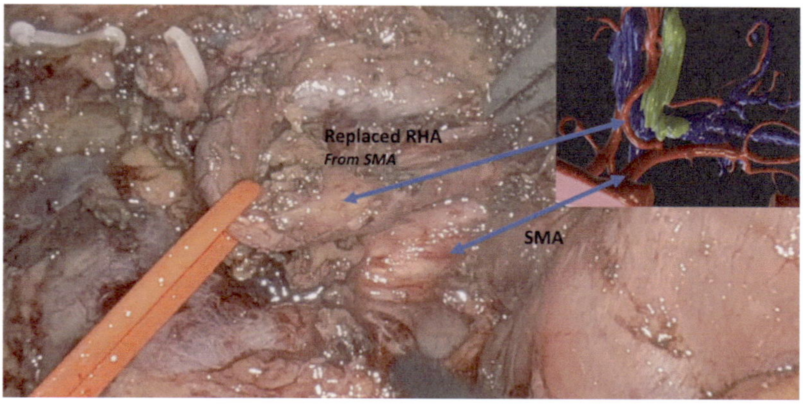

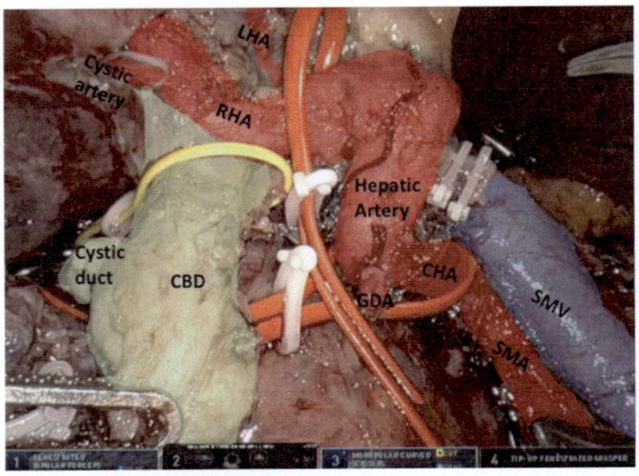

Fig. 7.4 Posterior/left renal vein approach: anatomical orientation after wide Kocherization and identification of origin of superior mesenteric artery

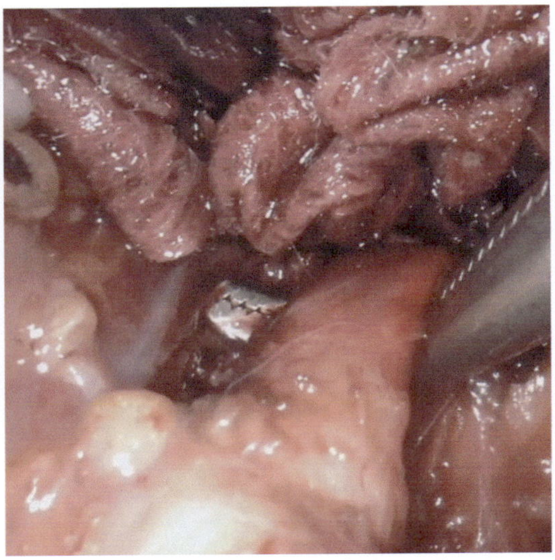

Fig. 7.5 Left/Treitz approach: identification of superior mesenteric artery

starting the dissection from the distal part of the inferior vena cava, as demonstrated in the video.

The posterior/left renal vein approach should be used for posteromedial tumours in the pancreatic head and neck, as well as periampullary tumours extending from the pancreatic body to the head. As shown in the video, this approach may be technically easier to be performed through robotic surgery as it allows for a greater degree of movement, more precise dissection, and is associated with a shorter learning curve.

7.4 Left Approach (Treitz Ligament Approach)

In this approach, the ligament of Treitz is first divided, after which the proximal jejunum is pulled to the left, exposing the first and second jejunal arteries. Next, the first and second jejunal arteries are divided at their origin from the SMA. The proximal jejunum should be retracted further to produce a counterclockwise rotation of the SMA, allowing for the identification and division of the inferior pancreaticoduodenal artery (IPDA). Additionally, traction of the proximal jejunum enables clearance of the posterior and right aspects of the SMA. Subsequently, the jejunum is divided, and the duodenum is transposed to the right, allowing for the exposure and division of the remaining connective tissue attached to the superior mesenteric pedicle.

The benefit of this approach is the ability to adequately assess the SMA without the need for mobilization of the duodenum or colon, in contrast to the right posterior approach. It allows for adequate dissection of the posterior and right aspects of the SMA (Fig. 7.5) [12]. However, unlike the right posterior approach, the approach should not be performed through robotic means due to the limited accessibility and view of the operating field.

This approach is best suited for tumours located along the uncinate process and ventral pancreas, but surgeons should take caution that it might be challenging in patients with fatty mesentery. For these cases, indocyanine green (ICG) fluorescence imaging can increase the ease of SMA localization.

7.5 Anterior Approach (After Pancreatic Neck Transection)

In the included video, the following vessels were first identified: portal vein, SMV, and SMA. Subsequently, the SMA was dissected from the right side, from the origin of the middle colic artery to the right side of the celiac trunk.

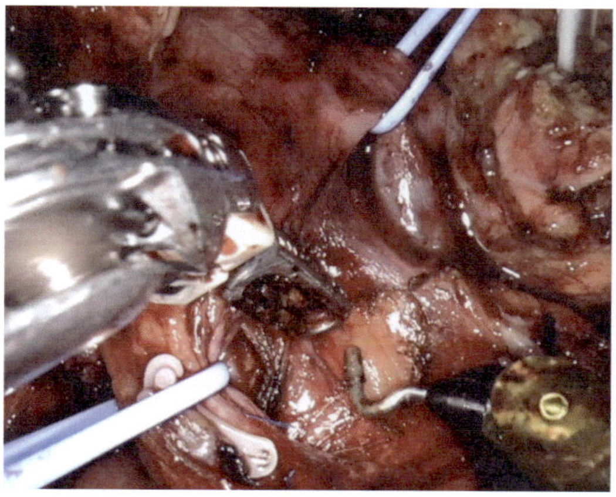

Fig. 7.6 Anterior/after pancreatic neck transection approach: identification of superior mesenteric vein and portal vein

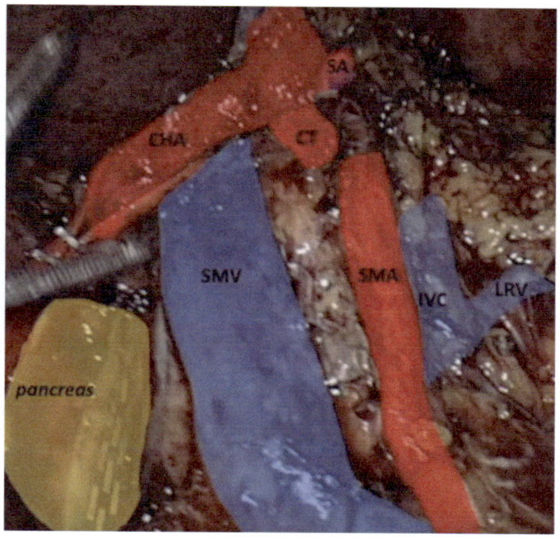

Fig. 7.7 Superior/after pancreatic neck transection approach: anatomical orientation after right-to-left dissection of the hepatoduodenal ligament with extension down the celiac trunk and inside the perineural and lymphatic tissue

The video shows both robotic and laparoscopic procedures performed for this approach, highlighting the flexibility of this technique. The anterior approach allows for direct access and clear visualization of the SMA and surrounding structures, facilitating precise dissection and vascular control (Fig. 7.6).

This approach should be performed for patients requiring major venous resection and reconstruction during a pancreaticoduodenectomy. It is particularly beneficial when dealing with complex vascular involvement, as it provides excellent exposure and control of the major vessels. It also allows for a thorough assessment of the SMA and SMV, which is crucial for ensuring oncological clearance and successful reconstruction.

7.6 Superior Approach (After Pancreatic Neck Transection)

This approach begins with the right-to-left dissection of the hepatoduodenal ligament to expose the common hepatic artery and the gastroduodenal artery, as well as the removal of the anterior lymph nodes. The dissection should also extend down the celiac trunk, inside the perineural and lymphatic tissue, and onto the aorta and the origin of the SMA. After pancreatic division, the SMA is dissected from the left side, from the origin of the middle colic artery to the right side of the celiac trunk (Fig. 7.7).

This approach is indicated for patients who require a radical antegrade modular pancreatosplenectomy (RAMPS) or a total pancreatectomy [13]. It provides comprehensive access to the vascular structures and the lymphatic tissues, allowing for thorough lymphadenectomy and ensuring clear surgical margins.

By enabling meticulous dissection of the SMA and associated vascular structures, this technique is advantageous for achieving oncological clearance, especially in cases involving extensive perineural and lymphatic spread. This approach also ensures that the surgeon can navigate the complex anatomy effectively, thereby enhancing the precision and safety of the procedure.

Overall, this approach is best suited for cases that demand extensive resection and meticulous handling of vascular and lymphatic structures, making it a vital technique in the surgical armamentarium for advanced pancreatic procedures.

7.7 Tips for SMA Dissection

To enhance the visualisation and safety of the SMA first approach in MIPD, two imaging adjuncts are often utilised.

First is the application of ICG fluorescence imaging. ICG fluorescence imaging can significantly improve the localisation of the SMA, reduce the complexity of the procedure, and increase the likelihood of a successful outcome. This was illustrated in the video during the left posterior approach, where the presence of mesenteric fat made it challenging to identify the SMA. ICG fluorescence imaging was utilised and aided in the localisation of the SMA.

Second, the use of three-dimensional (3D) reconstruction of preoperative imaging. As demonstrated in the video, 3D reconstruction is beneficial as it provides a comprehensive view of the patient's anatomy and helps identify vascular anomalies such as a replaced RHA (Fig. 7.8). This is especially important as vascular patterns differ greatly among different individuals. In a cohort of 155 patients, the IPDA and first jejunal artery were found to form a common trunk in 66% of patients, while IPDA originated from the SMA directly in 33% and, more rarely, from a replaced RHA [14]. Hence, this imaging technique is a powerful tool to identify vascular patterns and enhance surgical planning. When paired with a minimally invasive approach, it can help to minimise the risk of vascular injury.

Through the integration of these imaging adjuncts, surgeons can achieve superior visualization and anatomical orientation, which are crucial for the successful implementation of SMA dissection in MIPD.

7.8 Final Thoughts

The approaches and techniques elaborated in this chapter have been modified for the benefits of increased safety and simplicity. It is important to note that we do not routinely perform a complete SMA dissection but only its superior part. This is to begin the initial separation from the mesopancreatic tissue, as shown in Fig. 7.9. Once the manoeuvre is completed, even if only partially, the subsequent completion of mesopancreatic dissection becomes significantly easier.

Most of the approaches outlined in this chapter are not performed exclusively and are often used in combination, as SMA identification in real-life scenarios can be challenging. Knowledge of these different approaches will enable surgeons to identify the SMA correctly and safely.

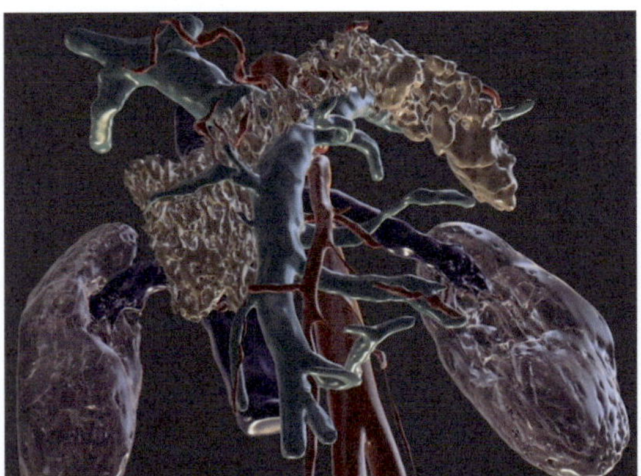

Fig. 7.8 Use of three-dimensional reconstruction of preoperative imaging to aid in identifications of vascular pattern and enhance surgical planning

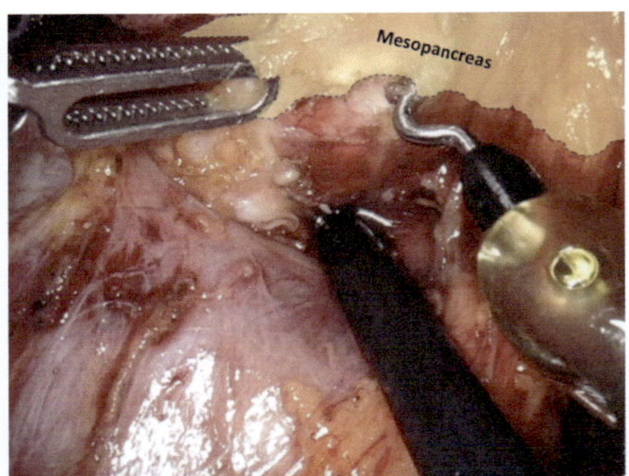

Fig. 7.9 Posterior/left renal vein approach: early identification of mesopancreas for dissection

Acknowledgements The authors thank Miss Flavia Ielpo Fuentes for drawing the picture.

References

1. Ironside N, Barreto SG, Loveday B, et al. Meta-analysis of an artery-first approach versus standard pancreatoduodenectomy on perioperative outcomes and survival. Br J Surg. 2018;105:628–36. https://doi.org/10.1002/bjs.10832.
2. Fernandes ESM, de Mello FPT, Braga EP, de Souza GO, Andrade R, Pimentel LS, Girão CL, Siqueira M, Moraes-Junior JMA, de Oliveira RV, Goldaracena N, Torres OJM. A more radical perspective on surgical approach and outcomes in pancreatic cancer-a narrative review. J Gastrointest Oncol. 2023;14(4):1964–81. https://doi.org/10.21037/jgo-22-763. Epub 2023 Mar 7. PMID: 37720458; PMCID: PMC10502544.
3. Ielpo B, Anselmo A, Masuda Y, Xuan MYH, Burdio F, De Blasi V, Sanchez-Velazquez P, Giuliani A, Azagra JS, Viola GM, Podda M, Pellino G, Rosso E. Superior mesenteric artery first approach for minimally invasive Pancreaticoduodenectomy: a step-by-step surgical technique video. Ann Surg Oncol. 2023;30(3):1500–3. https://doi.org/10.1245/s10434-022-12743-2. Epub 2022 Nov 5.
4. Ielpo B, d'Addetta MV, Anselmo A, Rosso E, de Blasi V, Sanchez-Velazquez P, Vellalta G, Podda M, Burdio F. Levels of robotic mesopancreas dissection according to malignancy and vascular anatomy: what surgeons need to know. Ann Surg Oncol. 2024;31(3):1916–8. https://doi.org/10.1245/s10434-023-14686-8. Epub 2023 Dec 10. PMID: 38071705; PMCID: PMC10838235.
5. Ielpo B, Caruso R, Duran H, Diaz E, Fabra I, Malavé L, Quijano Y, Vicente E. Robotic versus standard open pancreatectomy: a propensity score-matched analysis comparison. Updat Surg. 2019;71(1):137–44. https://doi.org/10.1007/s13304-018-0529-1. Epub 2018 Mar 26.
6. Ielpo B, Duran H, Diaz E, Fabra I, Caruso R, Malavé L, Ferri V, Nuñez J, Ruiz-Ocaña A, Jorge E, Lazzaro S, Kalivaci D, Quijano Y, Vicente E. Robotic versus laparoscopic distal pancreatectomy: a comparative study of clinical outcomes and costs analysis. Int J Surg. 2017;48:300–4. https://doi.org/10.1016/j.ijsu.2017.10.075. Epub 2017 Nov 6.
7. Strobel O, Hank T, Hinz U, et al. Pancreatic cancer surgery: the new R-status counts. Ann Surg. 2017;265:565–73. https://doi.org/10.1097/SLA.0000000000001731.
8. Martin DF. Computed tomography of the normal pancreatic uncinate process. Clin Radiol. 1988;39:195–6. https://doi.org/10.1016/S0009-9260(88)80024-2.
9. Zhu C, Ma L, Jia Z, et al. Novel morphological classification of the normal pancreatic uncinate process based on computed tomography. J Int Med Res. 2020;48:300060520957453. https://doi.org/10.1177/0300060520957453.
10. Ielpo B, Anselmo A, Koh Y, Burdio F, De Blasi V, Sanchez-Velazquez P, Azagra JS, Huscher C, Giuliani A, Pellino G, Rosso E. Minimally invasive pancreatic anastomosis after pancreaticoduodenectomy: multi-institutional step by step video description of the technique. Updat Surg. 2023;75(1):255–9. https://doi.org/10.1007/s13304-022-01389-0. Epub 2022 Nov 12.
11. Ielpo B, Sanchez P, Grande L, Burdio F. Laparoscopic pancreatoduodenectomy: how we have standardized the technique (with video). Updat Surg. 2022;74(4):1479–81. https://doi.org/10.1007/s13304-021-01235-9. Epub 2022 Feb 11.
12. Ielpo B, Burdio F, Martinez A, Sanchez-Velazquez P. Pancreatectomy with concomitant portal vein resection in the current neoadjuvant era. Hepatobiliary Surg Nutr. 2022;11(2):295–8. https://doi.org/10.21037/hbsn-21-547. PMID: 35464289; PMCID: PMC9023828.
13. Ielpo B, Pietrasz D, Torrent L, Tortajada P, Ciacio O, Pittau G, Adam R, Sa CA. Laparoscopic radical antegrade modular pancreatosplenectomy (RAMPS) technique: toward the standardization of the technique (with video). Surg Laparosc Endosc Percutan Tech. 2020;30(4):e23. https://doi.org/10.1097/SLE.0000000000000798.
14. Ishikawa Y, Ban D, Matsumura S, et al. Surgical pitfalls of jejunal vein anatomy in pancreaticoduodenectomy. J Hepatobiliary Pancreat Sci. 2017;24:394–400. https://doi.org/10.1002/jhbp.451.

8 Levels of Mesopancreas Dissection in Robotic Pancreatoduodenectomy

Mauro Podda and Benedetto Ielpo

8.1 Historical Context and Evolution of Mesopancreas Dissection

The concept of mesopancreas dissection has evolved significantly over the past few decades. Traditional open PD was the standard approach until minimally invasive techniques, including laparoscopic and robotic pancreatic head resection, emerged [1, 2]. The introduction of robotic systems has brought about a paradigm shift in pancreatic surgery, offering enhanced precision and control. The term "mesopancreas" was first introduced to describe the posterior attachment of the pancreatic head, a crucial area for achieving clear surgical margins in PD [2]. Early studies highlighted the importance of complete mesopancreas excision in improving oncological outcomes [3]. The classification of mesopancreas dissection into different levels based on tumour characteristics and vascular anatomy has refined surgical techniques, enabling tailored approaches for different clinical scenarios. In the late twentieth century, pancreatic surgery was fraught with high morbidity and mortality rates [4–6]. The advent of better imaging techniques, improved surgical instruments, and enhanced perioperative care has significantly improved patient outcomes. The development of minimally invasive techniques, particularly robotic surgery, represents a major advancement. The precision of robotic instruments allows for meticulous dissection of the mesopancreas, which is critical in avoiding complications and ensuring complete tumour removal [7]. The evolution of robotic surgery in PD has been marked by several milestones. Initial attempts at minimally invasive PD through laparoscopy were hampered by technical limitations and steep learning curves. However, with advancements in robotic platforms, including improved instrument dexterity and better visualization, surgeons can now perform complex dissections with greater accuracy. Studies have shown that robotic PD is associated with reduced blood loss, shorter hospital stays, and lower complication rates compared to traditional open surgery [8–13].

Supplementary Information The online version contains supplementary material available at https://doi.org/10.1007/978-3-031-99695-5_8. The videos can be accessed individually by clicking the DOI link in the accompanying figure caption or by scanning this link with the SN More Media App.

M. Podda
Department of Surgical Science, University of Cagliari, Cagliari, Italy
e-mail: mauropodda@ymail.com

B. Ielpo (✉)
HPB Unit, Hospital del Mar, Barcelona, Spain
e-mail: ielpo.b@gmail.com

B. Ielpo et al. (eds.), *Minimally Invasive Pancreatoduodenectomy in Cancer*,
https://doi.org/10.1007/978-3-031-99695-5_8

8.2 Anatomical Background

The mesopancreas is a pivotal structure in PD, comprising fatty tissue interspersed with vascular structures, nerves, lymph nodes, and lymphatic vessels. It serves as the posterior attachment of the pancreatic head and encompasses critical vascular and neural pathways. Understanding the boundaries and contents of the mesopancreas is crucial for safe and effective dissection. Anatomically, the mesopancreas is delineated:

(A) *Laterally*: by the medial and posterior border of the uncinate process.
(B) *Medially*: by the right border of the superior mesenteric vein (SMV) and superior mesenteric artery (SMA).
(C) *Proximally*: by the origin of the celiac trunk.
(D) *Distally*: by the beginning of the mesenteric root.
(E) *Posteriorly*: by the left renal vein.

This anatomical configuration makes the mesopancreas a complex and challenging area for surgical dissection, especially considering the variability in vascular anatomy among different patients (Fig. 8.1). The presence of crucial vascular structures like the SMA and SMV necessitates careful planning and precise execution during surgery to minimize the risk of bleeding and ensure complete tumour resection. The SMA and SMV play key roles in supplying blood to the intestines and draining blood from the pancreas and duodenum. Variations in the origins and courses of these vessels are common, which can complicate surgical planning. For instance, the presence of a replaced right hepatic artery originating from the SMA or variations in the branching pattern of the inferior pancreaticoduodenal arteries (IPDAs) must be carefully identified pre- or intraoperatively and managed during surgery (Fig. 8.2).

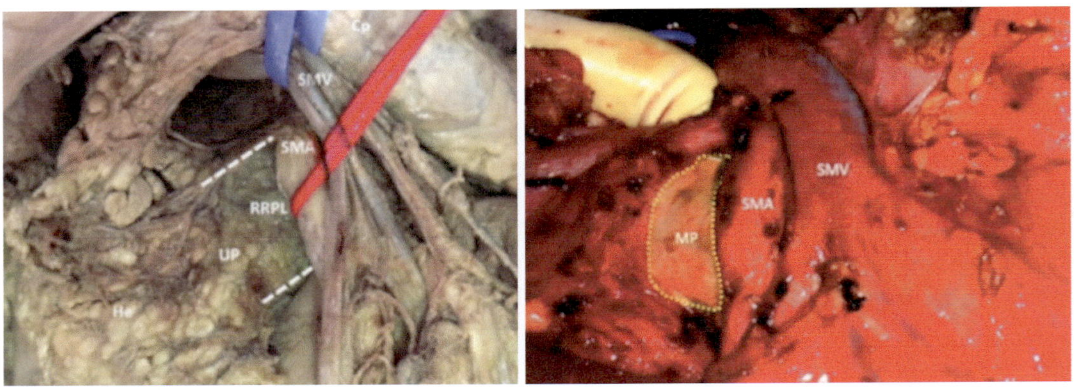

Fig. 8.1 Limits of the mesopancreas: medial and posterior border of the uncinate process (laterally), right border of the superior mesenteric vein (SMV) and superior mesenteric artery (SMA) (medially), origin of the celiac trunk (proximally), beginning of the mesenteric root (distally), left renal vein (posteriorly)

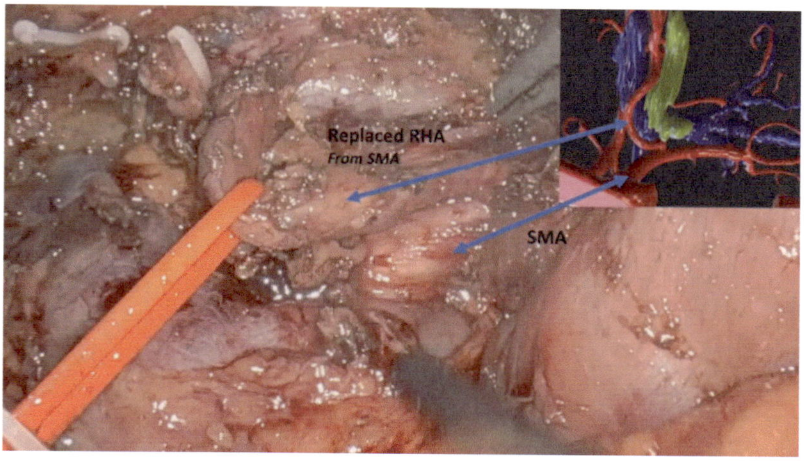

Fig. 8.2 The presence of a replaced right hepatic artery originating from the superior mesenteric artery (SMA) must be carefully identified pre- or intraoperatively and managed during surgery

8.3 Mesopancreas Dissection Main Steps

8.3.1 Initial Preparation and Exposure

(A) *Dissection of the SMA*: The procedure begins with the dissection of the SMA using a posterior approach (Fig. 8.3). The origin of the SMA is identified in the axilla between the inferior vena cava and the left renal vein. This early identification and dissection of the SMA are crucial for making subsequent steps safer and more controlled. The SMA is a critical vessel, and its early identification helps prevent inadvertent injury and ensures that the dissection proceeds safely, as shown in the video.

(B) *Jejunal Loop Management*: The first jejunal loop is dissected proximally to the Treitz ligament and then transected using a mechanical stapler. This step helps in mobilizing the small intestine and gaining better access to the mesopancreas. Proper management of the jejunal loop is essential to create a clear field for dissection and avoid tension on the bowel.

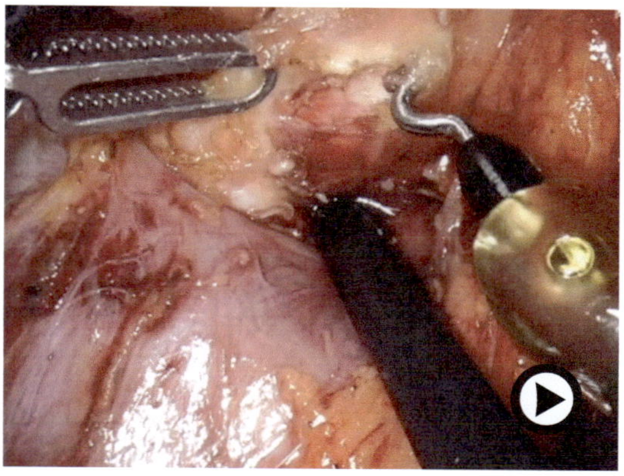

Fig. 8.3 Posterior approach to the superior mesenteric artery (SMA). The origin of the SMA is identified in the axilla between the inferior vena cava and the left renal vein (Posterior approach to superior mesenteric artery (▶ https://doi.org/10.1007/000-hen))

8.3.2 Dissection of the Uncinate Process

(A) *Separation from Mesentery*: The uncinate process is separated from the mesentery of the first jejunal loop (Fig. 8.4). The dissection proceeds in a vessel-free space between the uncinate process and the terminal branch of the SMV, which can be safely navigated using scissors. This step requires delicate handling to avoid injury to the SMV and its tributaries.

(B) *Exposure of SMA*: The first jejunal branch of the SMV is dissected and sacrificed to expose the SMA. The uncinate process is then dissected off the SMA in a caudal to cranial approach, ensuring clear visualization and control of the SMA. This dissection must be meticulous to avoid bleeding and ensure complete removal of the uncinate process, as shown in the video.

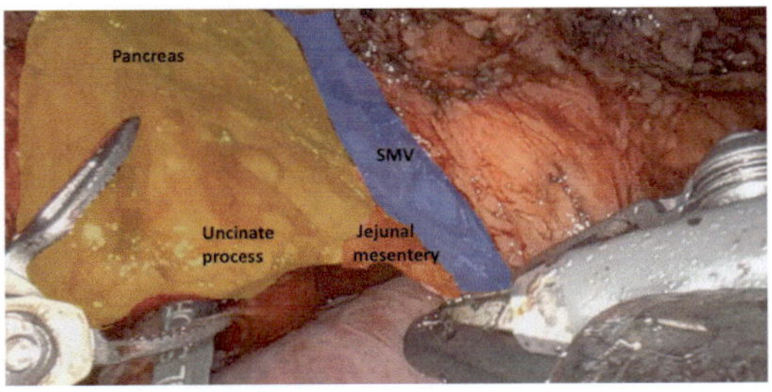

Fig. 8.4 The uncinate process is separated from the mesentery of the first jejunal loop. The dissection proceeds in a vessel-free space between the uncinate process and the terminal branch of the superior mesenteric vein (SMV)

8.3.3 Control of Key Vascular Structures

(A) *Inferior Pancreaticoduodenal Vein (IPDV)*: The IPDV is typically encountered early in the superficial dissection of the mesopancreas. Small veins are managed using LigaSure or similar devices, while larger veins may require hand-tied ligatures. The robotic platform provides enhanced precision for these delicate tasks. Control of the IPDV is crucial to prevent significant blood loss (Fig. 8.5).

(B) *Inferior Pancreaticoduodenal Arteries (IPDA)*: In the deep dissection of the mesopancreas, the IPDAs are transected. Robotic VesselSealer and radiofrequency devices are employed to control bleeding and ensure haemostasis. Managing the IPDAs is critical as these arteries supply blood to the pancreas and duodenum.

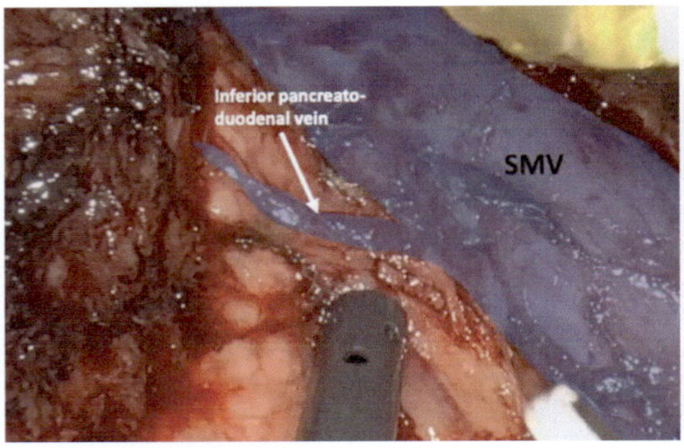

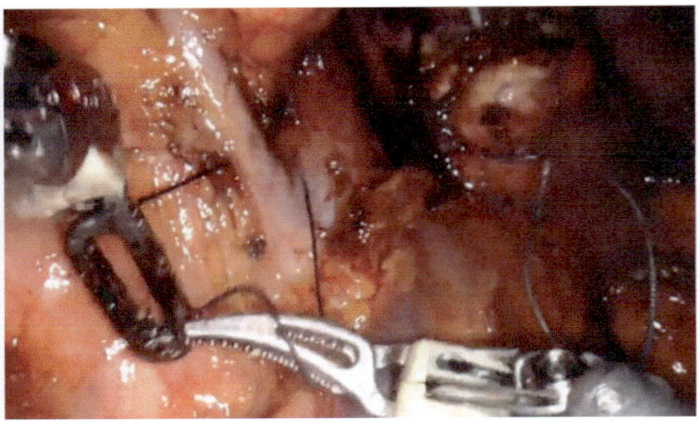

Fig. 8.5 Inferior pancreaticoduodenal vein (IPDV) encountered in the superficial dissection of the mesopancreas. Larger veins require hand-tied ligatures

8.4 Mesopancreas Dissection Levels

8.4.1 Level 1: Benign and Low-Grade Tumours

This level of dissection is indicated for benign and low-grade tumours, where a complete mesopancreas dissection is not necessary (Fig. 8.6). These tumours typically have limited invasiveness and do not require extensive removal of surrounding tissues. So, this type of dissection focuses on removing the tumour while preserving as much of the surrounding normal tissue as possible.

The SMV is dissected after sectioning Henle's gastrocolic trunk, the IPDV, and small pancreatic tributaries. The mesopancreas dissection is initiated caudally by retracting the SMV leftward. It ends anteriorly to the immediate right of the first jejunal artery, which is preserved. The first jejunal artery is preserved. Then, the inferior pancreaticoduodenal artery (IPDA) is exposed, ligated, and divided. The VesselSealer, radiofrequency instrument, and the "hook" cautery can be used for dissection. In this fashion, the SMV is isolated, leaving a posterior portion of mesopancreatic tissue, preserving the jejunal arteries and mesojejunum, and representing the limit of this type of mesopancreatic dissection.

During the dissection, it is essential to know the anatomical variations of the IPDV, which can arise directly from the first jejunal vein or the SMV. The aim is to isolate the SMV, leaving a posterior portion of mesopancreatic tissue intact, thereby preserving the jejunal arteries and mesojejunum. The use of these tools ensures precise dissection and minimal tissue damage.

8.4.2 Level 2: Malignant Tumours

This level is used for malignant tumours where a complete mesopancreas dissection is essential for oncological clearance. Malignant tumours require more aggressive removal to ensure that no cancerous cells are left behind (Fig. 8.7). Also in this case, it is vital to know the anatomical variations of arteries, such as the case of a direct origin of the IPDA from the SMA or the first jejunal artery. The SMV is isolated after dissection and sacrifice of its tributaries, including the IPDV, first jejunal vein, colic vein, and Henle's gastrocolic trunk. The IPDA and first jejunal artery are ligated and divided. The SMA is dissected while preserving its neurovascular bundle. This extensive dissection aims to remove all potentially cancerous tissues and achieve clear surgical margins. Then, the IPDA and first jejunal artery are ligated and divided. In this type of dissection, the SMA is dissected, preserving the neurovascular bundle of the artery. Different types of energy devices can be used in this step, such as the Maryland bipolar dissector to identify the arterial and venous branches and the VesselSealer for a smooth dissection of the peri-

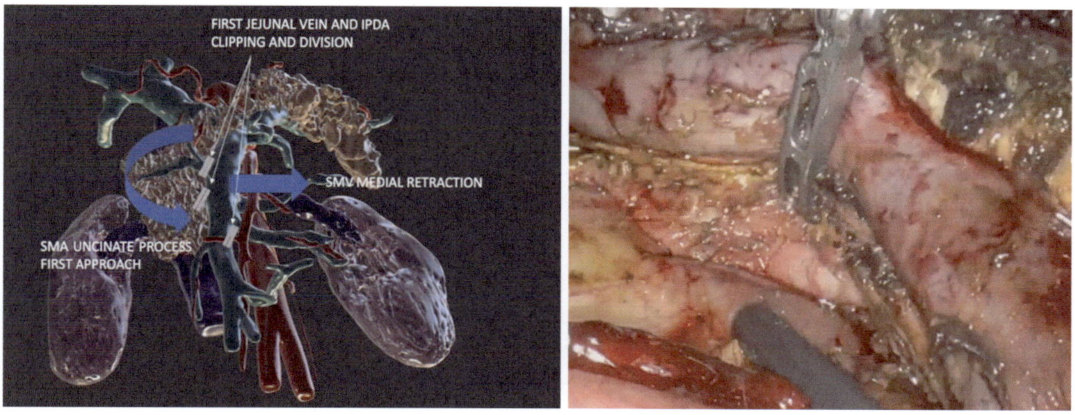

Fig. 8.6 Steps of the level 1 mesopancreas dissection and final view of the surgical field at the end of the resective step

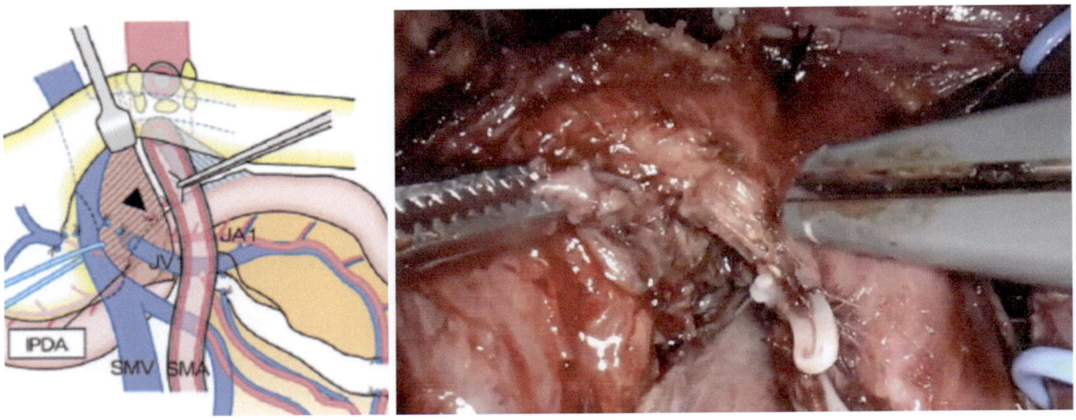

Fig. 8.7 Steps of the level 2 mesopancreas dissection and final view of the surgical field at the end of the resective step

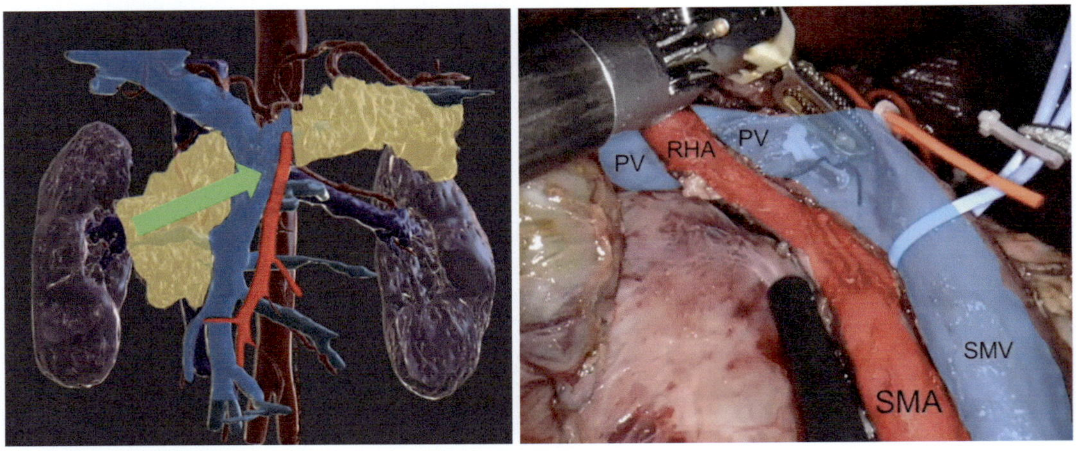

Fig. 8.8 Level 3 extended dissection with complete extirpation of the mesopancreas

arterial tissue. Thus, the mesopancreas and the mesojejunum are resected en bloc, ensuring complete removal of potentially malignant tissue. The use of advanced energy devices helps control bleeding and reduce operative time.

8.4.3 Level 3: Aggressive Malignant Tumours

Level 3 is the most extended dissection, in which the mesopancreas is completely extirpated en bloc with the tissue surrounding the SMA. This extensive dissection is reserved for aggressive malignant tumours, especially in cases where there is a suspicion of a certain grade of tissue infiltration, such as borderline cases that underwent neoadjuvant treatment. These tumours often invade surrounding tissues, requiring more radical surgical approaches (Fig. 8.8).

This anterior approach is conducted up to the left side of the SMV, which is reached using a VesselLoop to control it. Then, the IPDA and the first jejunal artery are ligated and divided, and the SMA is dissected just outside its adventitial plane. This is a technique described by Buchler's group called "*Triangle operation*" because it allows for a complete cleaning of the tissue between the SMV, the SMA, and the hepatic artery. This leads to the complete extirpation of the mesopancreas. The "*Triangle operation*" technique ensures thorough removal of all cancerous tissues, even those infiltrating the surrounding structures.

As shown in the video, preoperative three-dimensional imaging of vascular reconstructions is vital for identifying eventual anomalies and planning the safe and proper surgical approach. The use of BullDog clamps helps in controlling the proximal and distal portions of the SMV and splenic vein during venous resection, facilitating safe reconstruction.

8.5 Clinical Significance of Mesopancreas Dissection

The clinical significance of mesopancreas dissection lies in its impact on surgical outcomes, particularly in terms of oncological clearance and postoperative complications [7]. Incomplete dissection can lead to positive surgical margins, increasing the risk of tumour recurrence. On the other hand, meticulous dissection reduces the likelihood of residual disease and improves overall survival rates. Robotic PD, with its enhanced visualization and precision, has shown promising results in achieving clear margins and minimizing complications. The ability to perform delicate dissections in the confined space around the SMA and SMV, while controlling bleeding and preserving critical structures, underscores the importance of robotic technology in mesopancreas dissection. Studies have shown that patients undergoing robotic PD have lower rates of postoperative complications compared to those undergoing traditional open surgery [9]. This is attributed to the minimally invasive nature of robotic surgery, which results in less tissue trauma, reduced blood loss, and faster recovery times. Moreover, the enhanced precision of robotic instruments allows for more accurate dissection and preservation of vital structures, leading to better oncological outcomes [13].

8.6 Technical Nuances and Surgical Tips

Successful mesopancreas dissection in robotic PD requires a combination of technical proficiency, anatomical knowledge, and surgical judgment. Here are some key technical nuances and tips:

8.6.1 Preoperative Planning

(A) Utilize preoperative imaging, including CT angiography and 3D reconstructions, to map out the vascular anatomy and identify any anomalies. Preoperative planning is crucial for anticipating potential challenges and ensuring a smooth surgical procedure.

(B) Plan the surgical approach based on the tumour location, size, and involvement of surrounding structures. Tailoring the surgical plan to the individual patient's anatomy and tumour characteristics improves the likelihood of a successful outcome.

8.6.2 Robotic Setup and Instrumentation

(A) Ensure optimal positioning of the robotic system and trocars to facilitate access to the pancreatic head and mesopancreas. Proper setup minimizes the need for instrument exchanges and reduces operative time.

(B) Select appropriate robotic instruments, such as the VesselSealer, bipolar dissectors, and hook cautery, for precise dissection and haemostasis. Using the right instruments ensures precision and safety during the procedure.

8.6.3 Dissection Technique

(A) Begin with a thorough dissection of the SMA using a posterior approach to establish a safe working space. Early identification of the SMA sets the stage for a controlled and safe dissection.

(B) Employ traction and counter-traction techniques to expose the mesopancreas and identify key vascular structures. These techniques help in maintaining a dry surgical field and avoiding injury to critical structures.

(C) Use energy devices judiciously to control bleeding and avoid thermal injury to surrounding tissues. Proper use of energy devices ensures haemostasis while minimizing damage to adjacent tissues.

8.6.4 Management of Vascular Structures

(A) Carefully dissect and control the IPDV, IPDA, and other tributaries of the SMV to prevent excessive bleeding. Proper vascular control is essential for reducing intraoperative blood loss and preventing complications.

(B) In level 3 dissections, consider the use of BullDog clamps and other vascular control devices to manage venous resections and reconstructions (Fig. 8.9). These devices help in achieving precise control of blood vessels, facilitating safe and effective resections.

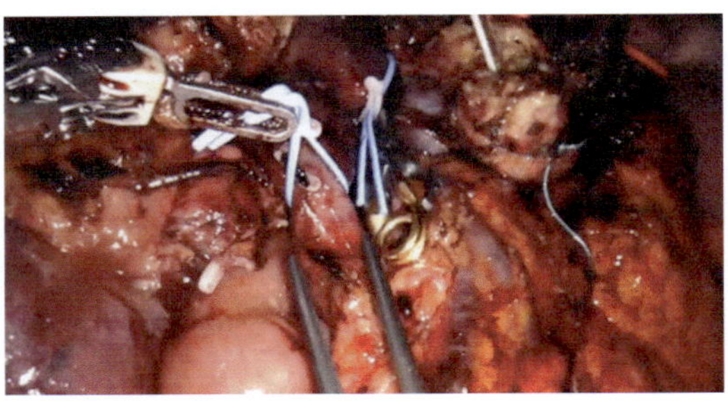

Fig. 8.9 Use of BullDog clamps to manage venous resections and reconstructions during level 3 mesopancreas dissection

8.6.5 Intraoperative Decision-Making

(A) Be prepared to adapt the surgical plan based on intraoperative findings, such as unexpected vascular anomalies or tumour involvement. Flexibility and the ability to make real-time decisions are crucial for handling unforeseen challenges.

(B) Maintain a focus on oncological principles, ensuring complete removal of the tumour and affected mesopancreas tissue. Adhering to oncological principles ensures that the primary goal of surgery, which is complete tumour removal, is achieved.

8.7 Complications and Management

While robotic PD has many advantages, it is not without potential complications. Understanding these complications and their management is crucial for improving patient outcomes.

8.7.1 Haemorrhage

(A) *Cause*: Haemorrhage can occur due to injury to major vessels like the SMA, SMV, or their branches during dissection. Vascular injuries can result in significant blood loss and require immediate intervention.

(B) *Management*: Immediate identification and control of the bleeding source using robotic instruments like the VesselSealer or suturing techniques are essential. Preoperative planning with detailed imaging can help anticipate vascular anomalies and plan accordingly. Proper vascular control during dissection minimizes the risk of haemorrhage.

8.7.2 Pancreatic Fistula

(A) *Cause*: Inadequate sealing of the pancreatic duct or disruption of the anastomosis can lead to pancreatic fistula. Pancreatic fistulas result in leakage of pancreatic enzymes, causing inflammation and infection.
(B) *Management*: Ensure meticulous anastomotic techniques during surgery. Postoperative management may include drainage, nutritional support, and, in some cases, surgical re-intervention. Proper post-operative care is essential for managing pancreatic fistulas and preventing complications.

8.7.3 Infection

(A) *Cause*: Surgical site infections or abscess formation can result from contamination or prolonged operative time. Infections can lead to delayed recovery and increased hospital stays.
(B) *Management*: Adherence to strict aseptic techniques, appropriate use of prophylactic antibiotics, and careful postoperative monitoring are critical. Preventive measures and early intervention are key to managing infections.

8.7.4 Delayed Gastric Emptying

(A) *Cause*: Disruption of normal gastric motility can occur due to surgical manipulation or nerve injury. Delayed gastric emptying results in prolonged nausea and vomiting, delaying recovery.
(B) *Management*: Supportive care, including nasogastric decompression, prokinetic agents, and nutritional support, is often necessary until normal function resumes. Early intervention and supportive care help manage this complication effectively.

8.7.5 Venous Thromboembolism

(A) *Cause*: Prolonged operative time and post-operative immobility increase the risk of deep vein thrombosis and pulmonary embolism. Venous thromboembolism is a serious complication that can lead to life-threatening conditions.
(B) *Management*: Prophylactic anticoagulation and early mobilization are essential preventive measures. Ensuring that patients are mobilized early and receive appropriate prophylaxis reduces the risk of thromboembolic events.

8.8 Recent Advancements and Future Directions

Advancements in robotic technology and surgical techniques continue to enhance the efficacy and safety of mesopancreas dissection in PD. Innovations such as enhanced imaging modalities, real-time navigation systems, and improved robotic instruments are poised to further refine surgical outcomes.

8.8.1 Enhanced Imaging Modalities

(A) Techniques like intraoperative fluorescence imaging and indocyanine green (ICG) angiography help in better visualization of vascular structures and tissue perfusion, reducing the risk of intraoperative complications. These imaging techniques provide real-time feedback, allowing for more precise dissection and better outcomes.

8.8.2 Real-Time Navigation Systems

(A) Integration of augmented reality (AR) and virtual reality (VR) in the operating room allows for real-time guidance during complex dissections, improving accuracy and safety. These technologies help surgeons visualize the anatomy in three dimensions, enhancing their ability to navigate complex structures.

8.8.3 Improved Robotic Instruments

(A) The development of more sophisticated robotic instruments with enhanced articulation, better haptic feedback, and advanced energy devices enhances the surgeon's ability to perform delicate dissections with greater precision. These improvements in instrumentation facilitate safer and more effective surgeries.

Future research is likely to focus on the integration of artificial intelligence (AI) and machine learning to assist in surgical planning and decision-making. AI-driven algorithms could analyse preoperative imaging data to predict optimal dissection planes and identify potential complications, thereby augmenting the surgeon's expertise. The use of AI in surgery has the potential to revolutionize surgical planning and execution, making procedures safer and more efficient.

Additionally, ongoing studies on the molecular and genetic profiling of pancreatic tumours may lead to personalized surgical approaches, tailoring the extent of mesopancreas dissection based on individual tumour biology and patient characteristics. Personalized medicine approaches can help identify the most effective surgical strategies for each patient, improving outcomes and reducing complications.

8.9 Conclusion

Robotic mesopancreas dissection in PD is a complex but essential procedure for achieving oncological efficacy and minimizing complications. By understanding the anatomical nuances and mastering the technical aspects of mesopancreas dissection, surgeons can improve patient outcomes and advance the field of pancreatic surgery. This chapter provides a comprehensive guide to the levels of mesopancreas dissection, emphasizing the importance of tailored approaches based on tumour type and vascular anatomy.

The continuous evolution of robotic technology and surgical techniques holds promise for further advancements in mesopancreas dissection, paving the way for more precise, effective, and personalized surgical interventions in pancreatic cancer treatment. As technology and techniques continue to advance, the future of pancreatic surgery looks promising, with the potential for even better patient outcomes and reduced complications.

References

1. Fuks D. Minimally invasive pancreatoduodenectomy. Br J Surg. 2020;107(6):630–1.
2. Yosuke I, et al. Pancreatoduodenectomy with systematic mesopancreas dissection using a supracolic anterior artery-first approach. Ann Surg. 2015;262(6):1092–101.
3. Papavasiliou P, et al. The anatomic course of the first jejunal branch of the superior mesenteric vein in relation to the superior mesenteric artery. Int J Surg Oncol. 2012;2012:538769.
4. Lupascu C, et al. Posterior approach pancreaticoduodenectomy: best option for hepatic artery anatomical variants. Hepato-Gastroenterology. 2011;58:2112–4.
5. Ielpo B, et al. Superior mesenteric artery first approach for minimally invasive pancreaticoduodenectomy: a step-by-step surgical technique video. Ann Surg Oncol. 2023;30(3):1500–3.
6. Ielpo B, et al. Minimally invasive pancreatic anastomosis after pancreatoduodenectomy: multi-institutional step by step video description of the technique. Updat Surg. 2023;75(1):255–9.
7. Ielpo B, d'Addetta MV, Anselmo A, Rosso E, de Blasi V, Sanchez-Velazquez P, Vellalta G, Podda M, Burdio F. Levels of robotic mesopancreas dissection according to malignancy and vascular anatomy: what surgeons need to know. Ann Surg Oncol. 2024;31(3):1916–8.
8. Pessaux P, et al. Pancreaticoduodenectomy: superior mesenteric artery first approach. J Gastrointest Surg. 2006;10:607–11.
9. Chen S, et al. Robot-assisted laparoscopic versus open pancreaticoduodenectomy: a prospective, matched, mid-term follow-up study. Surg Endosc. 2015;29:3698–711.

10. Popescu I, et al. Total meso-pancreas excision: key point of resection in pancreatic head adenocarcinoma. Hepato-Gastroenterology. 2011;58:202–7.
11. Kawabata Y, et al. Appraisal of a total meso-pancreato-duodenum excision with pancreaticoduodenectomy for pancreatic head carcinoma. Eur J Surg Oncol. 2012;38:574–9.
12. Kayahara M, et al. Surgical strategy for carcinoma of the pancreas head area based on clinicopathologic analysis of nodal involvement and plexus invasion. Surgery. 1995;117:616–23.
13. Hackert T, et al. The TRIANGLE operation: radical surgery after neoadjuvant treatment for advanced pancreatic cancer: a single arm observational study. HPB (Oxford). 2017;19(11):1001–7.

9 Intraoperative Management of the Gastroduodenal Artery

Sarah B. Hays, Sangrag Ganguli, Khaled Omar, and Melissa E. Hogg

9.1 Introduction

Bleeding events related to the gastroduodenal artery (GDA) are one of the most feared complications for pancreas surgeons. While post-pancreatectomy hemorrhage (PPH) is rare and observed in less than 10% of patients, it accounts for up to 38% of mortality following pancreatoduodenectomy, making it the leading cause of mortality following pancreatic resection [1, 2]. The incidence of GDA pseudoaneurysm (PSA) formation is 1.3%, and the presence of a PSA increases the risk for delayed PPH [3]. In the setting of a PSA, hemorrhage occurs roughly two weeks after surgery, which is frequently after the patient has been discharged. Sixty-seven percent of patients who present with PPH secondary to ruptured PSA have a preceding complication [3]. The development of a postoperative pancreatic fistula (POPF) significantly increases the risk of having a GDA-related bleeding event [4]. At high-volume pancreatic surgery centers, the incidence of PPH is low, at 5%, but despite this, mortality rates following PPH remain as high as 21–88%. Clearly, it is essential to identify techniques for management of the GDA to avoid the development of PSA and PPH. Here, we review the current literature on the intraoperative management of the GDA during pancreatoduodenectomy, with specific advice on how to approach the GDA using a MIS/robotic platform.

Supplementary Information The online version contains supplementary material available at https://doi.org/10.1007/978-3-031-99695-5_9. The videos can be accessed individually by clicking the DOI link in the accompanying figure caption or by scanning this link with the SN More Media App.

S. B. Hays · S. Ganguli
Department of Surgery, NorthShore University Health System, Evanston, IL, USA

Department of Surgery, University of Chicago Medical Center, Chicago, IL, USA
e-mail: Sarah.Hays@uchicagomedicine.org; Sangrag.Ganguli@uchicagomedicine.org

K. Omar · M. E. Hogg (✉)
Department of Surgery, NorthShore University Health System, Evanston, IL, USA
e-mail: k.omar.eras@gmail.com; mhogg@northshore.org

9.2 Classification of Post-pancreatectomy Hemorrhage

In 2007, the International Study Group of Pancreatic Surgery (ISGPS) defined PPH based on the time of onset, the location, and the severity of hemorrhage (Table 9.1) [5]. Based on these criteria, there are three grades of PPH (Table 9.2) with different diagnostic and therapeutic approaches [5]. In a pooled analysis of 43 randomized control trials, the reported rate of ISGPS Grade B/C PPH was 8.1%, a rare but serious complication [6].

B. Ielpo et al. (eds.), *Minimally Invasive Pancreatoduodenectomy in Cancer*,
https://doi.org/10.1007/978-3-031-99695-5_9

Table 9.1 International Study Group of Pancreatic Surgery (ISGPS) definition summary of PPH

Criteria	Definition	Clinical implication
Time of onset	Early: ≤24 h after the end of the index surgery	Coagulopathy, vascular resection, or inadequate hemostasis responsible for early PPH, whereas pancreatic fistulas responsible for late PPH
	Late: >24 h after the end of the index surgery	
Location	Intraluminal: intra-enteric bleeding	Could present as hematemesis, bleeding from nasogastric tube, or melena
	Extraluminal: bleeding into the abdominal cavity	Sanguineous abdominal drain output
Hemorrhage severity	Mild: decrease in hemoglobin concentration <3 g/dl	No need for angioembolization or reoperation
	Severe: >4–6 units of PRBC transfused over 24 h; decrease in hemoglobin concentration >4 g/dl	Need for angioembolization or relaparotomy

Table 9.2 Classification of PPH based on time of onset, location, and hemorrhage severity

Grade	Time	Location	Hemorrhage severity	Clinical condition	Diagnostic studies	Treatment approach
A	Early	Intra- or extraluminal	Mild	Well	CBC Ultrasound CT (if needed)	Observation
B	Early	Intra- or extraluminal	Severe	Well/intermediate	CBC Ultrasound CT Angiography Endoscopy	Transfuse, ICU care, endoscopy, embolization, relaparotomy (for early PPH)
	Late	Intra- or extraluminal	Mild			
C	Late	Intra- or extraluminal	Severe	Life-threatening	Angiography CT Endoscopy	Angioembolization Relaparotomy

9.3 Prevention and Treatment of Post-pancreatectomy Hemorrhage

Given the high rate of mortality, surgeons have been eager to identify ways to reduce the risk of PPH, including operative techniques and pre- and postoperative management [6]. In 2020 randomized control trial revealed that incorporating a smaller jejunal incision during a pancreaticojejunostomy was associated with decreased risk of PPH [7]. The specific type of anastomosis may also influence the risk of PPH. A large multicenter trial compared pancreatogastrostomy (PG) and pancreatojejunostomy (PJ) and revealed that the incidence of Grade A and B PPH is increased after PG. [8] Another technical consideration includes implementing a protective soft tissue "wrap" around the splanchnic vessels, which has been shown to reduce the risk of PPH [9]. With regards to preoperative management, Tarvainen et al. identified that patients who received perioperative hydrocortisone were at higher risk for PPH [10, 11]. Postoperatively, techniques to avoid POPF, thus decreasing the inflammation and erosion of splanchnic vessels, have been limited and ultimately not significantly changed the rate of PPH [12].

Once a bleeding event occurs, a surgeon has a few options for management. One approach to addressing GDA stump hemorrhage is covered stent placement. This has been shown to be successful in achieving hemostasis in 95% of patients [13, 14]. Trans-arterial embolization of the hepatic artery is also an effective treatment for PPH. Although hepatic complications are possible, particularly in patients with underlying liver disease or prior liver surgeries, embolization of the hepatic artery still provides a more enduring treatment effect compared to selective embolization of the GDA stump [15]. Finally, if minimally invasive interventions fail to control bleeding, a return to the operative room may be required.

9.4 Intraoperative Management of the Gastroduodenal Artery

Of course, addressing the GDA during the initial surgical resection is preferred in the prevention of PPH or PSA formation. Different surgical techniques have been proposed as ways to mitigate this risk. First, experts argue against the skeletonization the visceral arteries as this may result in an iatrogenic vascular injury, which can increase the risk of PSA and PPH [16]. Suture ligation of the GDA, especially in a minimally invasive approach, can also increase the risk of PSA/PPH [17]. One explanation is that suture ligation is often used instead of a stapler in cases where tumor involvement of the vessel limits the space required to use the stapler. In such cases, extensive dissection around the vessels is likely performed to achieve negative margins, increasing the risk of injury to the vessel.

Coverage of the GDA vessel stump has been the most popular proposed technique to decrease the risk of PPH and PSA [18]. GDA stump bleeding is thought to be correlated with local inflammation and erosion from pancreatic leak [19]. Coverage of the vessels separates them from the pancreatic and biliary anastomosis, preventing exposure to pancreatic enzymes or bile. The concept of flap coverage was first proposed in 2005 by Maeda et al. using an omental flap to cover the splanchnic vessels and found a reduction in postoperative intra-abdominal bleeding and infection [20]. The omental flap has also been shown to prevent the formation of postoperative PSA following pancreatoduodenectomy [21]. The teres hepatic ligament and the falciform ligament have been proposed as other suitable options for vessel wrapping, reducing the risk of PPH [22]. One group has also described the flooring technique, the formation of a tissue layer between the major vessels and pancreatic anastomosis using the falciform ligament, and demonstrated decreased incidence of stump-related PPH [23].

By far, the most popular coverage technique is wrapping of the splanchnic vessels using a falciform ligament flap. In 2021, a randomized, controlled, multicenter trial was published investigating the impact of the falciform ligament wrap, known as the PANDA trial [24]. In this trial, patients were randomized to open pancreatoduodenectomy with or without a falciform ligament wrap around the hepatic artery and GDA stump. The primary endpoint was clinically relevant PPH, and per protocol analysis demonstrated significant reduction in the falciform wrap group (2.0% vs 7.2%, odds ratio 0.26 [0.09–0.80], $p = 0.017$). Welsch et al. argue that a falciform ligament wrap should be considered for all pancreatoduodenectomy, especially in cases with high risk for POPF. Critics argue that while this may have decreased the rate of PPH, it did not decrease the mortality rate in the wrap group. Others remain skeptical of wrapping and argue that wrapping doesn't prevent the formation of POPF, the biggest risk factor for development of PPH [25].

9.5 Approach to the Gastroduodenal Artery in Minimally Invasive Pancreatoduodenectomy

As interest in minimally invasive pancreatoduodenectomy rises, it is equally important to understand the best approaches to mitigate risk of postoperative complications both laparoscopically and robotically. In two landmark laparoscopic pancreatoduodenectomy trials, the PADULAP and PLOT trials, there were no significant differences between the laparoscopic and open cohorts in postoperative complications including PPH [26, 27]. Notably, in the PADULAP trial, postoperative pancreatic complications were consistently lower in the laparoscopic cohort, but this did not reach significance. These findings have been replicated in smaller studies [28, 29]. The wrapping technique has been successfully implemented in laparoscopic pancreatoduodenectomy with the use of the teres hepatic ligament [30]. In one small single-center study, performing the teres hepatic ligament wrap significantly lowered the risk of PPH [31].

With the rise and implementation of robotic pancreas surgery, there were initially concerns of safety, including risk of PPH. Early studies reported a slightly higher rate of PPH in the robotic cohort compared to open. This led to the adoption of the "no-touch technique" during the dissection of the GDA and hepatic artery, because the absence of haptic feedback can cause unidentified injury to the vessel, increasing the risk of PSA and PPH [32]. Utilizing this no-touch approach, subsequent studies on the robotic pancreatoduodenectomy (RPD) have demonstrated PPH rates equivalent to historical open series [17]. Interestingly, in a Magge et al. 2018 study, the authors implemented the use of the falciform wrap halfway through the study and found it to be a negative predictor of PSA formation. Recent clinical trials comparing robotic pancreatoduodenectomy to open have found no significant difference in the rate of PPH between the two approaches [33, 34]. Results from the pending DIPLOMA-2 trial, which compared minimally invasive (robotic and laparoscopic) pancreatoduodenectomy to open, have also demonstrated no difference in rate of POPF leading to PPH (IHPBA Abstract/Presentation). As more surgeons turn towards using the robot in pancreatic surgery, our recommendations for minimally invasive management of the GDA are described below.

The GDA is addressed during the second step of the RPD. At this point, as shown in the video, the stomach is already transected and reflected, the hilum is retracted with a liver retractor, and the hepatoduodenal ligament is open (Fig. 9.1). The *setup* is important to keep clean tissue planes and allow for maximal exposure to the GDA:

1. Removal of the hepatic artery lymph node. *Tip*: Start at 6 o'clock and proceed counterclockwise to 12–3 o'clock trying to leave fat on the node as a handle (Fig. 9.2a, b). Then come posterior to node and take the 3–6 o'clock area with a vessel sealing device due to perforating veins (Fig. 9.3).
2. Identify the common hepatic artery (CHA) (Fig. 9.4). Between the CHA and superior neck of the pancreas, identify the portal vein (PV) and clean off the lymphatics on top to see the vein wall (Fig. 9.5). *Tip*: Open horizontally midway between the artery and the pancreas. If you are too close to the pancreas, it will bleed. Leave some of the lymphatics on the CHA so you can grab this tissue to lift is up.
3. On the transected stomach specimen find the right gastric artery and ligate (Fig. 9.6). *Tip*: This can be done first, second, or third in terms of sequencing.

Now, as shown in the video, it is time to approach the *dissection* of the GDA. It is important to have a "no-touch technique"—essentially do not grab the vessel itself. *Tip*: Avoid dissecting off adventitial tissue on the anterior surface of the GDA. It is enticing because it is easy, but it can also be a handle to avoid grabbing vessel directly.

1. Medial dissection—Dissect the CHA off the PV and lift it with the left hand using a "spatula technique" (Fig. 9.7). This allows posterior medial access to the GDA. Tip: Keep wrist bent upward and retract the hand toward 10 o'clock to maximize visualization.

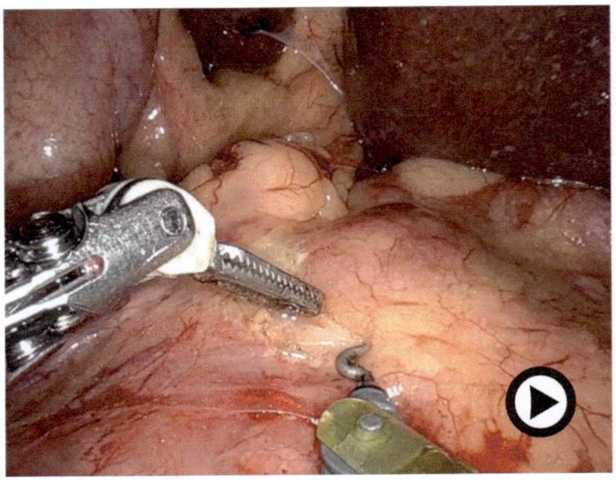

Fig. 9.1 Exposure at the beginning of dissection (Intraoperative management of the gastroduodenal artery (▶ https://doi.org/10.1007/000-hep))

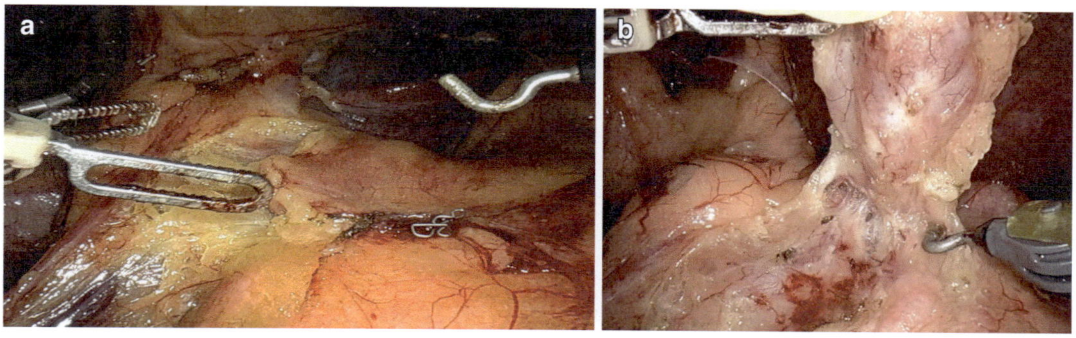

Fig. 9.2 (**a**) Initial dissection from 6 to 12 o'clock clockwise. (**b**) Dissection complete except for pedicle

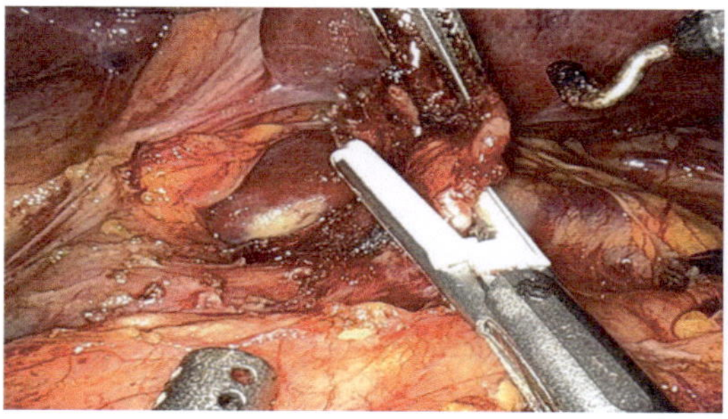

Fig. 9.3 Removal of the hepatic artery lymph node

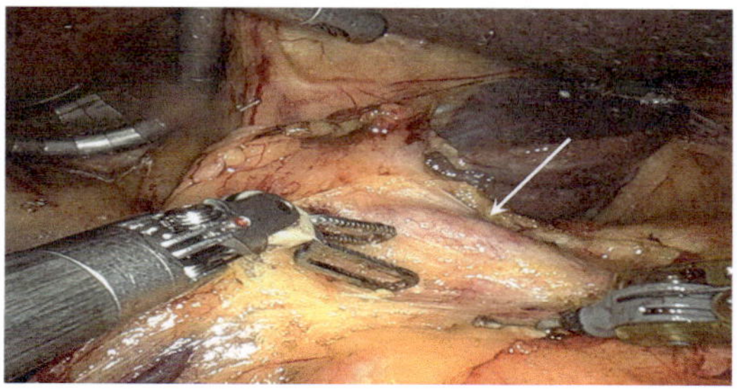

Fig. 9.4 Identifying the common hepatic artery (arrow)

2. Lateral dissection—There are several choledochal vessels, and it is helpful to try to coagulate these vessels to preempt any bleeding (Fig. 9.8a, b). Work to create a window toward the dissection that was performed medially and pass left hand to right then grab a vessel loop to retract (Fig. 9.9a, b). Tip: Find a window without a lot of perforating branches by being flexible to move the dissection cranial under the hepatic artery proper or more distal on the GDA.

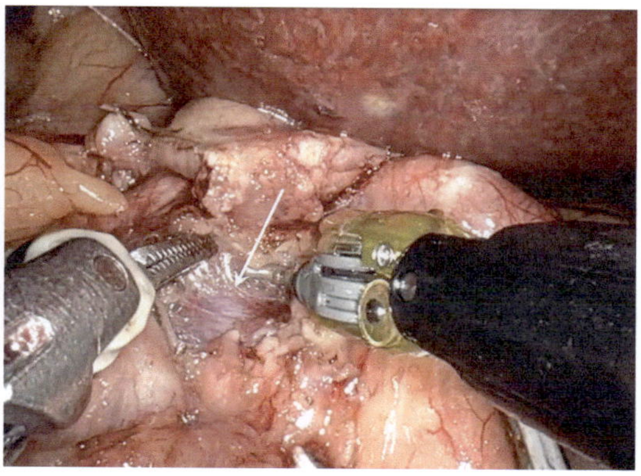

Fig. 9.5 Identifying the portal vein (arrow), found between the common hepatic artery and the superior neck of the pancreas

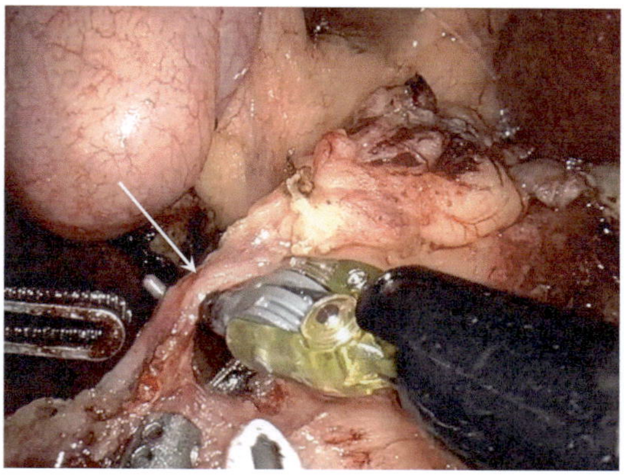

Fig. 9.6 Ligation of the right gastric artery (arrow)

3. Transection—The author's preference is a 30 mm vascular stapler with a curved tip. Ties or Hem-o-lok® clips are additional options. Tip: Bring the stapler in, open, reticulate it

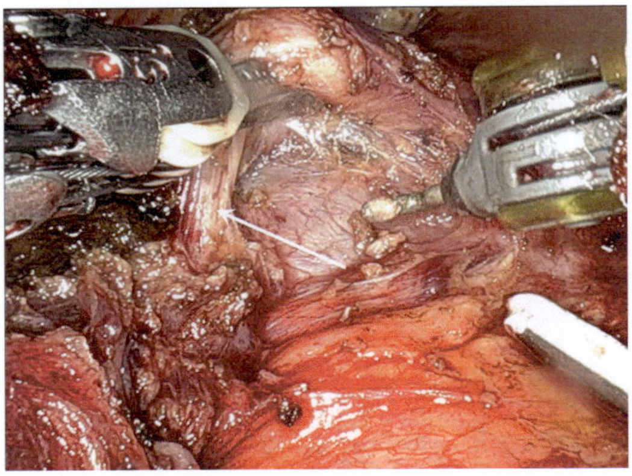

Fig. 9.7 Dissection of the common hepatic artery off the portal vein. Arrow points to the gastroduodenal artery

maximally to left, then place tip right under the vessel loop (Fig. 9.10a, b) and use a scooping motion. There are many ways to ligate the vessel including clips and suture ligation. The authors favor this approach because it is clean, atraumatic, and reproducible/consistent.

Tricks to stay out of trouble:

1. Check the lateral bile duct for aberrant artery (Fig. 9.11) or find the right hepatic artery prior to ligation of the GDA (Fig. 9.12).
2. Ultrasound or test clamp the GDA to assure flow in hepatic arteries prior to ligation (Fig. 9.13).

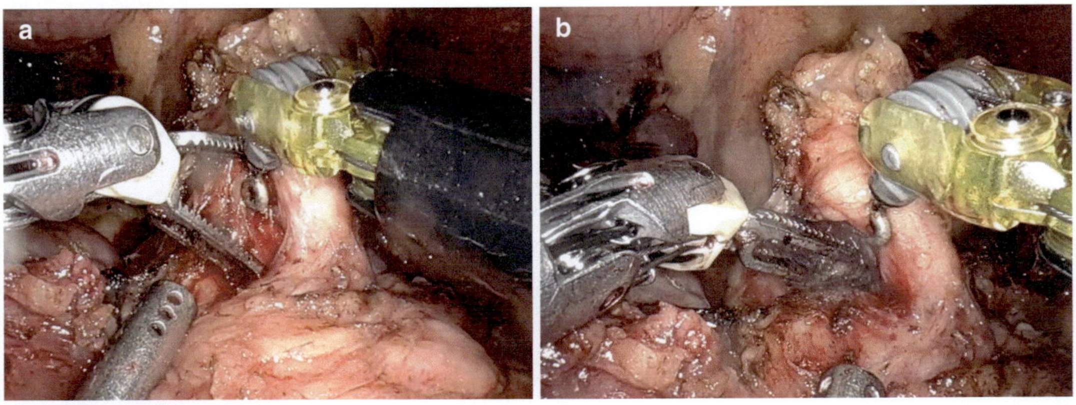

Fig. 9.8 (**a** & **b**) Lateral gastroduodenal artery dissection

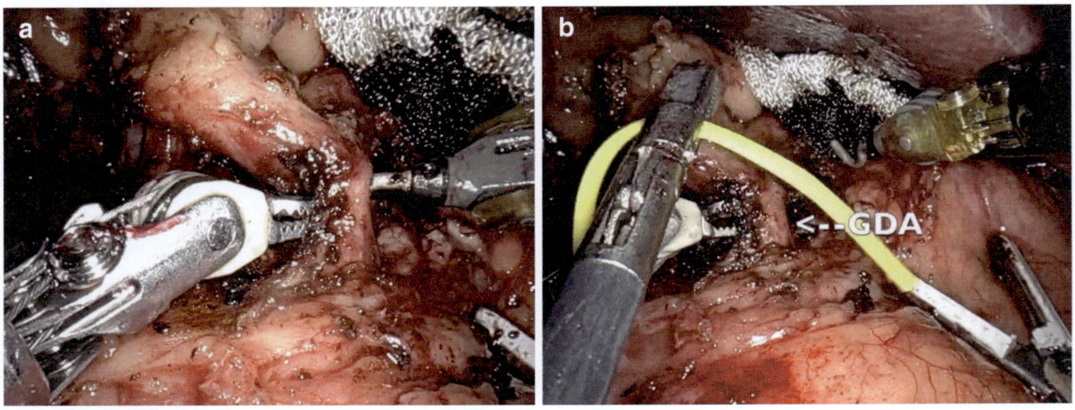

Fig. 9.9 (**a**) Posterior gastroduodenal artery dissection. (**b**) Pass vessel loop behind gastroduodenal artery

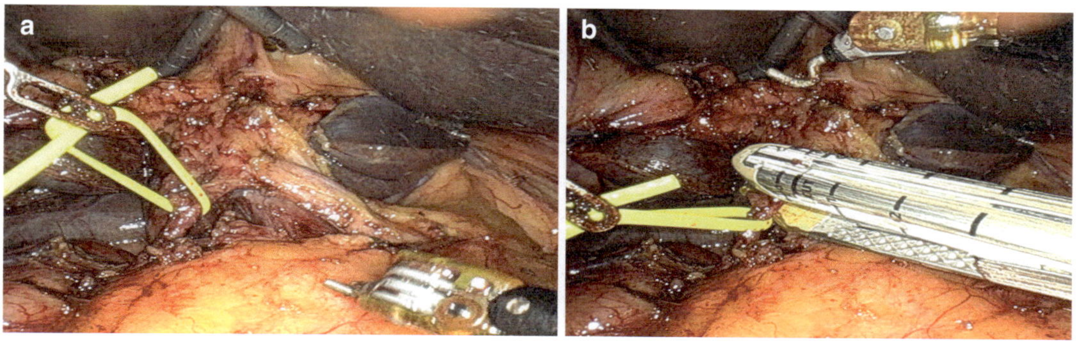

Fig. 9.10 Gastroduodenal artery ligation. (**a**) Vessel loop contains gastroduodenal artery. (**b**) Stapler for gastroduodenal artery ligation

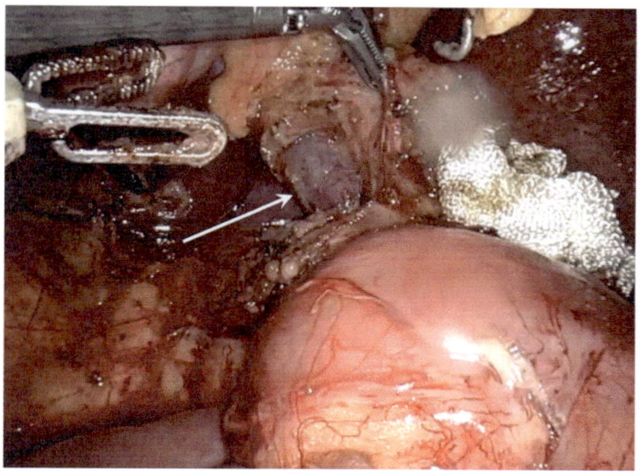

Fig. 9.11 Examine lateral bile duct for aberrant anatomy. Arrow indicates portal vein and robotic instrument retracts the common bile duct

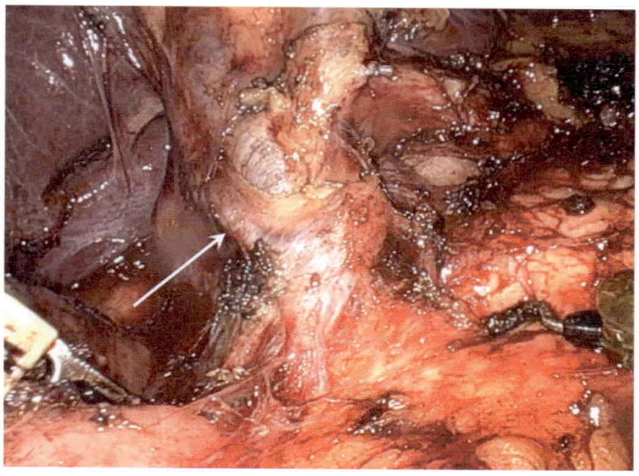

Fig. 9.12 Identify the right hepatic artery prior to gastroduodenal artery ligation. Arrow points to an anterior right hepatic artery "coming from" the gastroduodenal artery

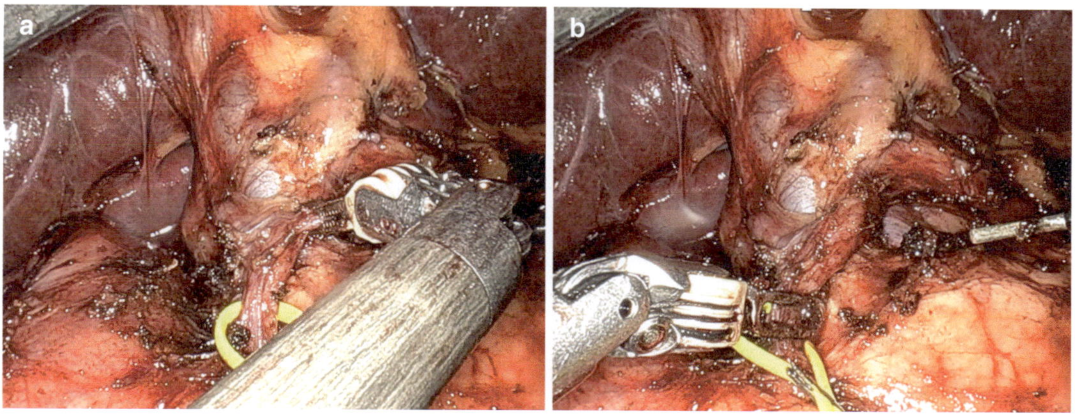

Fig. 9.13 Test clamp the gastroduodenal artery prior to ligation, vessel loop surrounds gastroduodenal artery (**a**) Common trunk to right hepatic artery and gastroduodenal artery clamped by robotic instrument. (**b**) GDA alone clamped by robotic instrument

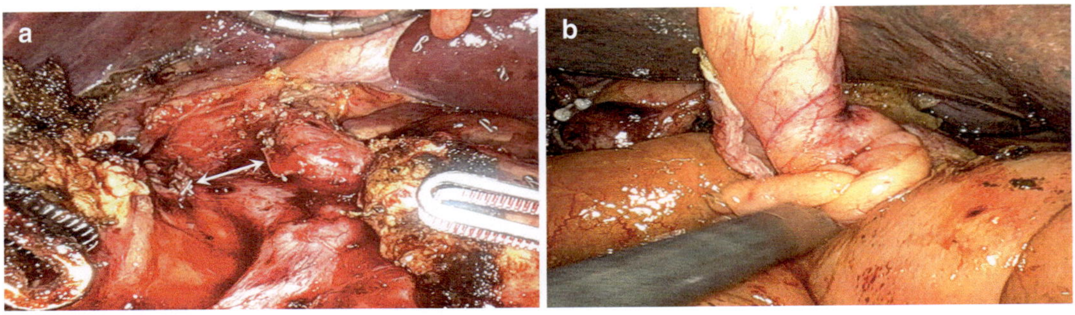

Fig. 9.14 Place falciform flap between the GDA stump and the pancreaticojejunostomy. (**a**) Double arrow points to GDA stump where falciform flap should lay. (**b**) Falciform flap

3. Place falciform between the GDA stump and the pancreaticojejunostomy (Fig. 9.14a, b). The senior author used to place a metal clip on the GDA stump to mark it for future imaging but has since moved away from that.

9.6 Conclusion

Post-pancreatectomy hemorrhage is a devastating complication of pancreatoduodenectomy, whether performed open or with a minimally invasive approach. Significant work has been done in attempt to decrease the rate of pseudoaneurysm formation and bleeding. The development of the falciform wrap is one successful example of an operative technique that can help to decrease this risk. As robotic pancreatoduodenectomy becomes more popular, effective management of the gastroduodenal artery to decrease the rate of associated complications is essential. Pancreas surgeons must be well trained in these techniques to provide their patients the best quality of life and chance of recovery.

References

1. Jagad RB, Koshariya M, Kawamoto J, Chude GS, Neeraj RV, Lygidakis NJ. Postoperative hemorrhage after major pancreatobiliary surgery: an update. Hepato-Gastroenterology. 2008;55:729–37.
2. Wolk S, Grützmann R, Rahbari NN, Hoffmann RT, Plodeck V, Weitz J, Welsch T, Distler M. Management of clinically relevant postpancreatectomy hemorrhage (PPH) over two decades – a comparative study of 1450 consecutive patients undergoing pancreatic resection. Pancreatology. 2017;17:943–50.
3. Brodie B, Kocher HM. Systematic review of the incidence, presentation and management of gastroduodenal artery pseudoaneurysm after pancreatic resection. BJS Open. 2019;3:735–42.
4. Ferguson BD. Toward better prediction of post-pancreatectomy hemorrhage. JAMA Netw Open. 2023;6:e2346069.
5. Wente MN, Veit JA, Bassi C, et al. Postpancreatectomy hemorrhage (PPH)–an international study group of pancreatic surgery (ISGPS) definition. Surgery. 2007;142:20–5.
6. Montorsi RM, Zonderhuis BM, Daams F, Busch OR, Kazemier G, Marchegiani G, Malleo G, Salvia R, Besselink MG. Treatment strategies to prevent or mitigate the outcome of post-pancreatectomy hemorrhage (PPH): a review of randomized trials. Int J Surg. 2023. https://doi.org/10.1097/JS9.0000000000000876.
7. di Mola FF, Grottola T, Panaccio P, Tavano F, De Bonis A, Valvano MR, Di Sebastiano P. End-to-side duct-to-mucosa pancreaticojejunostomy after pancreaticoduodenectomy a comparison trial of small versus larger jejunal incision. A single center experience. Ann Ital Chir. 2020;91:469–77.
8. Keck T, Wellner UF, Bahra M, et al. Pancreatogastrostomy versus pancreatojejunostomy for RECOnstruction after PANCreatoduodenectomy (RECOPANC, DRKS 00000767): perioperative and long-term results of a multicenter randomized controlled trial. Ann Surg. 2016;263:440–9.
9. Nour HM, Peristeri DV, Ahsan A, Shafique S, Khan PM, Sajid MS. Regional vessels wrapping following pancreaticoduodenectomy reduces the risk of post-operative extra-luminal bleed-

ing. A systematic review. Ann Med Surg (Lond). 2022;82:104618.
10. Tarvainen T, Sirén J, Kokkola A, Sallinen V. Effect of hydrocortisone vs pasireotide on pancreatic surgery complications in patients with high risk of pancreatic fistula: a randomized clinical trial. JAMA Surg. 2020;155:291–8.
11. Smits FJ, Henry AC, Besselink MG, et al. Algorithm-based care versus usual care for the early recognition and management of complications after pancreatic resection in The Netherlands: an open-label, nationwide, stepped-wedge cluster-randomised trial. Lancet. 2022;399:1867–75.
12. Harnoss JC, Ulrich AB, Harnoss JM, Diener MK, Büchler MW, Welsch T. Use and results of consensus definitions in pancreatic surgery: a systematic review. Surgery. 2014;155:47–57.
13. Chouliaras K, Kitano M. Pancreaticoduodenectomy (Whipple procedure). In: Karamanos E, editor. Common surgeries made easy: a quick guide for residents and medical students. Cham: Springer International Publishing; 2020. p. 169–75.
14. Min H, Yoon CJ, Lee JH, Choi WS, Yeo JB, Yoon Y-S, Cho JY, Lee HW, Lee JS. Covered stent placement for gastroduodenal artery stump hemorrhage after pancreaticoduodenectomy: long-term patency and risk factor of stent failure. Br J Radiol. 2022;95:20220022.
15. Wu C-C, Chen H-W, Lee K-E, Wong Y-C, Ku Y-K. Comparing the clinical efficacy of coil embolization in GDA stump versus common hepatic artery in postoperative hemorrhage after Pancreatoduodenectomy. J Pers Med. 2023;13:264.
16. Fujii Y, Shimada H, Endo I, Yoshida K, Matsuo K, Takeda K, Ueda M, Morioka D, Tanaka K, Togo S. Management of massive arterial hemorrhage after pancreatobiliary surgery: does embolotherapy contribute to successful outcome? J Gastrointest Surg. 2007;11:432–8.
17. Magge D, Zenati M, Lutfi W, Hamad A, Zureikat AH, Zeh HJ, Hogg ME. Robotic pancreatoduodenectomy at an experienced institution is not associated with an increased risk of post-pancreatic hemorrhage. HPB. 2018;20:448–55.
18. Xu C, Yang X, Luo X, Shen F, Wu M, Tan W, Jiang X. "Wrapping the gastroduodenal artery stump" during pancreatoduodenectomy reduced the stump hemorrhage incidence after operation. Chin J Cancer Res. 2014;26:299–308.
19. Koukoutsis I, Bellagamba R, Morris-Stiff G, Wickremesekera S, Coldham C, Wigmore SJ, Mayer AD, Mirza DF, Buckels JAC, Bramhall SR. Haemorrhage following pancreaticoduodenectomy: risk factors and the importance of sentinel bleed. Dig Surg. 2006;23:224–8.
20. Maeda A, Ebata T, Kanemoto H, Matsunaga K, Bando E, Yamaguchi S, Uesaka K. Omental flap in pancreaticoduodenectomy for protection of splanchnic vessels. World J Surg. 2005;29:1122–6.
21. Matsuda H, Sadamori H, Umeda Y, Shinoura S, Yoshida R, Satoh D, Utsumi M, Yagi T, Fujiwara T. Preventive effect of omental flap in pancreaticoduodenectomy against postoperative pseudoaneurysm formation. Hepato-Gastroenterology. 2012;59:578–83.
22. Zheng X, Jiang Z, Gao Z, Zhou B, Li G, Yan S, Mei X. Wrapping gastroduodenal artery stump with the teres hepatis ligament to prevent postpancreatectomy hemorrhage after pancreaticoduodenectomy. World J Surg Oncol. 2023;21:370.
23. Okada K, Murakami Y, Uemura K, Kondo N, Nakagawa N, Seo S, Otsuka H, Takahashi S. Flooring the major vessels with Falciform ligament to prevent post-pancreatectomy hemorrhage. World J Surg. 2020;44:3478–85.
24. Welsch T, Müssle B, Korn S, et al. Pancreatoduodenectomy with or without prophylactic falciform ligament wrap around the hepatic artery for prevention of postpancreatectomy haemorrhage: randomized clinical trial (PANDA trial). Br J Surg. 2021;109:37–45.
25. Tani M, Kawai M, Hirono S, Hatori T, Imaizumi T, Nakao A, Egawa S, Asano T, Nagakawa T, Yamaue H. Use of omentum or falciform ligament does not decrease complications after pancreaticoduodenectomy: nationwide survey of the Japanese Society of Pancreatic Surgery. Surgery. 2012;151:183–91.
26. Poves I, Burdío F, Morató O, Iglesias M, Radosevic A, Ilzarbe L, Visa L, Grande L. Comparison of perioperative outcomes between laparoscopic and open approach for pancreatoduodenectomy: the PADULAP randomized controlled trial. Ann Surg. 2018;268:731–9.
27. Palanivelu C, Senthilnathan P, Sabnis SC, Babu NS, Srivatsan Gurumurthy S, Anand Vijai N, Nalankilli VP, Praveen Raj P, Parthasarathy R, Rajapandian S. Randomized clinical trial of laparoscopic versus open pancreatoduodenectomy for periampullary tumours. Br J Surg. 2017;104:1443–50.
28. Kim SC, Song KB, Jung YS, et al. Short-term clinical outcomes for 100 consecutive cases of laparoscopic pylorus-preserving pancreatoduodenectomy: improvement with surgical experience. Surg Endosc. 2013;27:95–103.
29. Gumbs AA, Rodriguez Rivera AM, Milone L, Hoffman JP. Laparoscopic pancreatoduodenectomy: a review of 285 published cases. Ann Surg Oncol. 2011;18:1335–41.
30. Meng L, Cai H, Cai Y, Li Y, Peng B. Wrapping the stump of the gastroduodenal artery using the ligamentum teres hepatis during laparoscopic pancreaticoduodenectomy: a center's preliminary experience. BMC Surg. 2021;21:70.
31. Yu Z, Wu X, Zhou X, Hu X, Lu J, Fang S, Wang L, Ruan Y, Lu Y, Li H. Ligamentum teres hepatis wrapping of the gastroduodenal artery stump for protection in total laparoscopic pancreaticoduode-

nectomy: a single-center experience. J Int Med Res. 2023;51:3000605231188288.

32. Zeh HJ, Zureikat AH, Secrest A, Dauoudi M, Bartlett D, Moser AJ. Outcomes after robot-assisted pancreaticoduodenectomy for periampullary lesions. Ann Surg Oncol. 2012;19:864–70.
33. Klotz R, Mihaljevic AL, Kulu Y, et al. Robotic versus open partial pancreatoduodenectomy (EUROPA): a randomised controlled stage 2b trial. Lancet Reg Health Eur. 2024;39:100864.
34. Liu Q, Li M, Gao Y, Jiang T, Han B, Zhao G, Lin C, Lau WY, Zhao Z, Liu R. Effect of robotic versus open pancreaticoduodenectomy on postoperative length of hospital stay and complications for pancreatic head or periampullary tumours: a multicentre, open-label randomised controlled trial. Lancet Gastroenterol Hepatol. 2024;S2468-1253(24):00005–0.

Minimally Invasive Anastomosis After Pancreatoduodenectomy

10

Alberto García-Picazo, Benedetto Ielpo, Patricia Sánchez-Velázquez, and Fernando Burdio

10.1 Introduction

Minimally invasive pancreaticoduodenectomy (PD) is becoming an important surgical approach for pancreatic cancer, as described in the literature [1]. Nevertheless, it is a challenging procedure, not only due to the pancreatic resection but also because minimally invasive approach increases the complexity during the reconstruction phase. This procedure requires performing at least three different anastomoses (pancreas, bile duct, and stomach), but the most critical is the pancreatic anastomosis (PA).

PA is often considered the Achilles' heel of PD, which has led to the development of many techniques over the decades, each with varying degrees of technical difficulty, but without a universally accepted gold standard method [2, 3]. Moreover, each anastomosis must be adapted to the texture of the pancreatic parenchyma and the size of the pancreatic duct, which are key prognostic factors for developing postoperative pancreatic fistula (POPF). This is particularly true when the pancreas is soft and the duct is small and posteriorly located [1].

Several technical issues can increase the risk of POPF, such as improper suture tension, inadequate pancreas mobilization, pancreatic parenchyma tearing, an excessive diameter of the enteric orifice, or difficulties in controlling bleeding [1]. The significance of PA lies in the potential consequences of POPF, which include morbidity factors such as intra-abdominal collections, hemorrhage, delayed gastric emptying, prolonged hospital stay, and an increased risk of mortality [4].

The primary objective of performing a PA is to reduce the likelihood of developing POPF. Various techniques have been proposed, including invagination versus duct-to-mucosa pancreaticojejunostomy (PJ), pancreaticogastrostomy, the use of pancreatic duct stents (absorbable or non-absorbable), fibrin glue, and somatostatin analogs. However, according to the International Study Group of Pancreatic Surgery (ISGPS), no single technique has proven superior to the others [4]. The current recommendation is to perform a standardized technique at high-volume centers with experienced surgeons. Additionally, tools such as the Fistula Risk Score can help predict the risk of POPF [4].

Supplementary Information The online version contains supplementary material available at https://doi.org/10.1007/978-3-031-99695-5_10. The videos can be accessed individually by clicking the DOI link in the accompanying figure caption or by scanning this link with the SN More Media App.

A. García-Picazo · B. Ielpo (✉) ·
P. Sánchez-Velázquez · F. Burdio
HPB Unit, Hospital del Mar, Barcelona, Spain
e-mail: alberto.gpicazo@gmail.com; ielpo.b@gmail.com; psanchezvelazquez@psmar.cat; fburdio@hotmail.com

B. Ielpo et al. (eds.), *Minimally Invasive Pancreatoduodenectomy in Cancer*,
https://doi.org/10.1007/978-3-031-99695-5_10

Minimally invasive surgery for PD is becoming more common, although it involves additional technical difficulties, particularly in laparoscopic surgery due to the restricted range of instrument movement, which is more apparent during the reconstruction phase [5, 6]. These challenges have been mitigated with the advent of robotic surgery, which offers instruments with high degrees of freedom, three-dimensional (3D) stable vision, tremor suppression algorithms, and improved ergonomics for the surgeon, thereby reducing the complexity of the PD procedure.

The purpose of this chapter is to describe the most frequent anastomoses following minimally invasive PD, including step-by-step technical tips, indications, complications, and potential alternatives for each type of anastomosis.

10.2 Reconstruction

We recommend a single-loop reconstruction according to the Child technique, although a Roux-en-Y is also possible and recommended to avoid bile reflux.

10.3 Pancreatic Anastomosis

The most common types of PA are presented below, ordered by their technical complexity from low to high (Table 10.1).

Table 10.1 Different PA, ordered by their technical complexity

Level of complexity	Type of PA	Main indications
Low complexity	Barbed single-layer pancreaticojejunostomy	Prominent main pancreatic duct, hard pancreatic parenchyma
	Pancreatojejunostomy with coronary artery stent	High-risk patients of POPF, visible main pancreatic duct
Intermediate complexity	Blumgart PA	Dilated main pancreatic duct, soft pancreatic parenchyma
High complexity	Double purse-string pancreatico-gastrostomy	Non-visible main pancreatic duct, thick pancreatic parenchyma, large pancreatic size

Adapted by Ielpo et al. [1]

10.4 Barbed Single-Layer Pancreaticojejunostomy

The first step is placing a drain in the main pancreatic duct before beginning the anastomosis. The anastomosis is then performed with a full-thickness running barbed suture (3/0), divided into anterior and posterior walls. It is crucial that each layer of the suture includes the anterior and posterior walls of the main pancreatic duct to ensure a tight seal. The main advantage of this

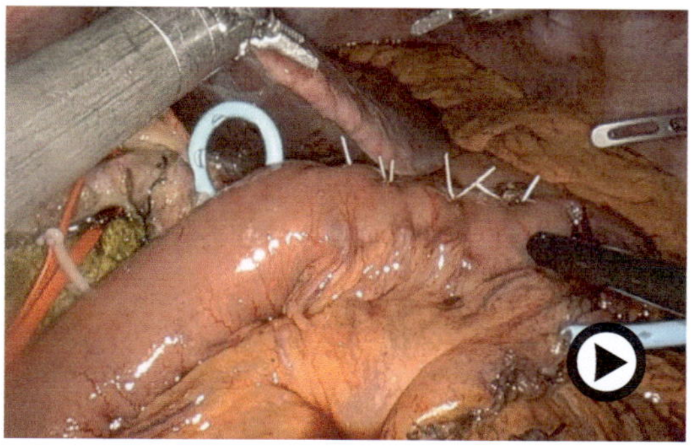

Fig. 10.1 The pancreatic drain is placed posterior to the PA (Blumgart anastomosis (▶ https://doi.org/10.1007/000-hes))

suture is its self-locking capacity, which minimizes pancreatic tissue damage due to suture traction, thereby reducing the risk of POPF.

Another important tip is to place a drain directly posterior to the PA (Fig. 10.1). This location is critical to prevent any possible collections associated with POPF, as placing a drain postoperatively can be particularly difficult [1].

This PA technique is indicated for straightforward cases with a prominent main pancreatic duct and hard pancreatic parenchyma.

10.5 Pancreatojejunostomy with Coronary Artery Stent

This technique was recently described by Huscher et al. for high-risk patients of POPF [7]. In this group, the use of an externalized trans-anastomotic stent can be an effective option. However, the issue arises when the stent malfunctions or becomes obstructed, which occurs in approximately 22% of cases, leading to increased morbidity [8]. Therefore, the specific characteristics of the coronary artery metal stent are key to preventing occlusion or displacement, making it a potentially useful tool for preventing POPF in high-risk patients [7].

The coronary artery stent, composed of a 75-mm cobalt–chromium strut with a double-spiral design and a titanium nitride oxide coating, is placed using the Seldinger technique [7]. This involves puncturing through the jejunal limb without the need for an enterotomy. The main pancreatic duct is intubated with a guidewire, after which the stent is advanced, expanded, and fixed to the main pancreatic duct. The stent has two radiopaque markers to confirm optimal placement via intraoperative fluoroscopy [7]. The proximal marker is placed on the intestinal side, and the distal marker 8–10 mm inside the main pancreatic duct. After confirming the placement, a 28 mm length and 25-mm-diameter stent is expanded (at a pressure of 8–10 bar), and the PJ is completed with capsule-serosa polypropylene running sutures [7].

This PA technique is not particularly difficult and is primarily indicated for high-risk patients of POPF with a visible main pancreatic duct.

10.6 Blumgart Anastomosis

Blumgart et al. described this technique in 2000, and it has since been standardized worldwide. It generally combines duct-to-mucosa anastomosis with a transpancreatic U-suture technique (Video 1) [9, 10]. Before starting the anastomosis, a pigtail drainage tube is placed posterior to the PJ, which is useful in case of POPF and is easier to place with this approach than percutaneously in the postoperative period. Moreover, this abdominal drain can be removed on postoperative day 5 (POD 5) if the amylase levels in the drain on POD 3 and 5 are less than three times the upper limit of blood amylase levels and there is no evidence of POPF (e.g., abnormal clinical course) [11–13].

The suture used is a double-needle 3/0 Gore-Tex, which is cut and knotted in the middle, resulting in a total length of 15 cm. This stitch is passed through the upper jejunal loop and then crossed over the pancreas with two transpancreatic stitches surrounding the main pancreatic duct (Fig. 10.2) [1]. These stitches are grasped by the tip-up robotic forceps with slight traction, allowing the jejunal loop to lie behind the posterior face of the pancreas (Fig. 10.3). Another 3/0 single-needle Gore-Tex suture is placed just posterior to the main pancreatic duct, between the

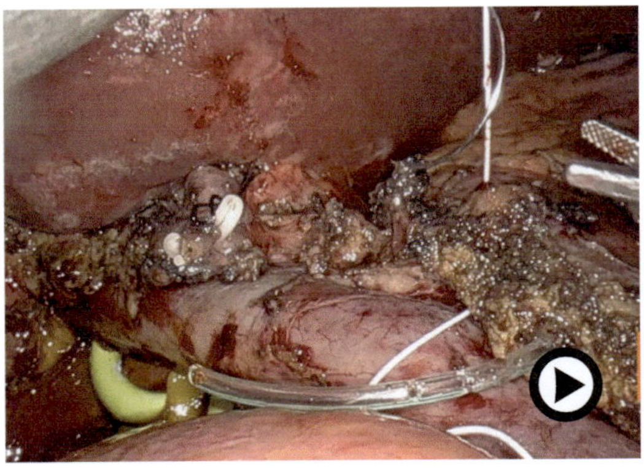

Fig. 10.2 Transpancreatic stitch, which pass through the upper jejunal loop and then cross over the pancreas (Transpancreatic stitches surrounding the main pancreatic duct (▶ https://doi.org/10.1007/000-her))

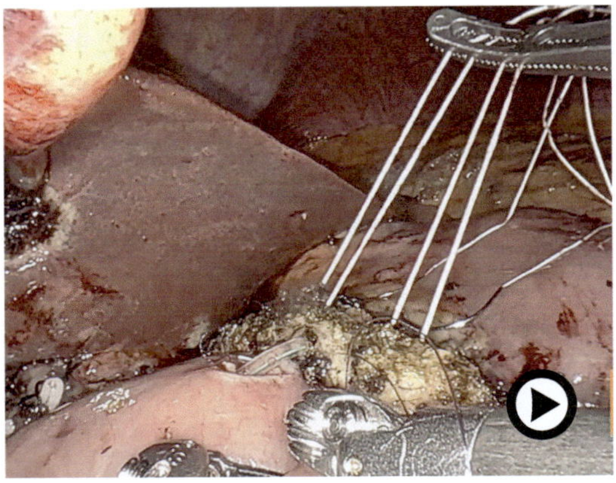

Fig. 10.3 Transpancreatic stitches are grasped by the tip-up robotic forceps with slight traction, allowing the jejunal loop to lie behind the posterior face of the pancreas (Stitches are grasped by the tip-up robotic forceps with slight traction (▶ https://doi.org/10.1007/000-heq))

pancreas and the jejunal loop, which is referred to as the Pittsburgh stitch (Fig. 10.4).

An enterotomy in the jejunum is created using monopolar energy applied to a PDS 5/0 needle, and a duct-to-mucosa anastomosis is performed with interrupted sutures (Fig. 10.5). At this stage, a pancreatic duct stent, typically biodegradable in our case, is usually placed after completing the posterior duct-to-mucosa wall [1]. The use of an internal-external pancreatic stent (absorbable or non-absorbable) can be an option in patients with high-risk factors for developing POPF, especially external ones. Once the sutures are passed, the two extremities are secured with a Hem-o-lok, which can be easily released later to avoid confusion among the different sutures. The posterior sutures are tied, except for the lateral ones, to avoid tension. After completing the duct-to-mucosa anastomosis, the two external transpancreatic sutures are passed through the anterior layer of the jejunum and tied, effectively sandwiching the pancreas neck within the jejunum [1].

Finally, sealants such as TachoSil® or Floseal®, biologic patches, or sutures can be applied to the PA, although there is no substantial evidence that these reduce the incidence of POPF [4].

This PA technique has moderate complexity due to the use of two transpancreatic sutures. It is indicated when the main pancreatic duct is dilated, and the pancreas is soft, as these transpancreatic stitches provide additional tensile strength in the pancreatic suture [1].

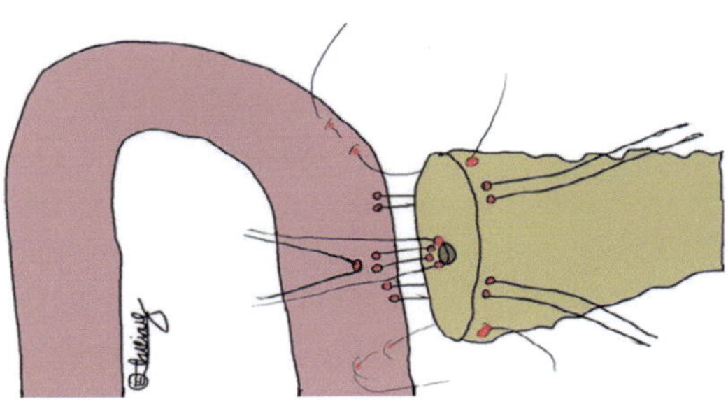

Fig. 10.4 Illustration of the Blumgart pancreaticojejunal anastomosis with transpancreatic and duct-to-mucosa stitches

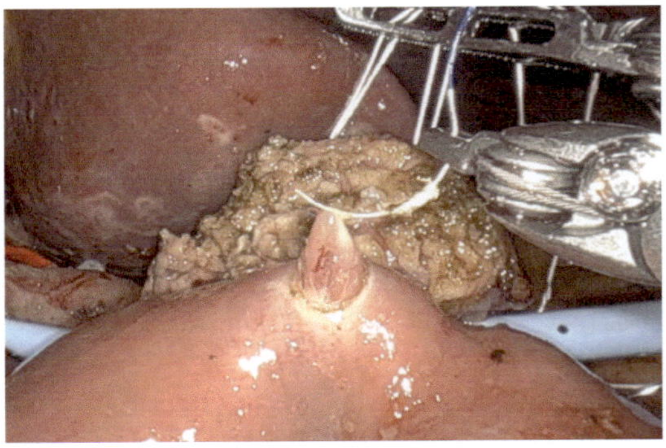

Fig. 10.5 Jejunum orifice made by the monopolar energy applied to the needle

10.7 Double Purse-String Pancreaticogastrostomy

In this PA, the critical step is to enhance the mobilization of the pancreatic stump, at least 3–4 cm. Two 2/0 polypropylene sutures are placed on the distal pancreatic stump at the superior and inferior edges of the pancreas. The pancreatic remnant is divided from the splenic artery/vein for 3–4 cm, as well as from the pancreatic body [1]. It is essential to preserve the anatomical structure of the pancreatic dorsal artery to minimize ischemia [1]. Once the pancreatic remnant is mobilized, the posterior stomach wall is moved laterally and lower to reach the superior pancreatic edge. A stomach incision is then made through the seromuscular layer, preserving the mucosa near the main pancreatic duct [1].

The first purse-string suture is applied with 2/0 absorbable Monocryl in a concentric fashion around the posterior gastric incision, involving the seromuscular layers. The second purse-string suture is then applied inside the stomach, including only the mucosa [1]. The posterior stomach wall incision is extended to the anterior wall, and the pancreatic remnant is positioned inside the stomach, allowing it to protrude 2–3 cm into the stomach lumen without external pressure [1]. The seromuscular purse-string suture is then tightened, followed by the mucosal one. Care must be taken not to overtighten the suture to avoid tearing the pancreas [1].

This PA technique is highly complex and is reserved for cases where the main pancreatic duct is inconspicuous. It can also be an option for cases with a thick and large pancreas, as the pancreatic body can be better adapted to the stomach. Adequate mobilization of the pancreas is the key to success. Some authors suggest that this PA has a lower incidence of POPF compared to PJ anastomosis, although strong evidence is lacking [14, 15].

10.8 Main Key Points for the PA

The following points were highlighted by the ISGPS [4]:

- The most crucial factor in avoiding POPF is performing a standardized PA technique and ensuring that PD is performed at high-volume centers by experienced surgeons.
- The use of internal-external pancreatic stents (absorbable or non-absorbable) may be beneficial for patients with high-risk factors for developing POPF, particularly external ones.
- Abdominal drains can be removed on POD 5 if the amylase levels in the drain on POD 3 and 5 are less than three times the upper limit of blood amylase levels and there is no evidence of POPF [11–13].
- There is no clear evidence that PJ or pancreaticogastrostomy is superior in terms of reducing POPF incidence.
- The use of tissue sealants, biologic patches, or special sutures has not shown substantial evidence of effectiveness.
- Tools such as the Fistula Risk Score can help predict the risk of POPF.

10.9 Biliary Anastomosis

The first step is assessing the bile duct diameter. If it is small, an anterior V-plasty may be a successful option, which involves making a longitudinal cut in the superior edge of the bile duct, as shown in Video 2. Minor hemorrhage in the bile duct wall may occur during manipulation and can be controlled either by thin stiches or with bipolar energy. The jejunal loop, located 20–40 cm from the PA, is then brought close to the bile duct, and an end-to-side hepaticojejunostomy is performed. The anastomosis begins with a double-layer suture using PDS 5/0, with running sutures for both the anterior and posterior layers. The first suture involves the posterior bile duct and bowel layer, without creating an enterotomy to prevent mucosa extrusion (Video 3).

Next, the bowel is opened using monopolar energy for precision, and the biliary stent or Kehr tube is placed through the anastomosis. The anterior wall is then closed with running sutures (PDS 5/0), and an additional anterior layer can be added for reinforcement.

Several factors can contribute to biliary leakage, the most common being a small or non-dilated bile duct, the absence of inflammation in the bile wall, short bile duct length, tension on the anastomosis, or tearing of the bile duct wall due to sutures. In most cases, these issues are technical, highlighting the importance of standardized techniques performed by experienced surgeons.

Several tips can help reduce the risk of leakage, including the use of biliary plasty, stents, tension-reducing sutures at each corner, interrupted sutures for the anastomosis, and, in some cases, the placement Kehr tube through the biliary anastomosis (Fig. 10.6). The Kehr tube is an interesting alternative for potentially reducing POPF morbidity, as bile decompression may play a role in maintaining pancreatic leaks, and the tube helps divert bile, thus improving PA healing. However, since it is a foreign body in the bile duct, it usually needs to be removed after 6 weeks during open surgery. In minimally invasive surgery, a small biliary leak may occur after the tube is removed due to the absence of inflammatory adhesions associated with the tube. Additionally, there is always a risk of creating a biliary leak during tube removal.

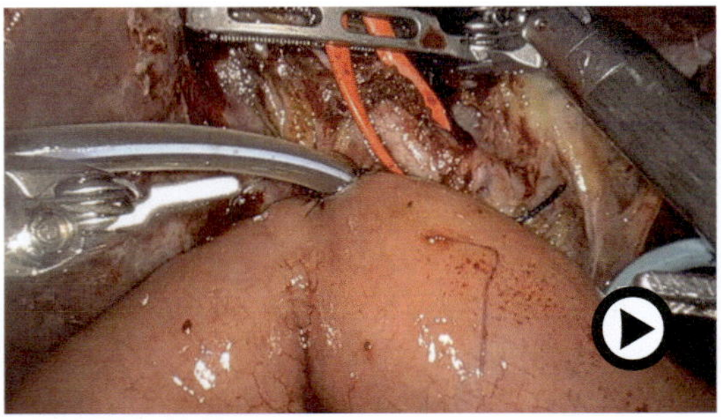

Fig. 10.6 Kehr tube placed in the biliary anastomosis (Gastrojejunal anastomosis (▶ https://doi.org/10.1007/000-het))

10.10 Gastrojejunal Anastomosis

The location of this anastomosis depends on whether the pylorus is preserved. In our case, we do not preserve it. We believe it is beneficial to remove the gastric antrum, where most parietal cells (gastrin producers) are located, as this may help reduce the incidence of marginal ulcers.

The same jejunal loop used for the previous pancreatic and hepatic anastomoses is utilized in an antecolic position, and it must be 30–40 cm away from the biliary anastomosis to prevent bile reflux. This approach is less complicated than the retrocolic one because it follows the previous intestinal loop without needing to locate the Treitz angle. We perform a side-to-side gastrojejunostomy (Video 4). The first step is to open the jejunum and the stomach in parallel lines, after which a stapler (60 mm) is introduced (Fig. 10.7). The entero-gastrostomy is then closed with a barbed 3/0 running suture.

Delayed gastric emptying (DGE) is one of the most common complications after PD, occurring in 10–45% of cases [16, 17]. Multiple non-surgical risk factors are associated with DGE, including patient age, preoperative biliary drainage, soft pancreatic texture, small pancreatic duct size, blood loss, POPF, bile leakage, intra-

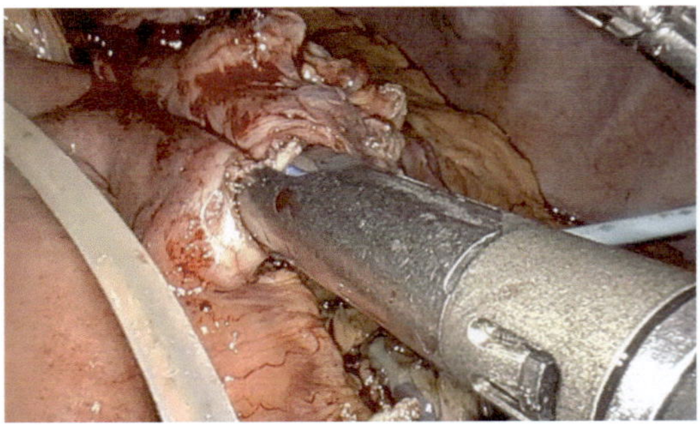

Fig. 10.7 Gastrojejunal anastomosis made by the Stapler

abdominal collections, and intra-abdominal abscesses [17]. On the surgical side, factors such as the gastrojejunostomy technique are significant, with the antecolic approach with a Braun digestive reconstruction being recommended. The relationship between pylorus preservation and DGE is controversial. Another technical tip to prevent DGE is to place the jejunal loop in a dependent position relative to the greater curvature of the stomach [18].

References

1. Ielpo B, Anselmo A, Koh Y, Burdio F, De Blasi V, Sanchez-Velazquez P, et al. Minimally invasive pancreatic anastomosis after pancreaticoduodenectomy: multi-institutional step by step video description of the technique. Updat Surg. 2023;75(1):255–9.
2. Tewari M, Mahendran R, Kiran T, Verma A, Dixit VK, Shukla S, et al. Outcome of 150 consecutive Blumgart's pancreaticojejunostomy after pancreaticoduodenectomy. Indian J Surg Oncol. 2019;10(1):65–71.
3. Hirono S, Kawai M, Okada KI, Miyazawa M, Kitahata Y, Hayami S, et al. Modified Blumgart mattress suture versus conventional interrupted suture in pancreaticojejunostomy during pancreaticoduodenectomy: randomized controlled trial. Ann Surg. 2019;269(2):243–51.
4. Shrikhande SV, Sivasanker M, Vollmer CM, Friess H, Besselink MG, Fingerhut A, et al. Pancreatic anastomosis after pancreatoduodenectomy: a position statement by the international study group of pancreatic surgery (ISGPS). Surgery. 2017;161(5):1221–34.
5. Ielpo B, Vincente E, Quijano Y, Duran H, Diaz E, Fabra I, et al. An organizational model to improve the robotic system among general surgeons. G Chir. 2014;35(1–2):52–5.
6. Ielpo B, Sanchez P, Grande L, Burdio F. Laparoscopic pancreatoduodenectomy: how we have standardized the technique (with video). Updat Surg. 2022;74(4):1479–81.
7. Huscher C, Perri G, Lazzarin G, Marchegiani G, Malleo G, Salvia R, et al. Coronary artery stent for securing high-risk pancreatico-jejunal anastomosis after pancreatoduodenectomy: a pilot series. Ann Surg. 2022;275(4):e665–8.
8. Andrianello S, Marchegiani G, Balduzzi A, Bastin A, Masini G, Esposito A, et al. Pros and pitfalls of externalized trans-anastomotic stent as a mitigation strategy of POPF: a prospective risk-stratified observational series. HPB. 2021;23(7):1046–53.
9. Li Z, Wei A, Xia N, Zheng L, Yang D, Ye J, et al. Blumgart anastomosis reduces the incidence of pancreatic fistula after pancreaticoduodenectomy: a systematic review and meta-analysis. Sci Rep. 2020;10(1):17896.
10. Blumgart LH, Fong Y. Surgery of the liver and biliary tract. 3rd ed. New York: Saunders Co Ltd; 2000.
11. Bassi C, Molinari E, Malleo G, Crippa S, Butturini G, Salvia R, et al. Early versus late drain removal after standard pancreatic resections: results of a prospective randomized trial. Ann Surg. 2010;252(2):207–14.
12. McMillan MT, Malleo G, Bassi C, Butturini G, Salvia R, Roses RE, et al. Drain management after pancreatoduodenectomy: reappraisal of a prospective randomized trial using risk stratification. J Am Coll Surg. 2015;221(4):798–809.
13. Malgras B, Dokmak S, Aussilhou B, Pocard M, Sauvanet A. Management of postoperative pancreatic fistula after pancreaticoduodenectomy. J Visc Surg. 2023;160(1):39–51.
14. Ma S, Li Q, Dai W, Pan F. Pancreaticogastrostomy versus pancreaticojejunostomy. J Surg Res. 2014;192(1):68–75.
15. Tittelbach-Helmrich D, Keck T, Wellner UF. Pankreatogastrostomie: wann und wie? [Pancreaticogastrostomy: when and how?]. Chirurg. 2017;88(1):11–7.
16. Wang TH, Lin AY, Mentor K, O'Grady G, Pandanaboyana S. Delayed gastric emptying and gastric remnant function after pancreaticoduodenectomy: a systematic review of objective assessment modalities. World J Surg. 2023;47(1):236–59.
17. Varghese C, Bhat S, Wang TH, O'Grady G, Pandanaboyana S. Impact of gastric resection and enteric anastomotic configuration on delayed gastric emptying after pancreaticoduodenectomy: a network meta-analysis of randomized trials. BJS Open. 2021;5(3):zrab035.
18. Dai S, Peng Y, Wang G, Yin L, Yan H, Xi C, et al. Risk factors of delayed gastric emptying in patients after pancreaticoduodenectomy: a comprehensive systematic review and meta-analysis. Int J Surg. 2023;109(7):2096–119.

Part III

Special Subjects

11 Complex Robotic Pancreaticoduodenectomy

Ahmad Abou Abbass and Emanuel Shapera

11.1 Preoperative Approach

Patient selection is key in Minimally Invasive Pancreaticoduodenectomy (MIPD), and this remains truer in those with complex anatomy. The patient must have the cardiopulmonary physiology to tolerate pneumoperitoneum for several hours. In those with frailty, age over 50 or a history of prior cardiac disease, risk stratification by a cardiologist is obtained. In those presenting with morbid obesity, any weight loss targeting fat while preserving lean muscle mass is ideal. Nonetheless, preoperative optimization must not delay a timely operation for malignancy unless neoadjuvant therapy is planned.

Imaging is essential, with triple-phase IV-contrasted CT scan of the abdomen and pelvis forming the basis of pre-procedure planning. Endoscopic ultrasonography can confirm the status of vessel involvement, though not every patient requires a biopsy for malignancy when the pretest probability is high. In patients with biliary-oriented diseases requiring MIPD, such as those with prior biliary cyst resection or biliary reconstruction, MRCP is warranted.

In the operating room, a surgical team familiar with robotic MIPD is critical. MIPD should not be performed in hospitals that frequently rotate operative staff for lack of retention, a problem increasingly more common in the post-COVID-19 pandemic era. This includes the scrub technician/nurse, circulator and first assistant, who performs bedside suctioning and retraction via a 12-mm laparoscopic port. Needless to say, the anesthesiologist must be prepared with central line and arterial line to resuscitate the patient should major bleeding occur, though this should be a rarity and will often warrant conversion to open technique.

Emergency sutures are prepared before incision with 4-0 and 5-0 polypropylene on a small half circle and reverse cutting needles, respectively, cut to 4 and 6 inches with a pre-tied knot or clip and pledget applied to the end (Fig. 11.1). This facilitates rapid suture ligation of vascular injuries with one robotic arm without needing a second arm to tie, which can be extremely useful in situations where two arms are being utilized for exposure, suctioning, or pressure.

Robotic port setup (Fig. 11.2) involves three 8-mm and one 12-mm trocars, along with the

Supplementary Information The online version contains supplementary material available at https://doi.org/10.1007/978-3-031-99695-5_11. The videos can be accessed individually by clicking the DOI link in the accompanying figure caption or by scanning this link with the SN More Media App.

A. A. Abbass (✉)
Hepatobiliary Surgery, Mission Hospital, Mission Viejo, CA, USA
e-mail: drahmid@hotmail.com

E. Shapera
Trinity Medical Multispecialty Group, Temecula, CA, USA
e-mail: emanuelshapera@gmail.com

B. Ielpo et al. (eds.), *Minimally Invasive Pancreatoduodenectomy in Cancer*,
https://doi.org/10.1007/978-3-031-99695-5_11

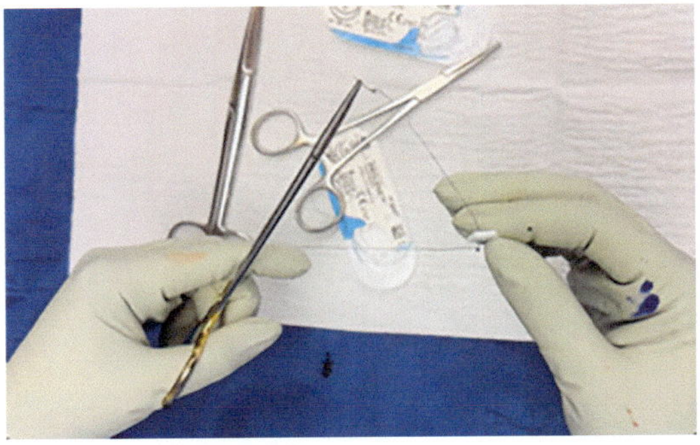

Fig. 11.1 Hemostatic suture

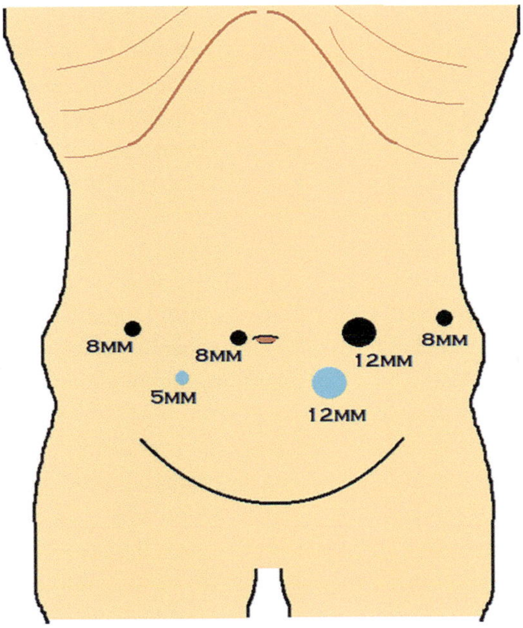

Fig. 11.2 Robotic port setup

aforementioned 12-mm assist port. These are placed roughly in a line corresponding to the umbilicus. The second port holds the 30-degree camera and is placed just to the right of the umbilicus. Patients with morbid obesity and altered skin anatomy from prior operations require some adjustment (Fig. 11.3). Entry is achieved by 5-mm Optiview trocar on a 0-degree laparoscope, which is then converted into either of the above mentioned ports. Pneumoperitoneum is maintained to 15 mm Hg of pressure. High flow or more "conventional" modalities of insufflation can be utilized; though the former may have advantages in creating a more reliable operating space even at

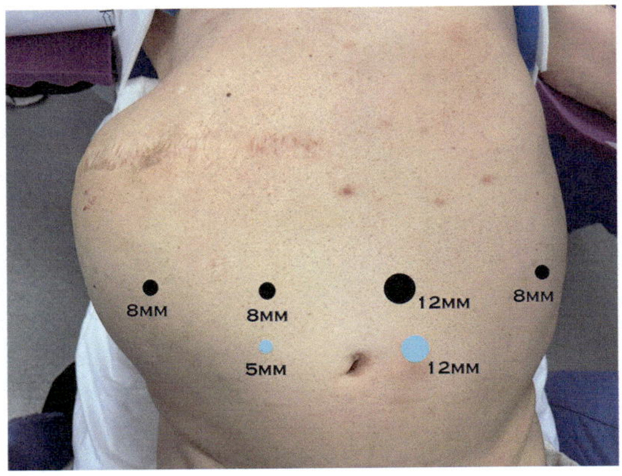

Fig. 11.3 Ports setup with obesity

lower pressures, potentially reducing postoperative pain, they can in certain circumstances increase the risk of air dissecting into nonoperative cavities, creating pneumothorax. Because air and not carbon dioxide is utilized, these can complicate the patient's postoperative course from an already complex MIPD mandating tube thoracostomy. Specimen extraction is completed by Pfannenstiel incision and skin suture closure is reinforced with Dermabond. Surgical drain is utilized routinely with a 19-Fr Blake and secured to the skin with 2–0 nylon suture.

Finally, predetermined criteria should be considered for when to convert to an open approach, and when to abort the operation entirely prior to crossing "points of no-return," such as parenchymal division of the pancreatic neck, ligation of the gastroduodenal artery, or transection of the bowel.

11.2 Patients with Elevated BMI

Given that both diabetes mellitus and morbid obesity—components of the increasingly more prevalent metabolic syndrome—are risk factors for the development of pancreatic cancer, MIPD in patients with an elevated BMI will become an increasingly more frequent operation in the near future (Fig. 11.5) [1]. In these patients, the umbilicus is no longer a reliable landmark, and it may result in ports placed more caudal than desired. Nonetheless, in robotic MIPD, ports placed slightly further away are more useful than ports placed too close, particularly when the robotic

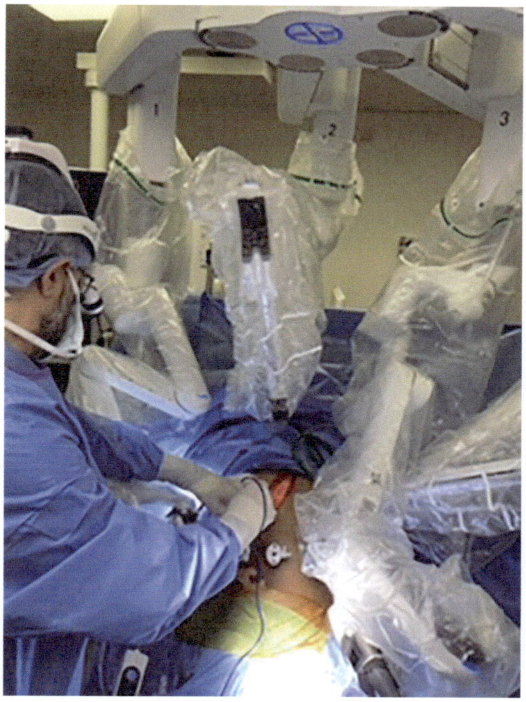

Fig. 11.4 Conversion to an open operation

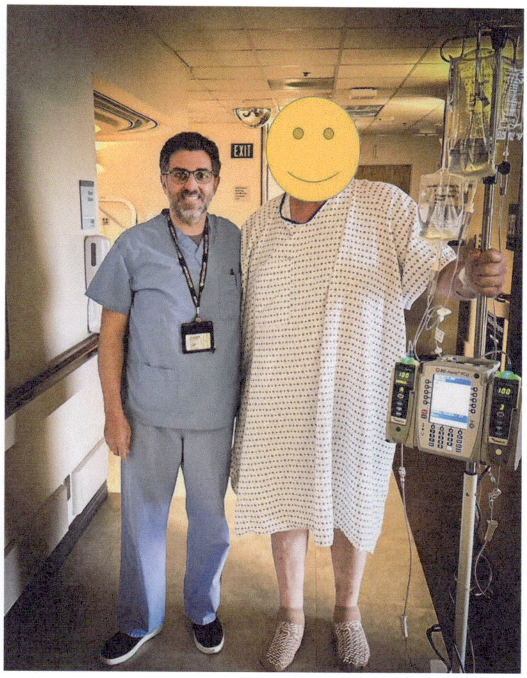

Fig. 11.5 A patient with obesity after MIPD on post operative day one

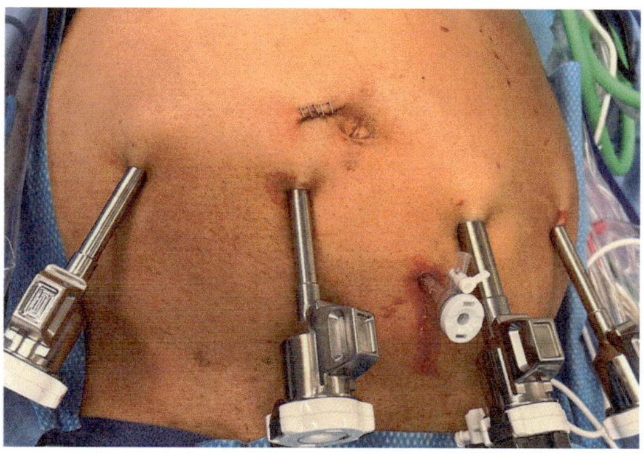

Fig. 11.6 Initial port placement just to the right of the umbilicus was determined early in this operation to be unsatisfactory. It was repositioned lower to accommodate the obese habitus and the skin stapled shut to maintain pnuemoperitoneum

stapler is utilized, which requires significant space. If the initial port placement is disadvantageous, the surgeon must utilize a different port placement to avoid unnecessary frustration in a complex MIPD (Fig. 11.6). An additional one or two small incisions may avoid the technical inferiority and operative frustration that could lead to an unplanned conversion with a large midline incision (Fig. 11.4).

Another cause for additional ports may be to increase bedside assistance and retraction due to the varying presence of visceral fat, though internal hammock suturing of the gallbladder and falciform ligament provide good exposure. Finally, a fatty pancreas increases the risk for postoperative pancreatic leak. In these circumstances, a small plastic 7-Fr tube fashioned as an ad hoc pancreatic stent can be useful. Post-surgery, patients should be educated on this placement so they are not alarmed when it passes in a bowel movement.

11.3 Patients with Complex or Altered Anatomy

The following is a compilation of MIPD performed in patients who have acquired variant or post-procedural altered anatomy (Fig. 11.7). Pertinent points are highlighted that the experienced hepatobiliary surgeon may apply in both complex and more "routine" MIPD.

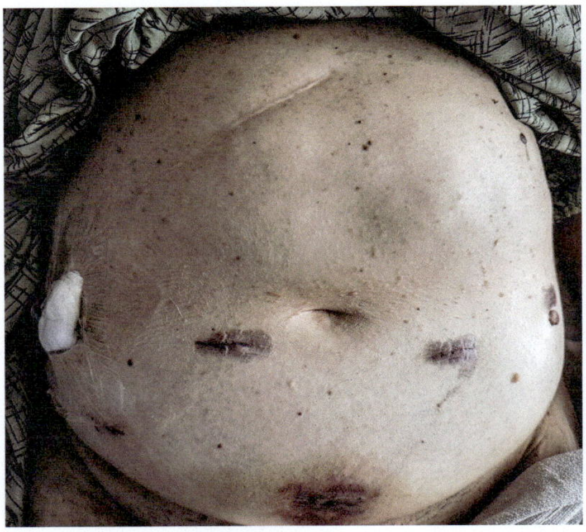

Fig. 11.7 An abdomen with the scar of a prior kocher incision. Despite the scar tissue, a MIPD was successful in this patient

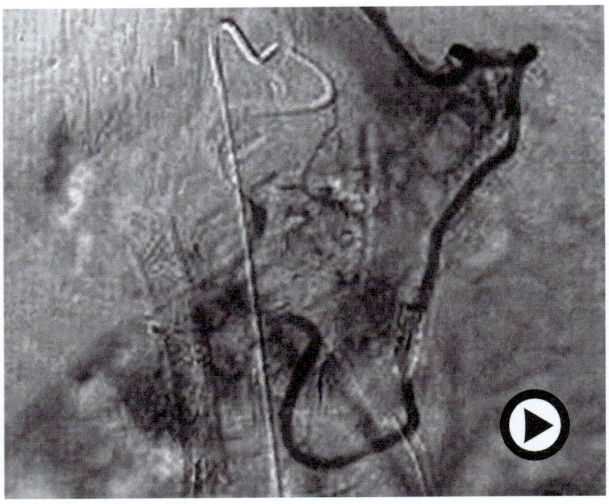

Fig. 11.8 Preoperative angiogram of a patient with a prior esophagectomy in preparation for MIPD (▶ https://doi.org/10.1007/000-hev)

11.3.1 A Patient with a Prior Ivor-Lewis Esophagectomy

Both esophageal and pancreatic cancer are rare diseases, with neither having screening protocols in the western world. Nonetheless, they also share similar risk factors such as tobacco abuse, alcohol abuse, and morbid obesity [2]. In the unfortunate patient who develops pancreatic cancer subsequent to curative resection for esophageal cancer, pancreaticoduodenectomy must be performed with preservation of the gastroduodenal artery (GDA), as it is the sole source of perfusion for the gastric conduit through the right gastroepiploic artery (GEA). In this case (Fig. 11.8), preoperative angiogram confirmed the singular necessity of the right GEA in the perfusion of the gastric conduit.

Because of the gastric pull up, the pancreatic head complex is pulled to the patient's left, mandating a port adjustment to reflect this. Dissection and exposure of the common hepatic artery beneath the gastro-hepatic ligament to identify the GDA is critical. It is preserved in its length up to the take-off of the right GEA. Indocyanine green confirms preservation and perfusion of the gastric conduit (Fig. 11.9). Distal to this, ligation flush to the head of the pancreas permits the MIPD to proceed in a more "routine" fashion (Fig. 11.11). The gastroepiploic vein (GEV) was diminutive and taken without edema of the stom-

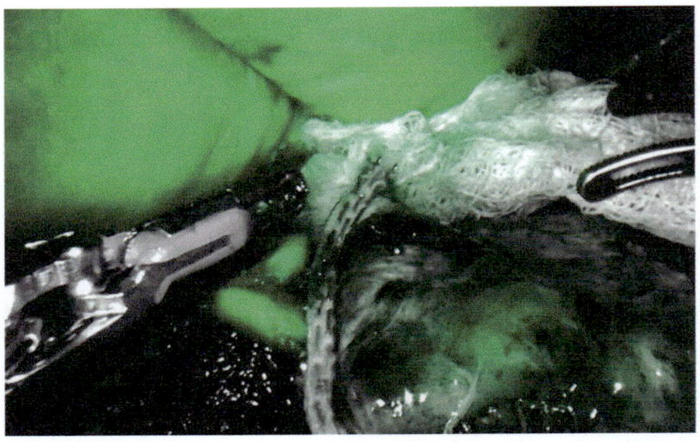

Fig. 11.9 ICG fluorescence confirming perfusion of the gastric conduit

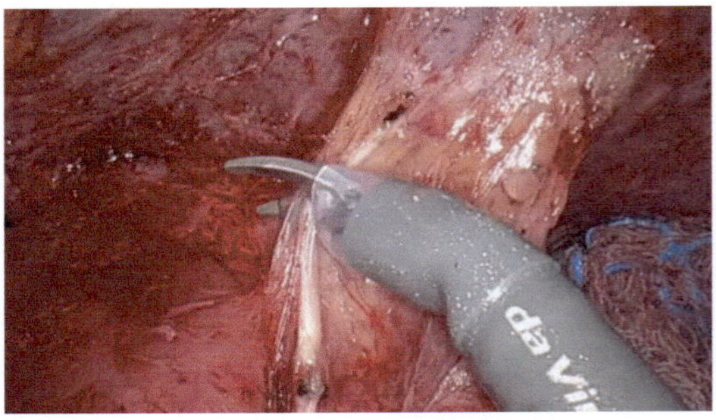

Fig. 11.10 Monopolar scissors utilized to dissect layer by layer adhesions between the liver and duodenum in a patient with a prior Hepatico-duodenostomy

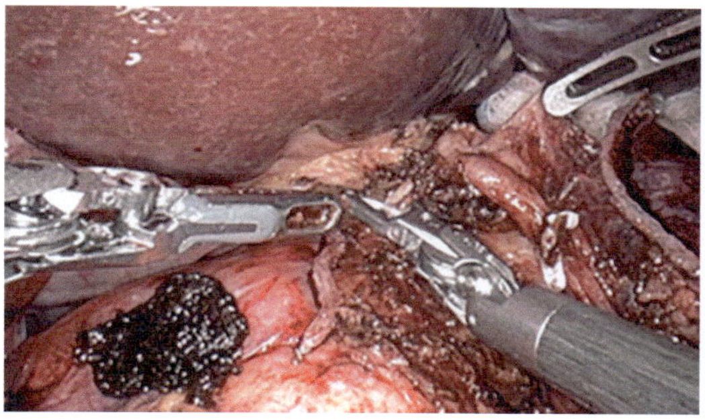

Fig. 11.11 Ligation of the GDA past the R GEA take-off

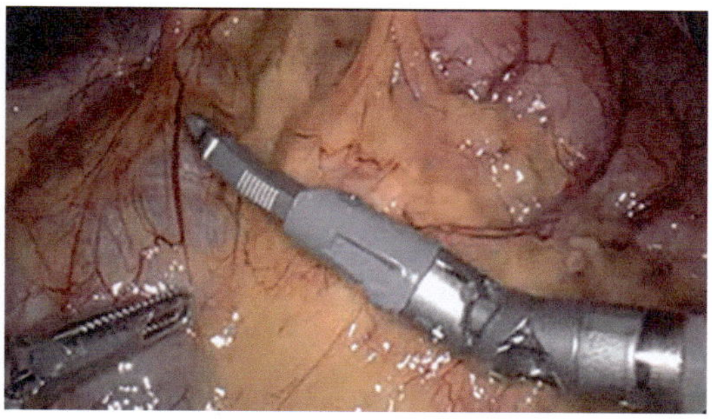

Fig. 11.12 The gallbladder fossa, pylorus and duodenum are adherent in this patient with a prior Hepatico-duodenostomy with remnant common bile duct stump stones

ach. Since a few years occurred between the index esophagectomy and the MIPD, venous collateralization had occurred, permitting accommodation of drainage that the GEV had managed. Intestinal, biliary, and pancreatic reconstruction proceeded as in other cases, and the patient was discharged without issue on postoperative day (POD) 5.

11.3.2 A Patient with a Prior Hepaticoduodenstomy for Choledocal Cyst Resection

A 25-year-old female had undergone choledochal cyst resection with hepaticoduodenostomy reconstruction 15 years prior to presentation. Due to the direct biliary-enteric anastomosis, the patient had recurrent ascending cholangitis and hepatic abscess. In addition, a long remnant common bile duct had via biliary stasis resulted in the formation of primary biliary and pancreatic duct stones with recurrent bouts of acute on chronic pancreatitis. An MIPD promised to resolve the pancreatitis, cholangitic abscesses and prevent the remnant bile duct from degenerating into cholangiocarcinoma. MRCP was sine qua non for this case, confirming the etiology of her presentation. Timing of the operation was critical as the patient had pancreatitis-induced portal vein narrowing which resolved with time prior to the resection.

As shown in the video, intraoperatively, the right colon was adherent to the gallbladder fossa and the duodenum expectedly fused to the hepatic hilum (Fig. 11.12). By mobilizing the right colon as in a "routine" MIPD and tracing the middle colic vein via the gastro-colic trunk, the superior mesenteric vein (SMV) was exposed and carefully separated from the pancreatic neck. A robotic bipolar Maryland grasper was particularly useful in bluntly dissecting the plane and also utilizing focused electrical energy to seal inflammatory attachments. This case highlights the utility of transecting the pancreas as the tunnel is developed, allowing exposure of the anterior surface of the SMV and permitting continued development of the plane cranially toward the PV. The hepatic hilum was tackled following Kocher maneuver and pancreatic neck dissection. Dense adhesions between the liver and duodenum were taken slowly, layer-by-layer, with a combination of monopolar scissors and bipolar sealer device (Fig. 11.10). The first portion of the duodenum was transected, preserving the pylorus, providing additional exposure from the medial aspect to dissect out the hepatico-duodenostomy (Fig. 11.13). Intraoperative ultrasonography, visualization of arterial pulsation, and injection of indocyanine green were critical adjuncts in discriminating between the branches of the common hepatic artery and the biliary anastomosis. Once the latter had been isolated and transected, the expendable branches of the common hepatic artery (right gastric, GDA) were more easily noted, ligated, and the pancreatic neck transected. This was followed by transection of the mesentery, with a more generous

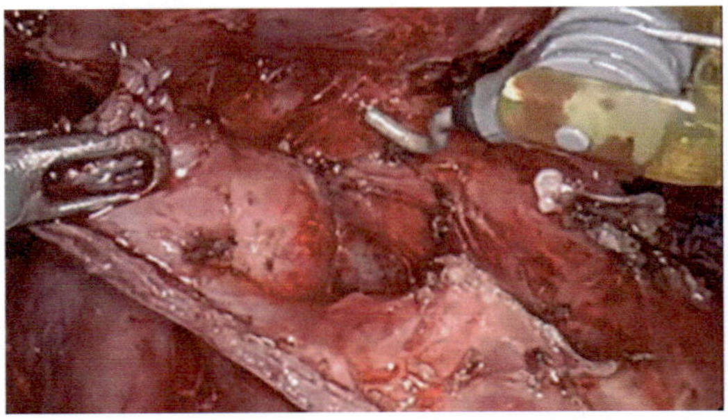

Fig. 11.13 Transection of first portion of Duodenum in a patient with a prior Hepatico-duodenostomy undergoing MIPD for retained distal common bile duct stones in common bile duct stump

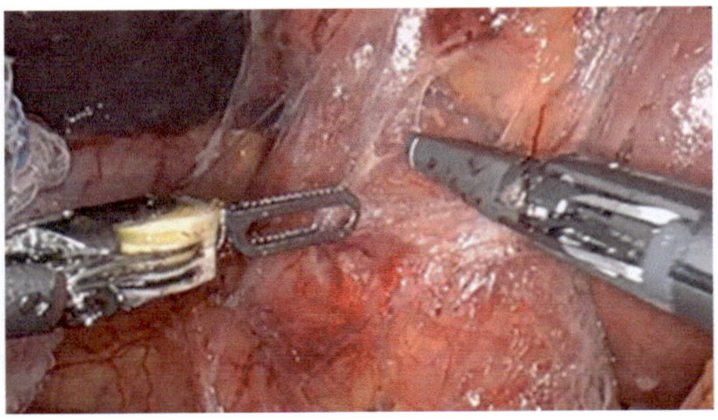

Fig. 11.14 Dissection of duodenum from aorta aneurysm is facilitated here by the AAA pushing the pancreatic head-duodenum complex anteriorly off the retroperitoneum

amount of tissue left on the SMA due to the noncancerous diagnosis. Transection of the ligament of Treitz completed removal of the specimen. Biliary, pancreatic, and intestinal reconstruction proceeded as usual. The patient recovered uneventfully with discharge home on POD 4.

11.3.3 Patient with Abdominal Aortia Aneurysm

Abdominal Aortic Aneurysm (AAA) and pancreatic cancer share many similar risk factors (elderly age, male sex, tobacco abuse, and diabetes mellitus); therefore, the probability of encountering both at the same time is not negligible [3]. The hepatobiliary and vascular surgeon should share the decision-making process, though usually this will favor tackling the pancreatic malignancy as it has a more certain prognosis of death if left untreated. AAA can pose numerous technical problems, such as anatomical distortion or adhesions—especially if a mycotic or inflammatory AAA has occurred. Conversely, as in the case presented by the authors, a degenerative AAA can stretch tissue planes anteriorly that must be entered during a Kocher maneuver, making MIPD slightly easier (Fig. 11.14). Carefully dividing the attachments between the duodenum and the AAA to avoid injury to the latter goes without saying (Fig. 11.15). This patient was discharged following an otherwise uneventful MIPD on postoperative day 4. Strong consideration should be given for endovascular repair of AAA following resection, since these lesions can balloon further should the patient undergo the oncologically necessary adjuvant chemotherapy that pancreatic cancer demands.

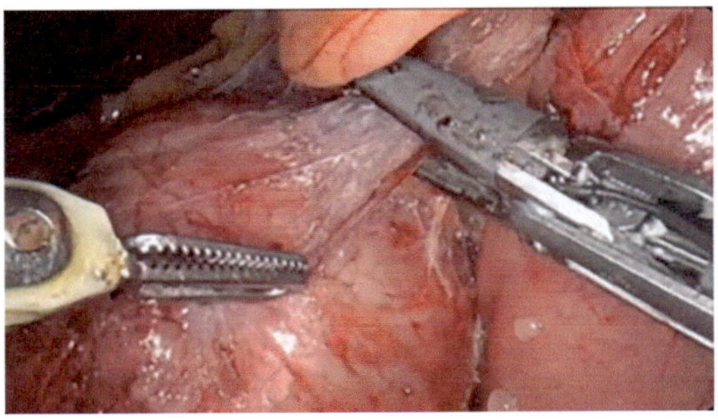

Fig. 11.15 The surgeon's left arm gently pushes the AAA to the patient's right, giving critical retraction for division with bipolar vessel sealing device

11.3.4 Patient with Small Pancreatic Duct

The pancreaticojejunostomy is fashioned by the Blumgart method. Transection of the pancreatic neck is performed with a purposeful 2-mm pancreatic duct stump, facilitating pancreaticojejunostomy anastomosis for easier suturing. In patients with a soft or fatty pancreas, or if preoperative imaging identifies a small (<3 mm) pancreatic duct, this maneuver is critical. The additional use of a 7-French plastic tube of any kind can help manage an expected postoperative pancreatic fistula (POPF). In very select cases where both factors are present, the stent, if fashioned long enough, can be externalized after

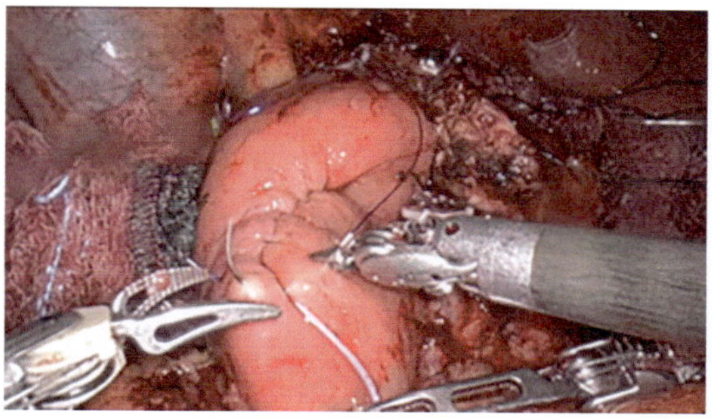

Fig. 11.16 A small caliber long length stent traverses the length of the pancreatico-jejunostomy anastomosis, protrudes through the jejunum at a seperate enterotomy and is then "wetzel'd" in place before being brought through the abdominal wall. Effectively it produces a controlled pancreatic leak, avoiding the complications of an uncontrolled leak

passing through the PJ anastomosis through a separate jejunostomy after it has been Wetzel'd, and then secured to the skin into a drainage bag (Fig. 11.16). Creating a controlled pancreatico-cutaneous fistula in this situation can mitigate the disaster of an unplanned one while permitting feeding, freedom from sepsis, and GDA stump aneurysm. This patient left on POD 8. External stent was removed 4 weeks later.

11.3.5 Patient with Aberrant Hepatic Duct Anatomy

Biliary reconstruction after MIPD often occurs at the level of the cystic duct following cholecystectomy. At this location, an aberrant right posterior hepatic duct is not an uncommon occurrence (Fig. 11.17). Although ducts smaller than 4 mm are often considered "safe" to ligate, intraoperative cholangiogram should be performed prior to any ligation (Fig. 11.18). These abberant ducts may represent the sole drainage of a particular segment or even sector of the liver, usually segments 6 and 7 (right posterior sector). Stent-guided hepaticojejunostomy should be considered in situations where this is the case. A ductoplasty between the main and aberrant hepatic ducts with monofilament suture is sewn so a single anastomosis is performed to minimize stricture risk, while interrupted sutures in place of a continuous one are thrown to prevent

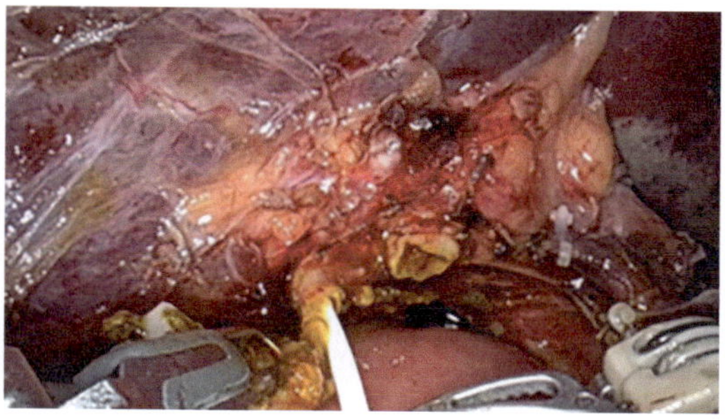

Fig. 11.17 Catheter insertion into a suspected right posterior hepatic duct

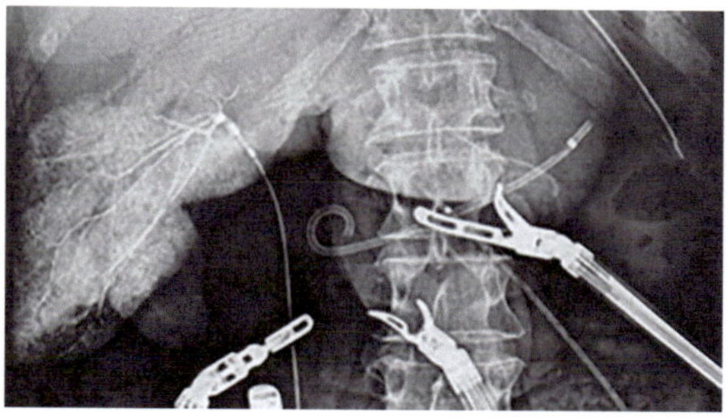

Fig. 11.18 Intraoperative cholangiogram of a confirmed right posterior hepatic duct

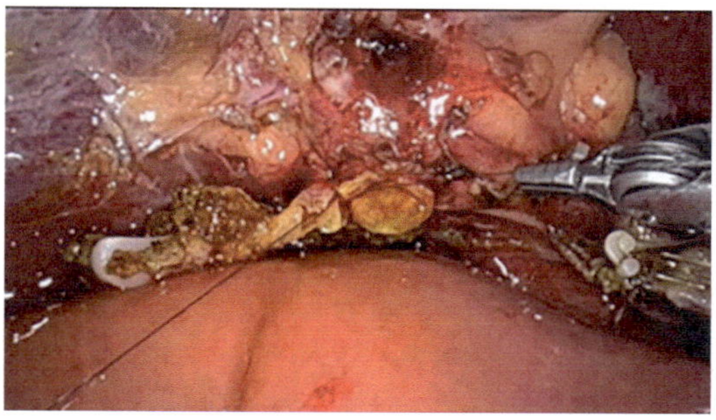

Fig. 11.19 Monofilament suture is utilized to sow the medial walls of the main and right posterior hepatic ducts, permitting a single hepatico-jejunostomy and reducing risk of stricture

narrowing (Fig. 11.19). Following MIPD, this patient left on POD 6.

11.3.6 Portal Venous Reconstruction

Although a separate chapter of this book is dedicated to venous reconstruction during MIPD, a chapter on complex MIPD cannot be complete without a discussion on this important topic.

Invasion of the portal venous (PV)-superior mesenteric venous (SMV) complex does not preclude resection, although neoadjuvant therapy offers an opportunity to test the biology of the disease and shrink the tumor [4]. The latter may permit a less involved patch or even primary vascular closure of a partial venous wall resection in place of a full segmental resection with primary anastomosis or interposition graft.

As shown in the video, dissection of the plane between the pancreatic neck and the PV-SMV complex is completed at the end of the procedure, although depending on where the invasion into the vein occurs, the more proximal and distal parts of the vein complex can be approached. Kocherization of the duodenum, uncinate dissection of the SMA, and division of the ligament of Treitz gives the specimen the mobility necessary to operate around the region between the pancreatic neck and the PV-SMV complex. Lymphadenectomy of the common hepatic artery exposes the proximal PV, permitting distal control (Fig. 11.20). SMV exposure for proximal control is obtained by tracing the gastro-colic branch (Fig. 11.23). Control of the first jejunal and splenic veins are attained as needed depending on how these veins join the PV-SMV complex. This is facilitated by dividing the stomach or proximal duodenum in a pyloric-preserving MIPD, followed by pancreatic neck transection once reconstruction has been determined to be feasible. Debakey bulldog clamps are introduced laparoscopically by

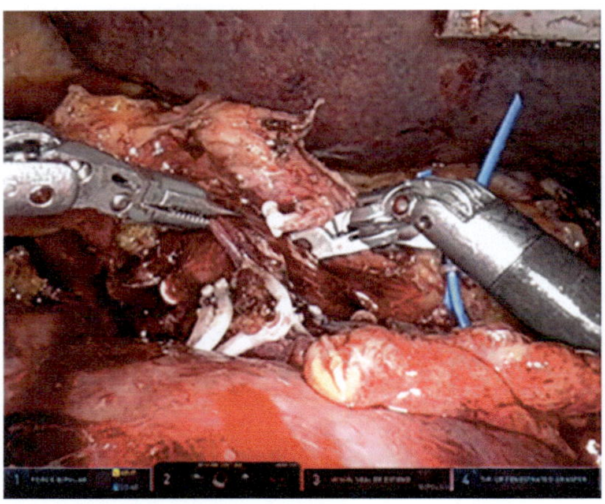

Fig. 11.20 Portal venous exposure at the porta hepatis

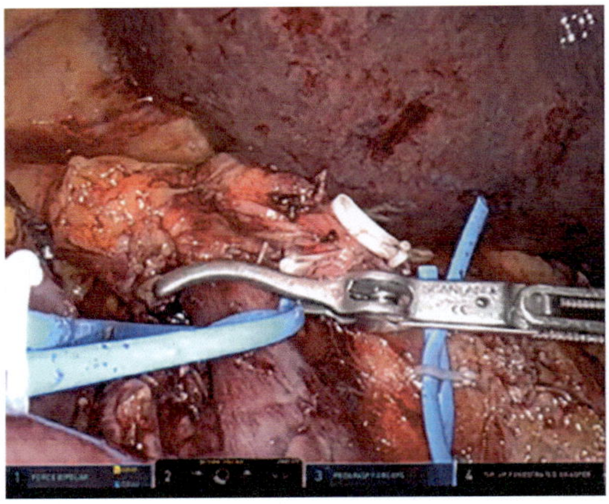

Fig. 11.21 Application of a Debakey bulldog clamp at the moment of vascular resection and reconstruction

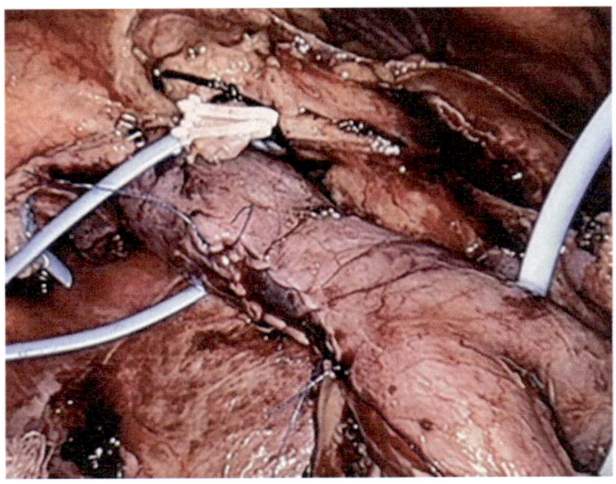

Fig. 11.22 A patch of the falciform ligament has been harvested and utilized as a patch in this reconstruction of the portal vein

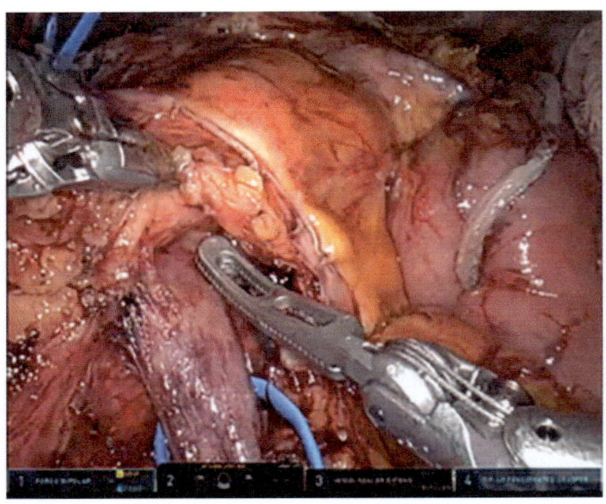

Fig. 11.23 Exposure of the SMV as it enters the neck of the pancreas, with the tunnel between the two structures already partly developed

the bedside assistant and manipulable by the console surgeon (Fig. 11.21).

Pericardial bovine patch is the preferred material for patch reconstruction, although falciform ligament patch has been used with success (Fig. 11.22). Primary closure with partial resection of the venous wall is usually avoided to prevent stenosis which may result in intestinal congestion, thrombosis, and/or eventual ischemia. If full segmental resection is required, a vascular surgeon assists in the case for saphenous vein harvesting and reconstruction. Only once the patch or conduit has been prepared to the planned size are the clamps applied to attain complete inflow and outflow control; then, the vein wall is transected with the pancreatic neck. Consciousness of the time spent clamped must be maintained. Although SMA clamping can increase the clamp time, this is usually not necessary. The choice of suture is Goretex™ 5-0; it is a non-absorbable monofilament with less of the frustrating memory of polypropylene suture. The robotic platform's wristed instruments, 4 working arms, and high-definition three-dimensional optics can make this nerve-wracking procedure not only enjoyable, but an introduction for the developing hepatobiliary surgeon to more complex MIPD. A small dose of daily aspirin in the postoperative period, in addition to enoxaparin for primary prophylaxis against venous thromboembolism, is sufficient to prevent mesenteric vascular events. In the case of the patient with the falciform patch, the patient left the hospital on POD 5.

11.4 Postoperative Management

Enhanced Recovery After Surgery (ERAS) protocols are utilized for all patients. This includes a combination of early ambulation, clear liquid diet, and oral analgesia after the operation. Nasogastric tube decompression is ended 24 h post-procedure. Drains are removed when the patient tolerates a full liquid diet without biochemical evidence of a pancreatico-intestinal leak. Operative time now averages 250 min, estimated blood loss at 200 ml, and the patient is most likely to endure a length of stay of just 4 days.

11.5 Conclusion

Complex MIPD offers a range of challenges, but whose solutions are built upon by performing more routine MIPD. The robotic platform provides the wristed instrumentation to tackle these difficult anatomical problems in a fashion even open approaches may find wanting, and the three-dimensional high-definition optics provides superior visualization. The combination of these two benefits is particularly useful in creating planes around critical vessels and identifying anatomy buried beneath scar tissue, the two most common difficulties in a complex MIPD. These cases can therefore be considered only after establishing proficiency on the robotic learning curve for more routine pancreaticoduodenectomy. The points highlighted in this chapter will allow the developing hepatobiliary surgeon to advance from more basic to more advanced MIPD safely.

11.6 Summary

- Robotic pancreaticoduodenectomy is itself a complex operation and to be tackled with caution
- Once proficiency is established on the learning curve for robotic pancreaticoduodenectomy, more complex cases can be tackled utilizing the basic principles learned from less complex cases
- Utilizing intraoperative ultrasonography, cholangiography, indocyanine green angiography, and appropriate port placement facilitates a safe and effective outcome.

References

1. Boutari C, Mantzoros CS. A 2022 update on the epidemiology of obesity and a call to action: as its twin COVID-19 pandemic appears to be receding, the

obesity and dysmetabolism pandemic continues to rage on. Metabolism. 2022;133:155217. https://doi.org/10.1016/j.metabol.2022.155217.
2. Karczewski J, Begier-Krasińska B, Staszewski R, et al. Obesity and the risk of gastrointestinal cancers. Dig Dis Sci. 2019;64:2740–9. https://doi.org/10.1007/s10620-019-05603-9.
3. Cho H-J, Yoo J-H, Kim M-H, et al. Risk of various cancers in adults with abdominal aortic aneurysms. J Vasc Surg. 2023;77:80–8.e2. https://doi.org/10.1016/j.jvs.2022.03.896.
4. Kim HS, Lee M, Han Y, et al. Role of neoadjuvant treatment in resectable pancreatic cancer according to vessel invasion and increase of CA19-9 levels. J Hepatobiliary Pancreat Sci. 2023;30:924–34. https://doi.org/10.1002/jhbp.1302.

Robotic Pancreaticoduodenectomy with Vascular Resection and Reconstruction

12

Niccolò Napoli, Emanuele F. Kauffmann, Michael Ginesini, and Ugo Boggi

12.1 Introduction

Despite recent advancements, largely due to the development of newer and more effective oncological treatments, radical resection of pancreatic cancer remains the only hope for a cure [1].

Pancreaticoduodenectomy, also known as the Whipple procedure, is used for tumors located in the head of the pancreas and the uncinate process. The goals of radical resection for ductal adenocarcinoma of the pancreas include the complete removal of the primary tumor, in the absence of distant metastasis, along with adequate lymphadenectomy. The likelihood of a margin-negative resection increases with the skeletonization of the lateral, posterior, and anterior borders of the superior mesenteric artery (SMA) down to the adventitia level, as well as the circumferential clearance of the common hepatic artery and the right lateral aspect of the celiac trunk. The radical removal of lymph nodes and extrapancreatic nerve tissue located between the celiac axis, the superior mesenteric artery, and the portal vein is known as the TRIANGLE operation [2].

Data supports an aggressive approach to partial or complete vein excision if tumor infiltration is suspected. Differentiating between tumor infiltration into the vein wall and tumor-related desmoplasia is often impossible [3]. Arterial resection may also be required. While further data is needed, the judicious use of this technique appears reasonable in very select populations [4, 5].

Robotic pancreaticoduodenectomy is gaining popularity due to the enhanced dexterity offered by the robotic system. This procedure can be performed while adhering to the same oncological principles established for the open procedure [6] and, in fact, outcomes are at least non-inferior [7, 8]. However, adding vascular resection to an already complex procedure significantly increases technical complexity, raising concerns about the safety of robotic pancreaticoduodenectomy with vascular resection and reconstruction. Consequently, this type of surgery has only been performed in a few centers [9–16]. Guidelines from Miami [17], Brescia [18], and Pisa [19] also indicate that minimally invasive pancreaticoduodenectomy with vascular resection and reconstruction should be performed only in the most experienced centers and that data should be recorded prospectively.

Supplementary Information The online version contains supplementary material available at https://doi.org/10.1007/978-3-031-99695-5_12. The videos can be accessed individually by clicking the DOI link in the accompanying figure caption or by scanning this link with the SN More Media App.

N. Napoli · E. F. Kauffmann · M. Ginesini · U. Boggi (✉)
Division of General and Transplant Surgery, University of Pisa, Pisa, Italy
e-mail: niccolo.napoli@unipi.it; ekauffmann@hotmail.it; m.ginesini1@gmail.com; u.boggi@med.unipi.it

B. Ielpo et al. (eds.), *Minimally Invasive Pancreatoduodenectomy in Cancer*,
https://doi.org/10.1007/978-3-031-99695-5_12

In this chapter, we present our experience with vascular resections during robotic pancreaticoduodenectomy. Additionally, we provide a summary of the available literature on this topic.

12.2 Indications and Center-Specific Experience

At our center, the indications for robotic pancreaticoduodenectomy have progressively expanded. However, evident vascular involvement, particularly with venous steno-occlusion, remains a contraindication. Despite this, vascular resection and reconstruction are feasible with a robotic approach. The increase in operative times and technical difficulty leads us to prefer the traditional approach in complex vascular scenarios. In a small series of five cases, including three pancreaticoduodenectomies, we demonstrated also the feasibility of arterial resection and reconstruction. However, in these patients, arterial resections were unplanned. Vascular procedures were eventually required because of intraoperative evidence of tumor abutment to peripancreatic arteries or iatrogenic injury during periadventilial dissections. It also important to consider that our center's extensive experience in vascular resection and reconstruction during pancreatectomy (over 1000 procedures) and solid organ transplantation (approximately 2500 kidney and/or pancreas transplants) makes this experience quite unique and possibly not widely duplicable.

Regarding venous resection, we have recently shown it to be feasible with results comparable to the traditional approach, especially in cases involving the superior mesenteric vein/portal vein less than 180°. In a recent article, we used propensity-score matched analysis to compare 35 patients who underwent venous resection during robotic pancreatectomy with 35 patients who underwent venous resection during open pancreatectomy. We found no statistically significant differences in the rates of vascular thrombosis, severe complications, and postoperative mortality. However, we observed lower blood loss and a reduced need for blood transfusions in the robotic group. Despite this, circumferential tumor involvement, particularly of the mesenteric-portal confluence, remains a challenging scenario for robotic surgery and a contraindication from our perspective. The inability to perform extensive intestinal mobilization, unlike in open surgery, makes direct reconstruction of the mesenteric-portal axis (type 3 reconstruction, according to ISGPS) less feasible, often requiring an interposition graft (type 4 reconstruction, according to ISGPS). Similarly, anastomosis of the splenic vein to the renal vein or inferior vena cava, useful in reducing the risk of segmental portal hypertension in cases of splenic vein ligation, is not easily achievable in robotic surgery, unlike in open procedures.

From January 1, 2008, to July 3, 2024, our center performed 1041 pancreaticoduodenectomies, 338 (32.4%) of which were robotic. During these robotic procedures, 44 vascular resections were performed: 40 (90.9%) were venous resections, 2 (4.5%) were arterial resections, and 2 (4.5%) were combined arterial and venous resections. Specifically, superior mesenteric vein/portal vein resection was performed in 58 patients: 4 (6.9%) were type 1, 13 (22.4%) were type 2, 27 (46.6%) were type 3, and 14 (24.1%) were type 4, according to the ISGPS classification.

12.3 Surgical Technique

The patient is prepared similarly to a standard pancreaticoduodenectomy, with the operative field including the inguinal regions and the left side of the neck to allow for possible vascular graft harvesting. Dissection proceeds along the peri-adventitial plane of the major peripancreatic arterial vessels, following the "cold TRIANGLE" technique. The specimen is detached from the retroperitoneum except in the area of suspected vascular involvement. Depending on the type of vascular involvement, the appropriate resection and reconstruction method is chosen. Expanded polytetrafluoroethylene (e-PTFE) is preferred for continuous suturing due to its tensile strength, with thin sutures (6-0, 7-0) being ideal. The superior mesenteric vein and portal vein are clamped with laparoscopic bulldog clamps, and the superior mesenteric artery is also clamped to reduce intestinal venous congestion. After opening the vessel, a flash of sodium heparin is injected via a Bracci's catheter connected to a syringe, operated by the surgeon at the table. Just before completing the suture, the proximal vascular clamp is briefly released. Afterwards, another sodium heparin flash is administered. If the clamping time exceeds 30 min, a bolus of unfractionated heparin is given to achieve an activated clotting time 200 and 250 s. Once the suture is completed, the downstream clamp is removed first to optimize hemostasis with separate polypropylene stitches at a lower pressure. A cellulose sheet (Tabotamp) can be used to promote hemostasis.

12.3.1 Types of Vein Resection and Reconstruction

Type 1 Vein Resection and Reconstruction Used for patients with "small" tumor abutment managed by limited sidewall resection. Vascular repair is performed by primary suture, ensuring the direction is perpendicular to the vein's longitudinal axis to prevent stenosis (Fig. 12.1a/b).

Type 2 Vein Resection and Reconstruction Applied when a larger side wall resection is performed, which would lead to vein stenosis with primary closure. A vascular patch is used for repair. During robotic pancreatoduodenectomy, if possible, type 2 resection is preferred over types 3 or 4 to avoid splenic reimplantation. The patch size must be carefully assessed. Rigid patches, such as a deceased donor arterial graft, are preferred for easier anastomosis, though autologous venous or peritoneal patches may be used (Fig. 12.2a/b/c). Biologic (e.g., bovine pericardium) or synthetic grafts can also be used.

Type 3 Vein Resection and Reconstruction After segmental vein resection, in robotic pancreatoduodenectomy, direct end-to-end anastomosis is challenging due to the anti-Trendelenburg position and consequently the limited intestinal mobility. Therefore, before trespassing the point of no return, a preemptive rescue strategy, like a jump graft, should be considered. The anastomosis is performed using two half-running sutures or a continuous suture by the parachute technique (Fig. 12.3a/b/c). The reverse Trendelenburg position can be adjusted, and the mesentery gently pushed closer to the liver using the fourth arm to facilitate the direct anastomosis.

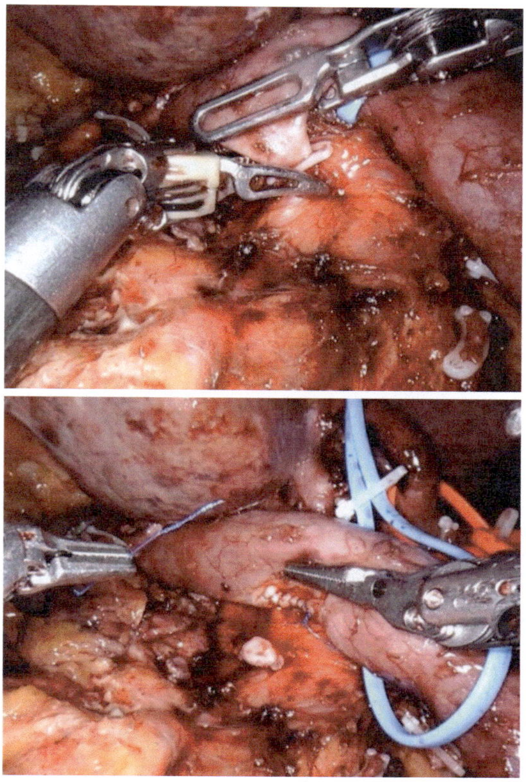

Fig. 12.1 Type 1 vein resection and reconstruction

Type 4 Vein Resection and Reconstruction When direct anastomosis is not feasible, a jump graft is used between vein stumps. We prefer the left internal jugular vein as a graft (Fig. 12.4a/b/c). If no autologous graft is available and the procedure is planned, a deceased donor graft can be used. If the resection involves the superior mesenteric vein, the first anastomosis allows some portal perfusion through the splenic vein (video 1). The distal anastomosis is performed under complete portal cross-clamping. The jump graft's length should be calibrated to avoid kinking when the reverse Trendelenburg position is removed.

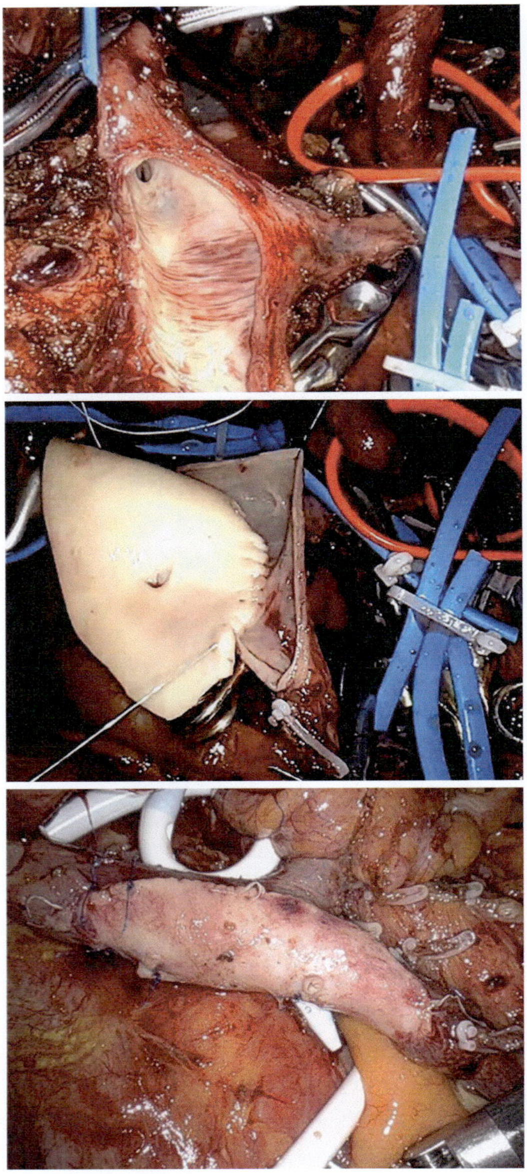

Fig. 12.2 Type 2 vein resection and reconstruction

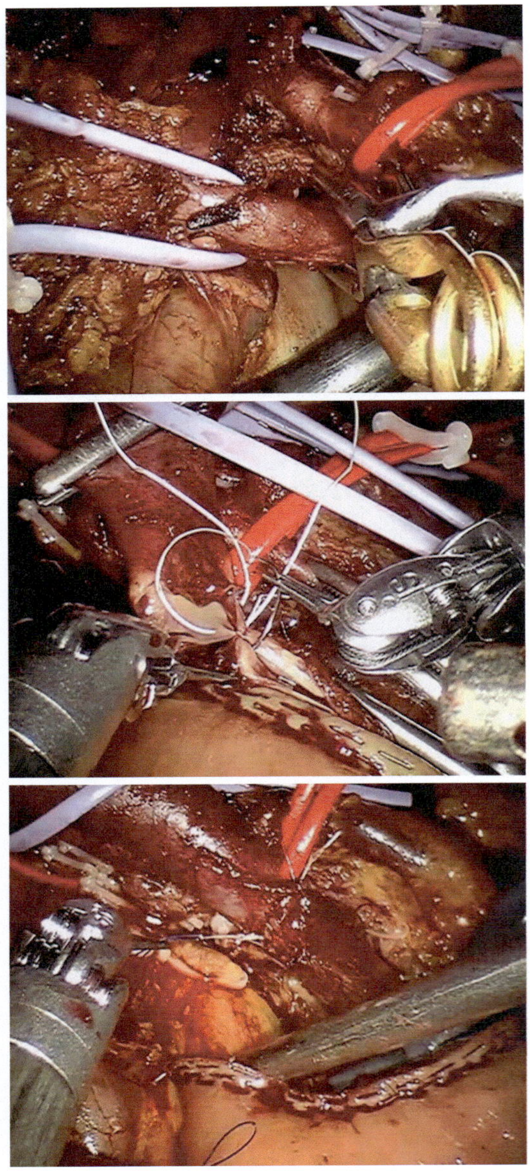

Fig. 12.3 Type 3 vein resection and reconstruction

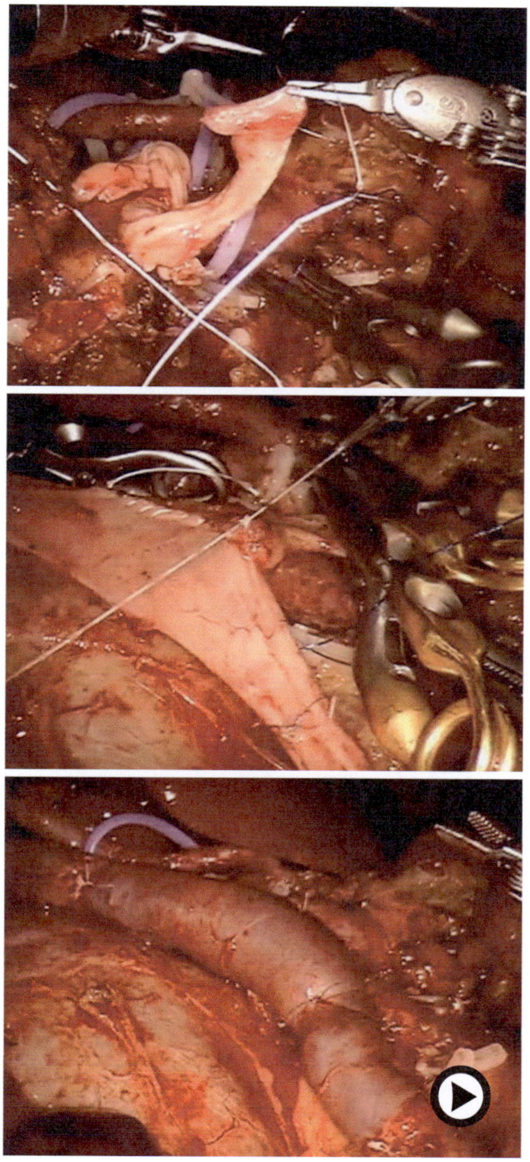

Fig. 12.4 Type 4 vein resection and reconstruction (▶ https://doi.org/10.1007/000-hew)

12.4 Arterial Repair of Resection

Arterial injuries during pancreatoduodenectomy require careful repair. The lack of tactile feedback in robotic surgery may increase iatrogenic vascular injuries. Careful bleeding control should be prioritized to avoid further injury. Arterial repair can be performed using the same techniques as planned resections.

Most arterial resections involve a vascular segment, and reconstruction is typically achieved by end-to-end anastomosis or interposing a graft. Synthetic grafts carry a higher thrombosis risk and necessitate chronic antiplatelet prophylaxis. The greater saphenous vein is a common interposition graft, with alternatives including internal iliac or superficial femoral arteries and deceased donor grafts. Small-caliber arteries may require interrupted sutures, but in general running sutures are preferred, leaving a shorter growth factor.

Intraoperative sodium heparin is usually administered for arterial reconstruction, followed by strict postoperative follow-up, including Doppler ultrasound examinations and laboratory tests (AST, ALT, and LDH). Doppler ultrasound is performed on the first and third postoperative days or as needed based on clinical conditions or lab results. Laboratory tests should be obtained every 12 h for the first five postoperative days, with lactate levels monitored especially during the initial hours post-surgery.

12.4.1 Results

Recently, our team published a study detailing 36 cases of robotic pancreatoduodenectomy with vein resection. In one instance (2.8%), conversion to open surgery was required due to retroperitoneal oozing, which proved difficult to manage using a minimally invasive approach. This patient had previously undergone a bone marrow transplant. The 90-day mortality rate in our series was 8.3%, with all deaths resulting from hemorrhagic complications. Additionally, one patient (2.8%) developed partial vein thrombosis, which was successfully treated with heparin therapy.

In 2011, Giulianotti et al. reported the first series of five patients undergoing pancreatectomy with vascular resection, including two cases of robotic pancreatoduodenectomy.

In 2019, the Pittsburgh group published their experience with 50 robotic pancreatoduodenectomies involving venous resection, 54% of which were classified as type 1 resections. Severe complications were observed in 14 patients (28%), with a 90-day mortality rate of 8%. Conversion to open surgery was necessary in five cases (10%): once due to bleeding and four times due to an inability to proceed with the robotic approach.

In 2022, Marino et al. reported on 10 robotic pancreatoduodenectomies involving venous resection (8 planned and 2 unplanned vascular resections) and compared the outcomes of this group with a matched cohort undergoing standard robotic pancreatoduodenectomy. In the vein resection group, one procedure required conversion to open surgery (10%), two patients needed repeat surgery (20%), and one patient died within 90 days (10%). Compared to the standard procedure, robotic pancreatoduodenectomy with vein resection was associated with longer operative times but resulted in lower blood loss, and had similar morbidity rates, with a lower incidence of severe complications, and comparable mortality. Also in 2022, a group from Shanghai published a series of 14 robotic pancreatoduodenectomies with vein resection, reporting a 90-day mortality rate of 7.1%. The study also found a 14% conversion rate to open surgery and a 7% thrombosis rate. Additionally, a study by Shyr et al., examining 11 cases of robotic pancreatoduodenectomy, noted that conversion to open surgery was required in over one-third of patients (36.4%) due to challenges in robotic vascular reconstruction.

It is important to highlight that recent difficulty scores for minimally invasive pancreatoduodenectomy and robotic pancreatoduodenectomy indicate that the anticipated need for vein resection significantly increases the risk of postoperative complications, classifying the procedure as complex. Therefore, this surgery should be performed exclusively in highly experienced centers and by the most proficient surgeons.

12.4.2 Conclusions

Vascular resections and reconstructions during robotic pancreatoduodenectomy are feasible when performed by highly experienced surgeons in high-volume centers. Extensive experience with open pancreatoduodenectomy, including vein resection, is crucial to overcoming the additional challenges posed by the minimally invasive technique. These procedures require meticulous planning and should only be attempted once the surgical team has gained proficiency with standard robotic pancreatoduodenectomy.

Conflicts of Interest and Source of Funding The authors have no conflict of interest to disclose. This study received no funds.

References

1. Mizrahi JD, Surana R, Valle JW, Shroff RT. Pancreatic cancer. Lancet. 2020;395(10242):2008–20. https://doi.org/10.1016/S0140-6736(20)30974-0.
2. Schneider M, Strobel O, Hackert T, Büchler MW. Pancreatic resection for cancer-the Heidelberg technique. Langenbeck's Arch Surg. 2019;404(8):1017–22. https://doi.org/10.1007/s00423-019-01839-1.
3. Boggi U, Kauffmann EF, Napoli N, et al. REDISCOVER guidelines for borderline-resectable and locally advanced pancreatic cancer: management algorithm, unanswered questions, and future perspectives. Updates Surg. Published online April 29, 2024. https://doi.org/10.1007/s13304-024-01860-0.
4. NCCN Clinical Practice Guidelines in Oncology (NCCN Guidelines®) for Guideline Name V.2.2024. © National Comprehensive Cancer Network, Inc. 2024. All rights reserved. Accessed [June 13rd, 2024]. To view the most recent and complete version of the guideline, go online to NCCN.org.
5. Napoli N, Kauffmann E, Cacace C, et al. Factors predicting survival in patients with locally advanced pancreatic cancer undergoing pancreatectomy with arterial resection. Updat Surg. 2021;73(1):233–49. https://doi.org/10.1007/s13304-020-00883-7.
6. Kauffmann EF, Napoli N, Ginesini M, et al. Feasibility of "cold" triangle robotic pancreatoduodenectomy. Surg Endosc. 2022;36(12):9424–34. https://doi.org/10.1007/s00464-022-09411-7.
7. Klotz R, Mihaljevic AL, Kulu Y, et al. Robotic versus open partial pancreatoduodenectomy (EUROPA): a randomised controlled stage 2b trial. Lancet Reg Health Eur. 2024;39:100864. Published 2024 Feb 22. https://doi.org/10.1016/j.lanepe.2024.100864.
8. Liu Q, Li M, Gao Y, et al. Effect of robotic versus open pancreaticoduodenectomy on postoperative length of hospital stay and complications for pancreatic head or periampullary tumours: a multicentre, open-label randomised controlled trial. Lancet Gastroenterol Hepatol. 2024;9(5):428–37. https://doi.org/10.1016/S2468-1253(24)00005-0.
9. Jin J, Yin SM, Weng Y, et al. Robotic versus open pancreaticoduodenectomy with vascular resec-

tion for pancreatic ductal adenocarcinoma: surgical and oncological outcomes from pilot experience. Langenbeck's Arch Surg. 2022;407(4):1489–97. https://doi.org/10.1007/s00423-021-02364-w.
10. Shyr BU, Chen SC, Shyr YM, Wang SE. Surgical, survival, and oncological outcomes after vascular resection in robotic and open pancreaticoduodenectomy. Surg Endosc. 2020;34(1):377–83. https://doi.org/10.1007/s00464-019-06779-x.
11. Marino MV, Giovinazzo F, Podda M, et al. Robotic-assisted pancreaticoduodenectomy with vascular resection. Description of the surgical technique and analysis of early outcomes. Surg Oncol. 2020;35:344–50. https://doi.org/10.1016/j.suronc.2020.08.025.
12. Beane JD, Zenati M, Hamad A, Hogg ME, Zeh HJ 3rd, Zureikat AH. Robotic pancreatoduodenectomy with vascular resection: outcomes and learning curve. Surgery. 2019;166(1):8–14. https://doi.org/10.1016/j.surg.2019.01.037.
13. Giulianotti PC, Addeo P, Buchs NC, Ayloo SM, Bianco FM. Robotic extended pancreatectomy with vascular resection for locally advanced pancreatic tumors. Pancreas. 2011;40(8):1264–70. https://doi.org/10.1097/MPA.0b013e318220e3a4.
14. Napoli N, Kauffmann EF, Ginesini M, et al. Robotic versus open Pancreatoduodenectomy with vein resection and reconstruction: a propensity score-matched analysis. Ann Surg Open. 2024;5(2):e409. Published 2024 Mar 26. https://doi.org/10.1097/AS9.0000000000000409.
15. Kauffmann EF, Napoli N, Cacace C, et al. Resection or repair of large peripancreatic arteries during robotic pancreatectomy. Updat Surg. 2020;72(1):145–53. https://doi.org/10.1007/s13304-020-00715-8.
16. Machado MAC, Mattos BH, Lobo Filho MM, Makdissi FF. Robotic resection and reconstruction of the superior mesenteric vein without graft during Pancreatoduodenectomy (with video). J Gastrointest Surg. 2021;25(11):3010–2. https://doi.org/10.1007/s11605-021-05043-9.
17. Asbun HJ, Moekotte AL, Vissers FL, et al. The Miami international evidence-based guidelines on minimally invasive pancreas resection. Ann Surg. 2020;271(1):1–14. https://doi.org/10.1097/SLA.0000000000003590.
18. Abu Hilal M, van Ramshorst TME, Boggi U, et al. The Brescia internationally validated European guidelines on minimally invasive pancreatic surgery (EGUMIPS). Ann Surg. 2024;279(1):45–57. https://doi.org/10.1097/SLA.0000000000006006.
19. Boggi U, Kauffmann E, Napoli N, et al. REDISCOVER international guidelines on the peri-operative Care of Surgical Patients with Borderline-resectable and Locally Advanced Pancreatic Cancer. Ann Surg. 2024;280(1):56–65. https://doi.org/10.1097/SLA.0000000000006248.

13 Barbed Sutures for Pancreato Jejunum Anastomosis

Luca Morelli, Annalisa Comandatore, Gregorio Di Franco, Simone Guadagni, and Niccolò Furbetta

13.1 Introduction

Pancreatoduodenectomy (PD) is a complex surgical procedure that is now typically performed following standardized approaches. The resective phase of the surgery largely mirrors the original technique outlined by Whipple [1], albeit with various modifications noted in diverse case studies. On the other hand, the reconstructive phase, especially concerning the handling of the pancreatic stump, continues to lack consistent standardization [2–4].

Thus far, there is no unanimous agreement on the most effective method for performing this anastomosis, widely regarded as the most challenging aspect. Various techniques for minimally invasive pancreato-jejunostomy (PJ) have been suggested [5–8].

The use of barbed sutures has been shown to be safe and time-saving in general surgery and urology [9–12]. However, until now, their application has been documented only in a few cases of minimally invasive pancreatic surgery. While some publications have discussed the use of barbed sutures in laparoscopic and robotic lateral PJ for chronic pancreatitis [13, 14], only three have mentioned their use in laparoscopic PJ after PD [7, 8, 15], and one in robotic PJ after PD [16]. Furthermore, its application has not been included in recent systematic reviews of PJ techniques [17–19].

The laparoscopic use of barbed sutures in performing PJ has been described passing through the pancreatic parenchyma [15] or in performing a single-layered running suture [7, 8]. The reported advantages are primarily related to the fact that simply pulling the suture through the tissue creates an appropriate amount of coiling tension to avoid excessive laxity or tension on the suture line. This allows visualization of the required tension and maintains the desired tension without cracking or traumatizing the pancreas. Additionally, advantages include reduced operating times with outcomes similar to those obtained in open surgery.

Robotic-assisted surgery (RAS) is viewed as a progression from traditional laparoscopy, offering solutions to some of the inherent limitations

Supplementary Information The online version contains supplementary material available at https://doi.org/10.1007/978-3-031-99695-5_13. The videos can be accessed individually by clicking the DOI link in the accompanying figure caption or by scanning this link with the SN More Media App.

L. Morelli (✉) · A. Comandatore · G. Di Franco · S. Guadagni · N. Furbetta
General Surgery Unit, Department of Surgery, Translational Research and New Technologies in Medicine, University of Pisa, Pisa, Italy
e-mail: luca.morelli@unipi.it; a.comandatore@libero.it; gregorio.difranco@med.unipi.it; simone.guadagni@med.unipi.it; n.furbetta@hotmail.it

B. Ielpo et al. (eds.), *Minimally Invasive Pancreatoduodenectomy in Cancer*,
https://doi.org/10.1007/978-3-031-99695-5_13

of manual laparoscopy. The benefits offered by RAS include the provision of seven degrees of freedom for instruments, stable and immersive stereoscopic high-definition imaging of the operating field, restoration of eye-hand coordination, and improved surgical dexterity. These advantages have contributed to a steadily growing adoption of robotic pancreatic surgery.

However, although the enabling features of RAS technology have facilitated the uptake of minimally invasive approaches, even in pancreatic surgery, the lack of haptic feedback is a significant drawback. This absence of tactile feedback can lead to issues such as excessive tension during suturing, iatrogenic tissue tearing, or suture rupture [20]. Visual feedback may partially address this challenge, particularly for experienced surgeons [21], but it remains a limitation of current robotic technologies.

The challenges posed by the lack of tactile feedback in pancreatic surgery are particularly pronounced, as tight knots on the pancreatic parenchyma can result in pancreas tears, potentially leading to postoperative leaks and the development of postoperative pancreatic fistula (POPF). To mitigate this issue, the use of barbed sutures can help maintain the necessary suture tension after each pass, thus enhancing the safety of RAS pancreatic procedures. The progressive tightening of running sutures through the jejunal passages ensures consistent optimal tension, reducing the risks of parenchymal and capsule lacerations.

13.2 Barbed Sutures

A barbed suture is a particular type of monofilament suture whose main characteristic is to have anchors protruding outward, allowing the sutures to slide in only one direction and therefore, once passed through the tissue, to maintain the tension applied to the suture. Barbed sutures are available in various calibers and with anchors of various shapes, for example formed within the core of the device, in a spiral pattern. The advantages of their use are mainly related to the ease with which tension can be evenly distributed along the entire suture, ensuring better long-term holding, and the lack of necessity to tie knots, which in some way improves the overall workflow of the procedure. In the execution of PJ, it is advisable to use 3/0 absorbable sutures, with anchors formed within the core of the device and slow absorption time (e.g., polydioxanone—PDS).

13.3 Technical Description

In detail, as shown in the video, we describe a technique characterized by the use of barbed sutures for all layers of the anastomosis, useful in robotic surgery for performing PJ [16], and applicable to laparoscopic surgery as well. In this section, we report not only the technique itself but also the necessary precautions in its preparation and tips to achieve the best results. The anastomosis consists of a double layer of monofilament, absorbable, running barbed suture, with stenting of the small jejunal enterotomy and the pancreatic duct. The external layer is fashioned to partial invaginate the pancreatic stump, while the internal one is created to be waterproof on the pancreatic edge of the cut surface. The main steps of the procedure are outlined below:

- *Transection of the Pancreas and Preparation of the Jejunal Limb*

The pancreas is transected vertically using monopolar scissors, ensuring careful hemostasis with the help of bipolar Maryland forceps. The pancreatic stump is freed to a distance of approximately 1–2 cm from the splenic artery and vein (Fig. 13.1). This limited mobilization prevents devascularization of the pancreatic stump, leaving just enough space on the posterior surface for the intended invagination.

The segment of the jejunum with the largest diameter is obtained by transecting it just distal to the Treitz ligament, approaching from the right side (Fig. 13.2). This wider segment of the jejunum facilitates an easier termino-lateral invagination of the pancreatic stump. This is a crucial aspect for the success of the invagination technique, enabling the jejunum to wrap around the pancreatic stump and fold over it. While the extent of invagination may vary based on indi-

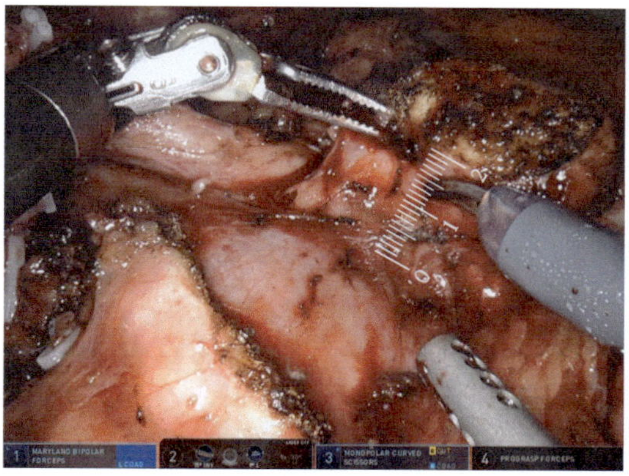

Fig. 13.1 Transection and preparation of the pancreatic stump

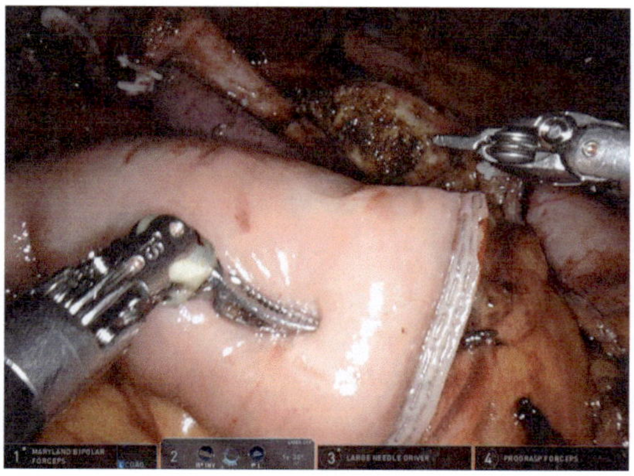

Fig. 13.2 Preparation of the jejunal limb

vidual jejunum size differences, it typically proves sufficient to achieve the desired outcome.

The initial step involves determining the optimal position for invaginating the jejunal limb, positioning it in front of the freed 1–2 cm pancreatic stump.

– *First Posterior (Outer) Layer*

As shown in the video, the anastomosis begins with a monofilament absorbable running barbed suture, initiating at the postero-inferior surface of the pancreas. The posterior surface of the pancreas is sutured to the seromuscular layer of the jejunum about 10 mm from the transection of the pancreas, the sutures are placed transversally through the pancreas and jejunum. The running suture is incrementally tightened following each pass through the jejunum (Fig. 13.3).

– *Second Posterior (Inner) Layer*

Another posterior layer, also using barbed suture, is positioned between the posterior transected surface of the pancreas (capsule and parenchyma) and the seromuscular layer of the jejunum slightly above the prior suture. The suture on the posterior wall is gradually tightened, with the barbed suture ensuring consistent tension across each suture bite (Fig. 13.4).

– *Enterotomy and Stent Positioning*

Upon finishing the posterior layer, monopolar scissors are employed to create a small enterotomy in the jejunum matching the size of the pancreatic duct, ensuring precise alignment opposite the pancreatic duct. A cut ureteral stent (typically 5 French) is then inserted, with the straight end in the Wirsung duct and the pigtail end in the jejunal lumen (Fig. 13.5). The stent can be secured to the anastomosis with a stitch (e.g., PDS) to prevent early dislocation.

The absence of suturing the Wirsung duct to the jejunum, stenting it instead, characterizes this approach. This method combines the benefits of duct-to-mucosa and invagination techniques. Unlike the stent in the duct-to-mucosa technique, the stent in this technique functions to align the Wirsung duct with the small incision in the jejunal wall. While RAS generally simplifies duct-to-mucosa anastomosis over open surgery, a known limitation of duct-to-mucosa is the challenge posed by small diameter pancreatic ducts, increasing the risk of obstruction or fistula formation. This technique circumvents such issues by avoiding a traditional Wirsung-jejunostomy.

Concerns may arise regarding stent dislocation or delayed retention. Despite several studies not reporting specific clinical issues following PJ [18, 22], we have yet to encounter any stent-related clinically significant complications, suggesting minimal impact on clinical outcomes.

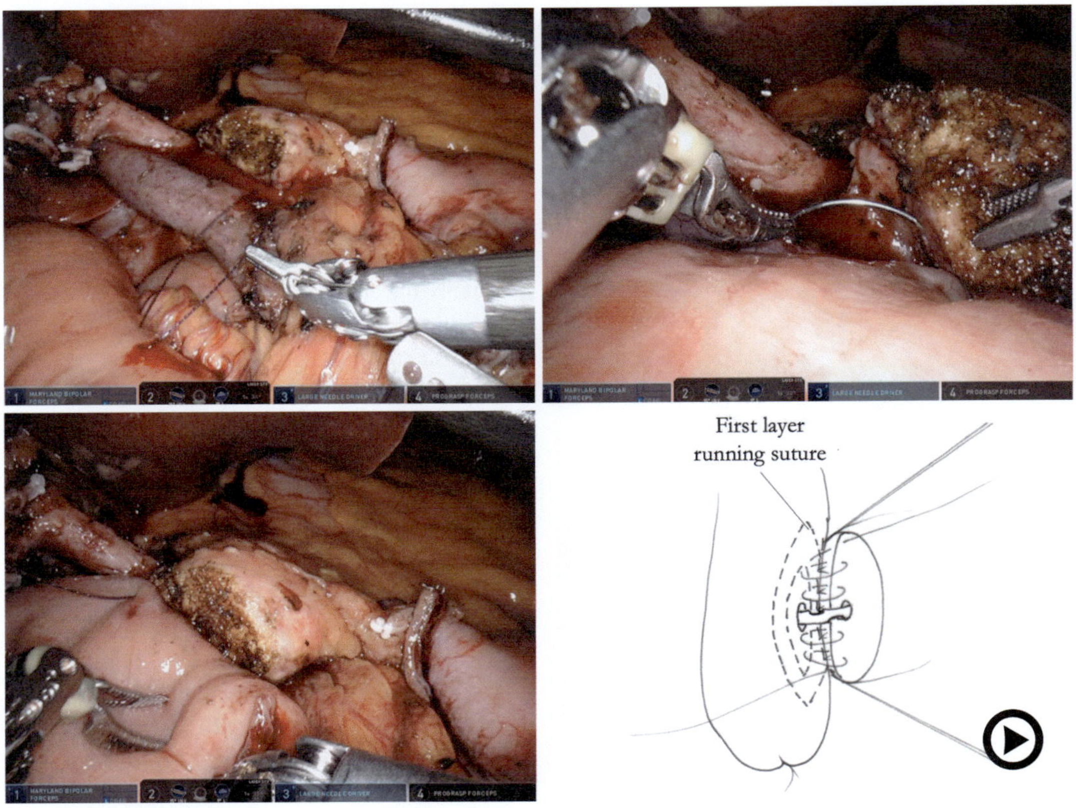

Fig. 13.3 First posterior (outer) layer. Illustration (Barbed sutures for pancreato jejunum anastomosis (▶ https://doi.org/10.1007/000-hex)). (Courtesy of Giulio Di Candio)

Nonetheless, further evaluation on larger cohorts with long-term monitoring is necessary to draw definitive conclusions on this specific aspect.

– *First Anterior (Inner) Layer*

Subsequently, the inner anterior layer is created with a continuous running suture connecting the anterior pancreatic transected surface (capsule and parenchyma) to the anterior seromuscular layer of the jejunum. The suture is gradually tightened after each pass through the jejunum. At the halfway mark, it is possible to start a new running suture from the upper apex of the anastomosis. This approach is necessary as the corners are the most critical points, and continuous tightening of the suture would obstruct visibility of the upper corner. The elliptical line of the inner layer is completed in this manner (Fig. 13.6).

– *Second Anterior (Outer) Layer*

Finally, the anastomosis is completed with the external anterior invaginating layer, using the last row of a running barbed suture. Each stitch begins with the needle entering the anterior pancreas (capsule and parenchyma) approximately 10 mm from the anterior transected surface. The needle should exit the pancreas 5 mm away from the initial entry point into the organ, and the suture is then passed through the jejunum. This technique allows the jejunum to roll over onto the pancreas as the sutures are adequately tensioned and tightened. These sutures are spaced approximately 3–5 mm apart to ensure that they overlap the anterior seromuscular layer of the jejunum over the pancreas (Fig. 13.7).

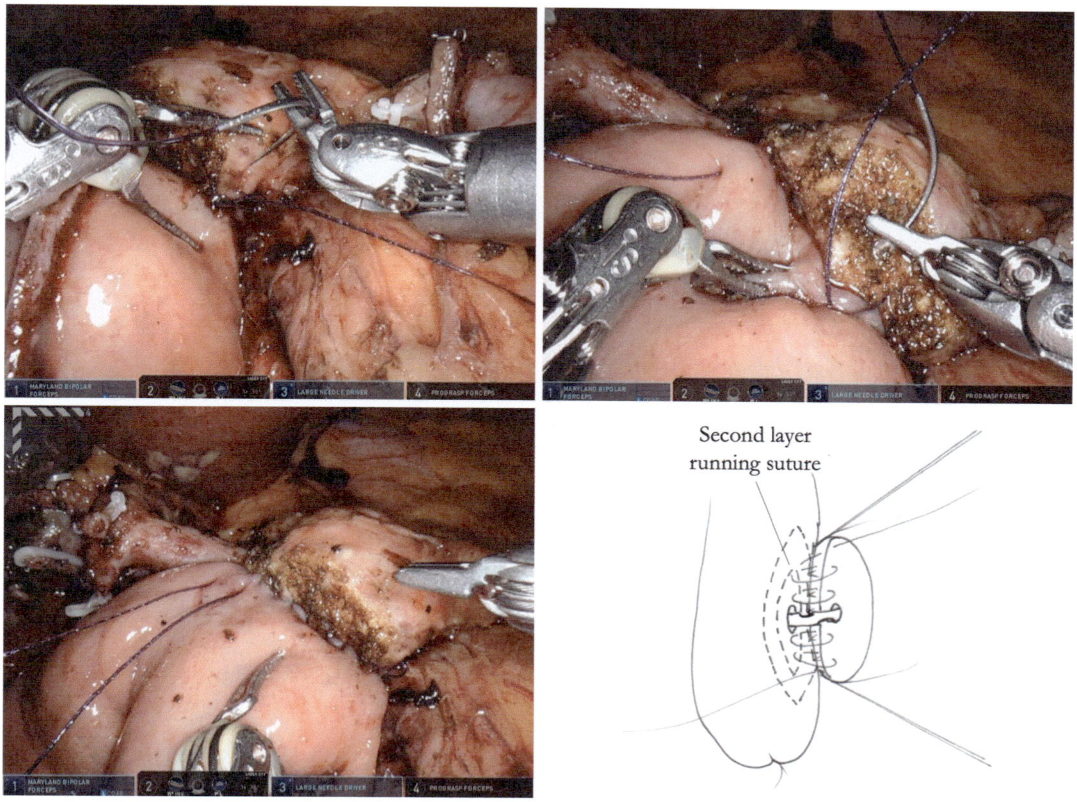

Fig. 13.4 Second posterior (inner) layer. Illustration. (Courtesy of Giulio Di Candio)

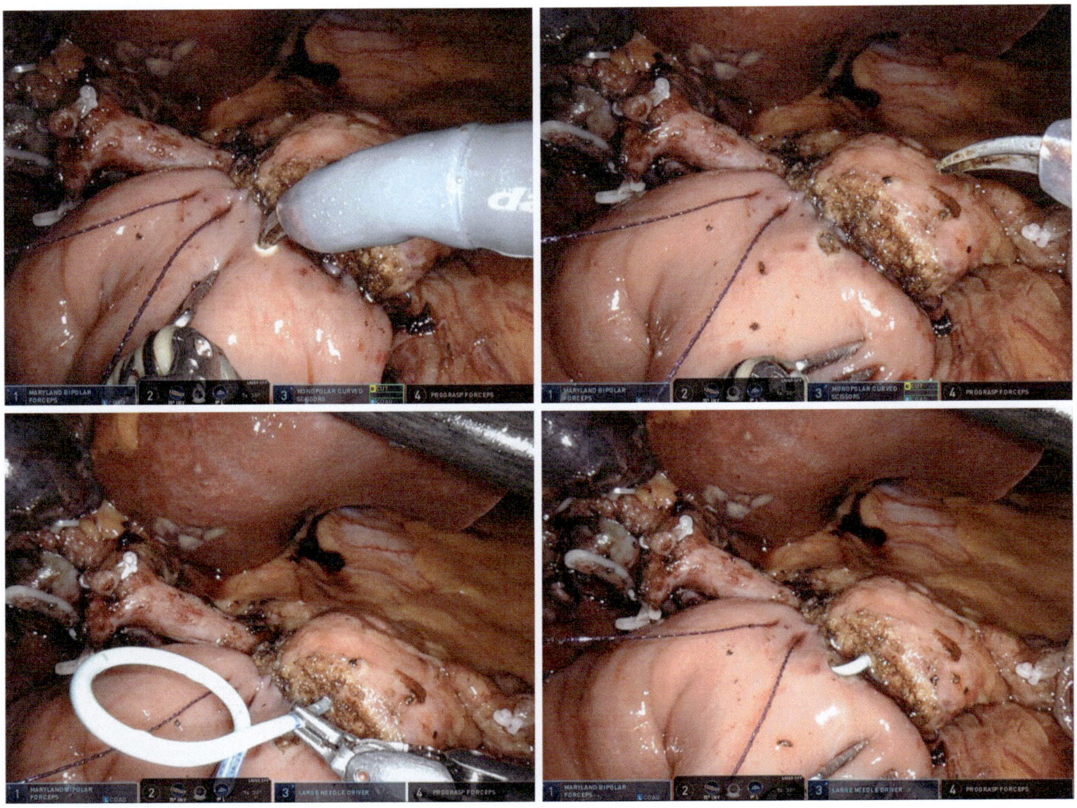

Fig. 13.5 Enterotomy and stent positioning

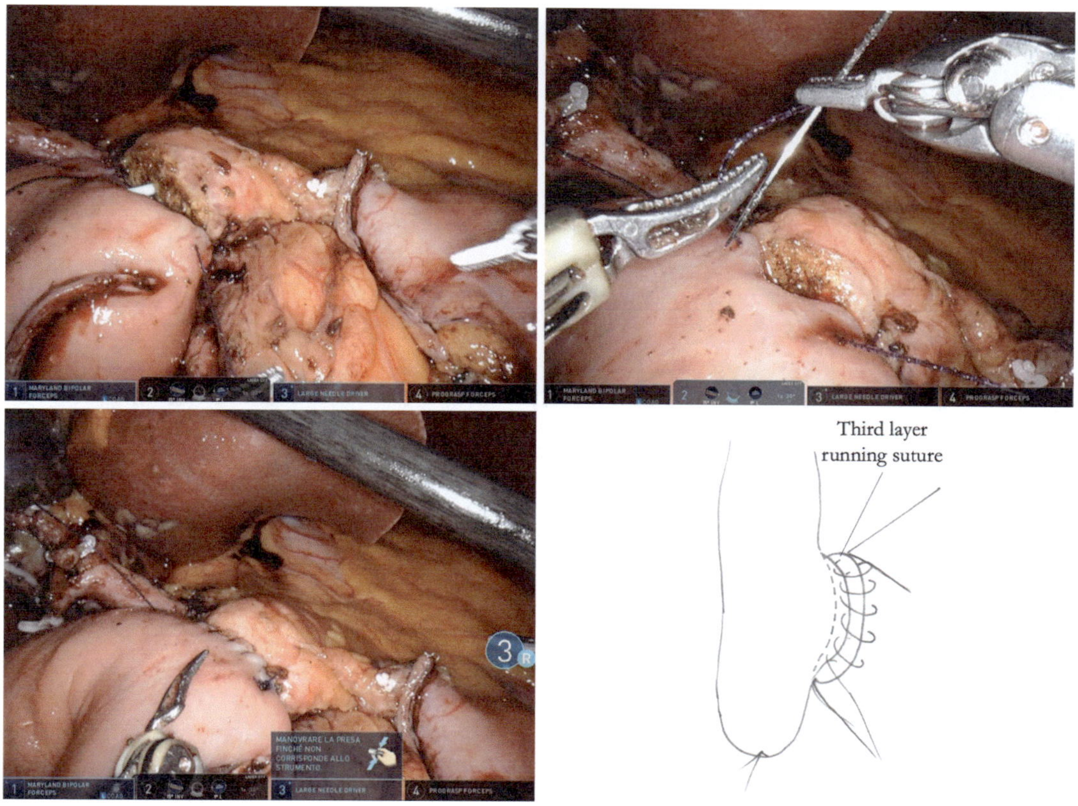

Fig. 13.6 First anterior (inner) layer. Illustration. (Courtesy of Giulio Di Candio)

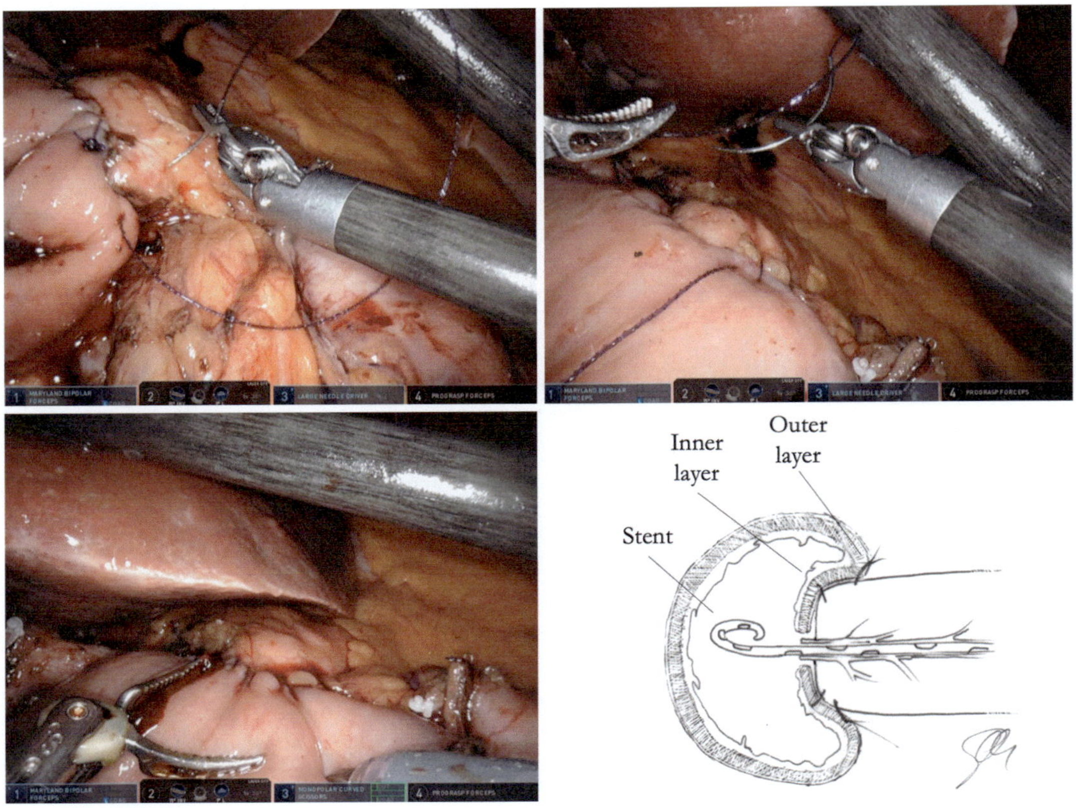

Fig. 13.7 Second anterior (outer) layer. Illustration. (Courtesy of Giulio Di Candio)

13.4 Comments

Barbed sutures have the potential to be utilized across all four layers of the anastomosis, particularly to address the robotic challenge of the lack of tactile feedback during suture tightening.

Certain surgeons have expressed concerns about utilizing barbed sutures on delicate tissues due to their thickness and the potentially more traumatic needle, particularly in cases involving soft pancreas. There are apprehensions about the increased risk of tissue lacerations and potential leaks of pancreatic juice. Despite these reservations, using barbed sutures also on soft gland textures, in the authors' experience, has not resulted in any lacerations [16]. Furthermore, due to the secure tightening of the suture, the jejunum appeared to adhere to the pancreas, creating a visually robust anastomosis that conveys a sense of strength.

Additionally, these sutures possess the necessary tensile strength that is seldom compromised by ongoing traction or manipulation with robotic instruments. This sets them apart from other monofilament sutures like polypropylene, which are more susceptible to breakage. Moreover, as continuous sutures, they not only save time but also have the potential to streamline the surgical process, enhancing the overall workflow compared to the interrupted sutures commonly utilized in most anastomotic techniques.

The reproducibility in every kind of pancreatic texture and pancreatic duct is one of the key points of the described technique. Rarely and in selected cases, with a particularly thick pancreas or intestinal loop with small diameter, the anastomosis might be done in a double posterior layer and single anterior layer, or even in a single layer for both anterior and posterior sides, therefore avoiding invagination of the pancreatic stump. In such instances, using a double layer could potentially increase the tension on the pancreatic parenchyma excessively, risking laceration.

Interestingly, recent papers have reported a decrease in clinically relevant pancreatic leaks when barbed sutures are utilized for open [23] and laparoscopic PJ after PD. This emphasizes the suggestion to use this kind of suture and to extend the use of barbed sutures to the robotic technique as well, since this may represent an important further specific advantage.

13.5 Conclusion

The use of barbed suture for PJ without performing the classical Wirsung-jejunostomy is viable and consistent regardless of pancreatic duct size and parenchyma, offering improvements to the surgical process in this procedure. More specifically, employing barbed sutures enables the realization of the potential benefits of RAS while mitigating the drawback associated with the lack of tactile feedback in robotic procedures. This is achieved by maintaining consistent tension on the continuous suture lines, particularly crucial during the reconstructive phase of the operation.

13.6 Summary

Barbed suture can be used to perform PJ anastomosis. The proposed technique, characterized by the use of barbed suture, is feasible and reproducible irrespective of pancreatic duct size and parenchyma and is applicable also to laparoscopic surgery. Main key points of the technique are as follows: 1—the 3/0 PDS barbed suture, is used for all the four layers of the anastomosis; 2—running sutures are tightened progressively, after each passage through the jejunum; 3—the small enterotomy is placed exactly opposite to the location of the pancreatic duct, without placing any sutures in the pancreatic ductal epithelium, but instead opposing and stenting them.

References

1. Whipple AO, Parsons WB, Mullins CR. Treatment of carcinoma of the ampulla of Vater. Ann Surg. 1935;102:763–79. https://doi.org/10.1097/00000658-193510000-00023.
2. Grobmyer SR, Kooby D, Blumgart LH, Hochwald SN. Novel pancreaticojejunostomy with a low rate of anastomotic failure-related complications. J Am Coll Surg. 2010;210:54–9. https://doi.org/10.1016/j.jamcollsurg.2009.09.020.
3. Kakita A, Takahashi T, Yoshida M, Furuta K. A simpler and more reliable technique of pancreatojejunal anastomosis. Surg Today. 1996;26:532–5. https://doi.org/10.1007/BF00311562.
4. Keck T, Wellner UF, Bahra M, Klein F, Sick O, Niedergethmann M, Wilhelm TJ, Farkas SA, Borner T, Bruns C, Kleespies A, Kleeff J, Mihaljevic AL, Uhl W, Chromik A, Fendrich V, Heeger K, Padberg W, Hecker A, Neumann UP, Junge K, Kalff JC, Glowka TR, Werner J, Knebel P, Piso P, Mayr M, Izbicki J, Vashist Y, Bronsert P, Bruckner T, Limprecht R, Diener MK, Rossion I, Wegener I, Hopt UT. Pancreatogastrostomy versus pancreatojejunostomy for reconstruction after PANCreatoduodenectomy (RECOPANC, DRKS 00000767): perioperative and long-term results of a multicenter randomized controlled trial. Ann Surg. 2016;263:440–9. https://doi.org/10.1097/SLA.0000000000001240.
5. Cai Y, Luo H, Li Y, Gao P, Peng B. A novel technique of pancreaticojejunostomy for laparoscopic pancreaticoduodenectomy. Surg Endosc. 2019;33:1572–7. https://doi.org/10.1007/s00464-018-6446-z.
6. Poves I, Morató O, Burdío F, Grande L. Laparoscopic-adapted Blumgart pancreaticojejunostomy in laparoscopic pancreaticoduodenectomy. Surg Endosc. 2017;31:2837–45. https://doi.org/10.1007/s00464-016-5294-y.
7. Azagra JS, Makkai-Popa ST, Pascotto B, Arru L, De Blasi V, Ramia JM, Ibanez-Aguirre FJ, Goergen M. Laparoscopic pancreaticojejunal anastomosis using knotless barbed absorbable sutures are simple, safe and effective: an experience with 34 procedures. Laparosc Surg. 2020;4:7–12. https://doi.org/10.21037/ls.2020.03.07.
8. Ielpo B, Anselmo A, Koh Y, et al. Minimally invasive pancreatic anastomosis after pancreaticoduodenectomy: multi-institutional step by step video description of the technique. Updates Surg. 2023;75(1):255–259. https://doi.org/10.1007/s13304-022-01389-0. Epub 2022 Nov 12. PMID: 36371550.
9. Lin Y, Liao B, Lai S, Huang J, Du L, Wang K, Li H. The application of barbed suture during the partial nephrectomy may modify perioperative results: a systematic review and meta-analysis. BMC Urol. 2019;19:5.

10. Manigrasso M, Velotti N, Calculli F, Aprea G, Di Lauro K, Araimo E, Elmore U, Vertaldi S, Anoldo P, Musella M, Milone M, Maria Sosa Fernandez L, Milone F, Domenico De Palma G. Barbed suture and gastrointestinal surgery. A retrospective analysis. Open Med. 2019;14:503–8. https://doi.org/10.1515/med-2019-0055.
11. Wiggins T, Majid MS, Markar SR, Loy J, Agrawal S, Koak Y. Benefits of barbed suture utilisation in gastrointestinal anastomosis: a systematic review and meta-analysis. Ann R Coll Surg Engl. 2020;102:153–9. https://doi.org/10.1308/rcsann.2019.0106.
12. Facy O, De Blasi V, Goergen M, Arru L, De Magistris L, Azagra JS. Laparoscopic gastrointestinal anastomoses using knotless barbed sutures are safe and reproducible: a single-center experience with 201 patients. Surg Endosc. 2013;27:3841–5. https://doi.org/10.1007/s00464-013-2992-6.
13. Kim EY, Hong TH. Laparoscopic longitudinal Pancreaticojejunostomy using barbed sutures: an efficient and secure solution for pancreatic duct obstructions in patients with chronic pancreatitis. J Gastrointest Surg. 2016;20:861–6. https://doi.org/10.1007/s11605-015-3053-3.
14. Balduzzi A, Zwart MJW, Kempeneers RMA, Boermeester MA, Busch OR, Besselink MG Robotic lateral Pancreaticojejunostomy for chronic pancreatitis. J Vis Exp. 2019. https://doi.org/10.3791/60301.
15. De Pastena M, van Hilst J, de Rooij T, Busch OR, Gerhards MF, Festen S, Besselink MG. Laparoscopic pancreatoduodenectomy with modified Blumgart pancreaticojejunostomy. J Vis Exp. 2018;2018 https://doi.org/10.3791/56819.
16. Morelli L, Furbetta N, Gianardi D, Guadagni S, Di Franco G, Bianchini M, Palmeri M, Masoni C, Di Candio G, Cuschieri A. Use of barbed suture without fashioning the "classical" Wirsung-jejunostomy in a modified end-to-side robotic pancreatojejunostomy. Surg Endosc. 2020. https://doi.org/10.1007/s00464-020-07991-w.
17. Olakowski M, Grudzińska E, Mrowiec S. Pancreaticojejunostomy—a review of modern techniques. Langenbeck's Arch Surg. 2020;405:13–22. https://doi.org/10.1007/s00423-020-01855-6.
18. Kawaida H, Kono H, Hosomura N, Amemiya H, Itakura J, Fujii H, Ichikawa D. Surgical techniques and postoperative management to prevent postoperative pancreatic fistula after pancreatic surgery. World J Gastroenterol. 2019;25:3722–37. https://doi.org/10.3748/wjg.v25.i28.3722.
19. Kornaropoulos M, Moris D, Beal EW, Makris MC, Mitrousias A, Petrou A, Felekouras E, Michalinos A, Vailas M, Schizas D, Papalampros A. Total robotic pancreaticoduodenectomy: a systematic review of the literature. Surg Endosc. 2017;31:4382–92. https://doi.org/10.1007/s00464-017-5523-z.
20. Bethea BT, Okamura AM, Kitagawa M, Fitton TP, Cattaneo SM, Gott VL, Baumgartner WA, Yuh DD. Application of haptic feedback to robotic surgery. J Laparoendosc Adv Surg Tech Part A. 2004;14:191–5. https://doi.org/10.1089/1092642041255441.
21. Meccariello G, Faedi F, AlGhamdi S, Montevecchi F, Firinu E, Zanotti C, Cavaliere D, Gunelli R, Taurchini M, Amadori A, Vicini C. An experimental study about haptic feedback in robotic surgery: may visual feedback substitute tactile feedback? J Robot Surg. 2016;10:57–61. https://doi.org/10.1007/s11701-015-0541-0.
22. Shin YC, Jang JY, Chang YR, Jung W, Kwon W, Kim H, Kim E, Kim SW. Comparison of long-term clinical outcomes of external and internal pancreatic stents in pancreaticoduodenectomy: randomized controlled study. HPB. 2019;21:51–9. https://doi.org/10.1016/j.hpb.2018.06.1795.
23. Guzowski AA, Gabra J, Ali NS. Updated barbed suture for pancreatic anastomosis during pancreaticoduodenectomy decreases incidence of clinically significant pancreatic fistula; our first 50 patients. HPB. 2019;21:S182–3. https://doi.org/10.1016/j.hpb.2019.03.336.

3D Virtual Surgical Planning in Pancreatic Cancer Surgery

14

Emilio Vicente, Yolanda Quijano, Valentina Ferri, Riccardo Caruso, and Pablo Ruiz

14.1 Introduction

Surgery for pancreatic tumors is notably complex and often poses significant challenges for surgeons. The pancreas' retroperitoneal location, its vascular connections, and the frequent invasion of nearby venous and arterial structures contribute to these challenges [1–3]. In recent years, minimally invasive surgery has increasingly played a role in treating pancreatic cancer, particularly with the introduction of robotic surgery.

The success of surgical treatment for pancreatic cancer is influenced by several factors, including the surgeon's experience, preoperative planning, and real-time decision-making [4]. To deliver optimal treatment for each patient in specific situations, a comprehensive diagnostic model is necessary, extending beyond the surgeon's deductive reasoning, and personal judgment during surgery. Thus, conducting a thorough and accurate preoperative assessment is essential. The insights gained from this assessment should guide precise preoperative planning to achieve of maximum surgical accuracy. However, a critical question arises: Are conventional imaging techniques sufficient to establish an appropriate therapeutic strategy? Likely not, as these methods have limitations in providing accurate preoperative staging of the disease and in predicting vascular involvement.

Innovations in three-dimensional (3D) imaging and advanced digital industrial technology have driven progress in medical imaging. Recently, traditional axial and two-dimensional views of anatomy in radiological studies have been enhanced by a 3D approach that allows for planes in any spatial direction, thereby improving depth perception and spatial orientation. Additionally, merging 3D radiological images [5, 6] with metabolic images [7, 8] enhances study quality and clinical relevance, aiding in the understanding of the patient's anatomy and the potential loco-regional spread of the tumor.

This study was supported by the Foundation for Development and Investigation in Surgical Oncology of Madrid.

Supplementary Information The online version contains supplementary material available at https://doi.org/10.1007/978-3-031-99695-5_14. The videos can be accessed individually by clicking the DOI link in the accompanying figure caption or by scanning this link with the SN More Media App.

E. Vicente (✉) · Y. Quijano · V. Ferri · R. Caruso · P. Ruiz
Sanchinarro University Hospital, Clara Campal Oncological Center, Service of General and Digestive Surgery, Health Sciences Faculty HM Hospitals, Camilo José Cela University, Madrid, Spain
e-mail: correo@emiliovicente.es; yolandaquijanosigloxxi@gmail.com; valenpeglio@gmail.com; ricaruso2@gmail.com; pabloruizquijano@gmail.com

B. Ielpo et al. (eds.), *Minimally Invasive Pancreatoduodenectomy in Cancer*,
https://doi.org/10.1007/978-3-031-99695-5_14

14.2 Next-Generation 3D Modeling by Cella Medical Solutions (3D MPS)

To create 3D models (3DM), data is acquired from computed tomography (CT), magnetic resonance imaging (MRI), PET (positron emission tomography)-CT, or PET-MRI scans. The data is exported in DICOM (Digital Imaging and Communication in Medicine) format and anonymized before being integrated into the PACS (picture archiving and communication system). Image coregistration techniques allow for the merging of different functional and anatomical modalities (e.g., PET-MRI and CT), assigning varying amounts of information accordingly. Registration algorithms employ linear or rigid transformations for global lesion characteristics and elastic or non-rigid transformations for local image deformations. In the initial phase of image processing, noise and artifacts are minimized using anisotropic diffusion filters, and intensity is normalized with the N3 algorithm (non-parametric non-uniform intensity normalization) to facilitate clear delineation of structural edges. The standard protocol involves segmenting the tumor, pancreatic duct, common bile duct, vascular structures, and surrounding organs as needed for surgical planning. If requested by the patient or surgeon, reconstructions of protheses, lymph nodes, and cysts can also be performed. Segmentation algorithms utilize active contour techniques and adaptive region growth. Moreover, Laplacian filters help reduce segmentation discrepancies from varying imaging techniques. The pancreatic parenchyma is then categorized into its components (body, uncinate process, tail, and head). Finally, the models are enhanced with interactive features, such as vascular resection with a 5-mm margin and intraluminal navigation to assess the degree of infiltration.

14.3 Information Obtained from 3D Reconstruction in Pancreatic Surgery

14.3.1 Vascular Anatomy of the Pancreatic Region

Understanding the vascular anatomy in pancreatic surgery is crucial for several reasons: (1) to prevent vascular injuries during the procedure due to anatomical variations, (2) to assess the potential for tumor infiltration, and (3) to reduce the risk of postoperative hemorrhagic or thrombotic complications [9].

The second most common variant is the presence of an accessory or replaced right hepatic artery (RHA), which originates from the superior mesenteric artery [9]. An accessory RHA provides a dual arterial supply to the right hepatic lobe from both the celiac trunk and the superior mesenteric artery, whereas a replaced RHA solely supplies the right hepatic lobe, affecting 10–24% of patients [10]. This anomaly is critical in the surgical technique for pancreatic cancer. The presence of an aberrant RHA does not appear to affect long-term survival or hepatic recurrence following resection for ductal adenocarcinoma of the pancreatic head [11–13]. Although no differences have been observed in the rates of major postoperative complications [11], the presence of an aberrant RHA significantly complicates the surgical approach. This artery often exhibits significant pathological changes due to compression and/or infiltration, and its resection and reconstruction are typically associated with a moderate to high risk of postoperative thrombosis.

The 3DM study is valuable for accurately identifying potential vascular anomalies, enabling the selection of appropriate strategy for vessel liberation, resection, and reconstruction.

14.3.2 Tumor Staging: Characterization of "T"

The size of the pancreatic tumor (Fig. 14.1) and the lesion's growth characteristics are clearly outlined in 3DM. For tumors situated within the pancreatic gland without significant perineural involvement, dissection is usually straightforward. However, this is not the case for lesions exhibiting considerable extraglandular growth (Fig. 14.2), where vascular infiltration is common, as shown in the video. When a lesion is located in the uncinate process, it often extends to the mesenteric root, leading to vascular infil-

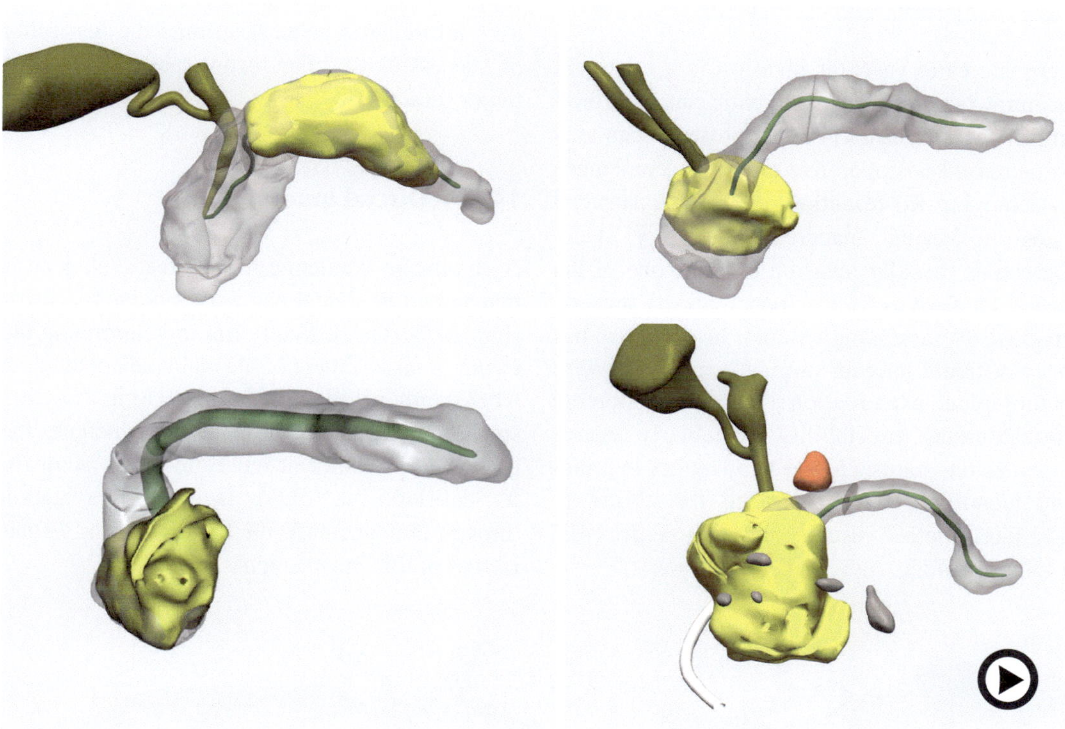

Fig. 14.1 Size and location of pancreatic tumor (3D reconstruction in pancreatic surgery (▶ https://doi.org/10.1007/000-hey))

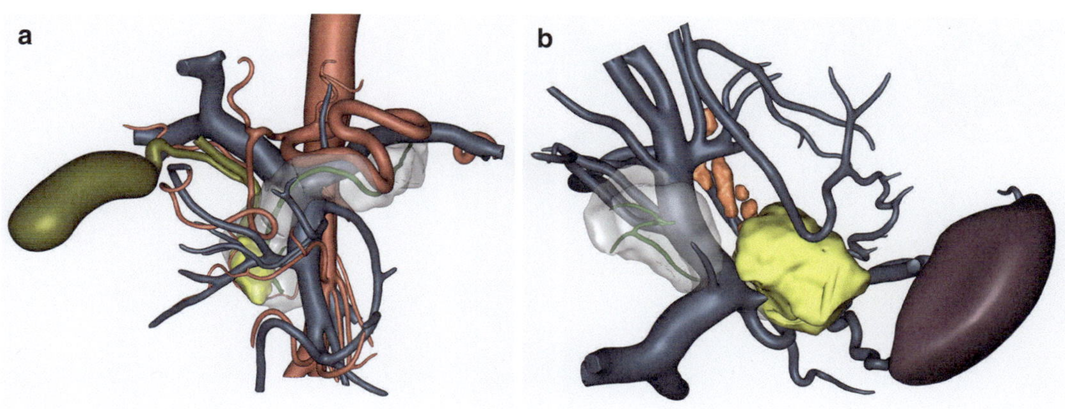

Fig. 14.2 (**a**) Intra pancreatic growth unusual vascular invasion (**b**) Extra pancreatic growth vascular invasion

tration (venous and/or arterial) in a high number of patients. In such instances, resecting the tumor along with the affected mesenteric vascular structures and performing subsequent reconstruction can be very complex and, at times, impossible.

14.3.3 Vascular Involvement

Peripancreatic vascular invasion is a relatively common occurrence in pancreatic cancer, affecting 21–64% of cases [14]. Its presence can lead to increased postoperative mortality, challenges in achieving R0 resection, and poorer survival rates following pancreatic surgery [15]. Detecting vascular invasion remains one of the key challenges in pancreatic surgery. Historically, assessing vascular involvement has been difficult, making surgical exploration with pathological examination the critical moment for evaluating resectability, particularly regarding vascular status. However, advances in imaging techniques have enhanced the ability to accurately detect vascular invasion (Figs. 14.3, 14.4, and 14.5).

As shown in the video, 3DM provides precise information on [1] the area and extent of vascular involvement, [2] the differentiation between tumor compression and actual vessel infiltration through intraluminal navigation, [3] the proximal and distal patency of the affected venous or arterial vessel, and [4] the potential presence of vascular thrombosis, along with associated collateral supply and hemodynamic changes, Fig. 14.6. This information helps determine the feasibility of successful vascular reconstruction following tumor resection.

14.3.4 Ductal Involvement

A significant challenge in pancreatic surgery is managing intraductal papillary mucinous tumors (Fig. 14.7). The difficulty lies in determining the extent of involvement of the main pancreatic duct when a tumor is identified, as well as in detecting small intraductal nodules that may indicate the presence of a tumor or represent a risk factor for its development. 3DM facilitates navigation through the pancreatic duct, allowing for visualization of this involvement.

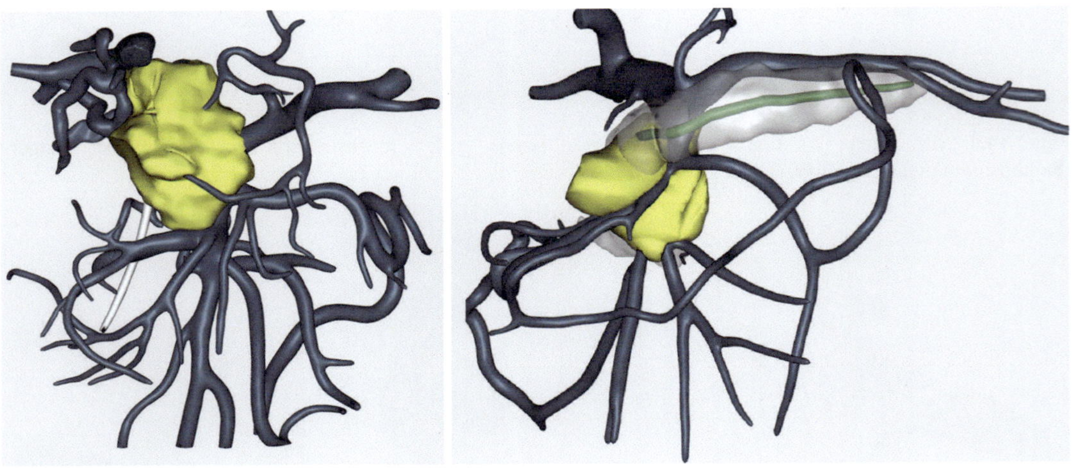

Fig. 14.3 Superior mesenteric vein invasion

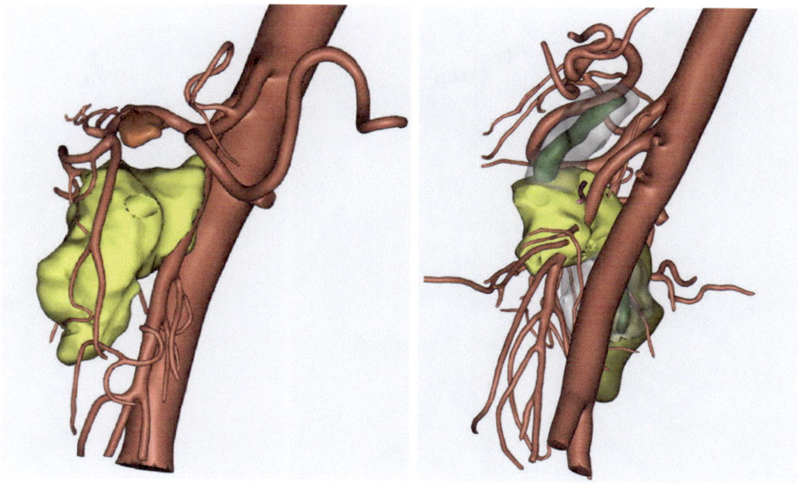

Fig. 14.4 Superior mesenteric artery invasion

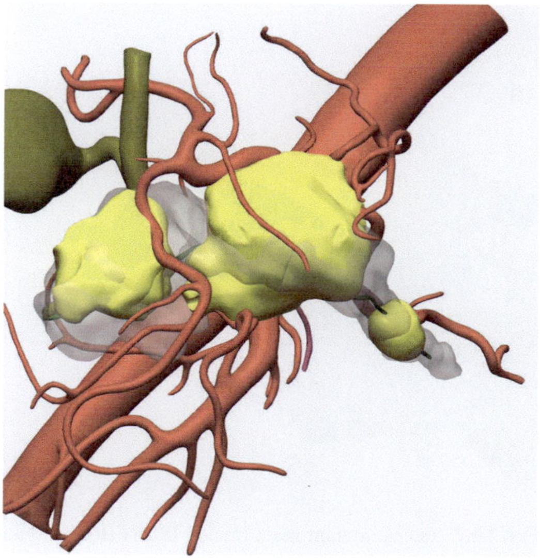

Fig. 14.5 Celiac axis invasion

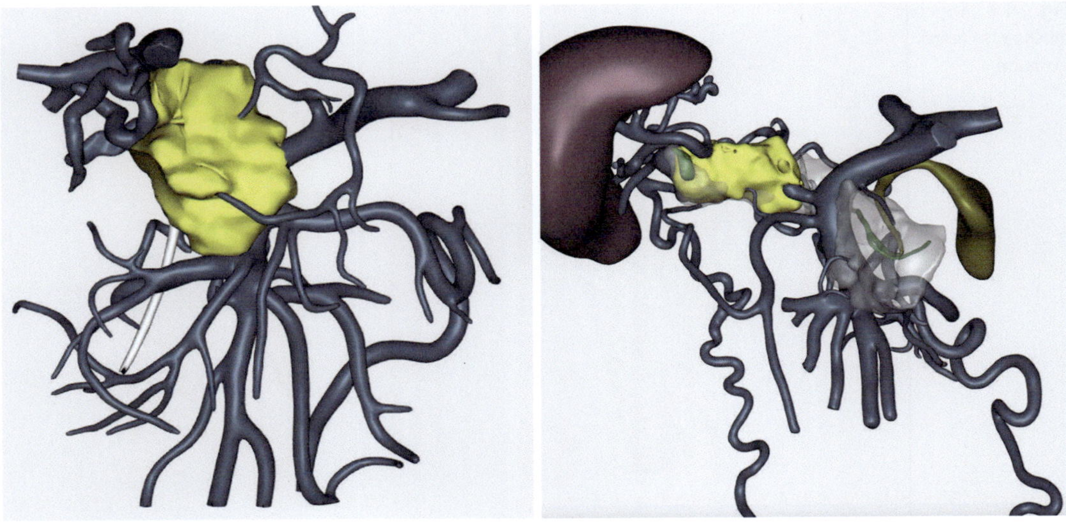

Fig. 14.6 Portal hypertension: *Proximal* collateral circulation/possibility of *anatomical* restoration of venous flow

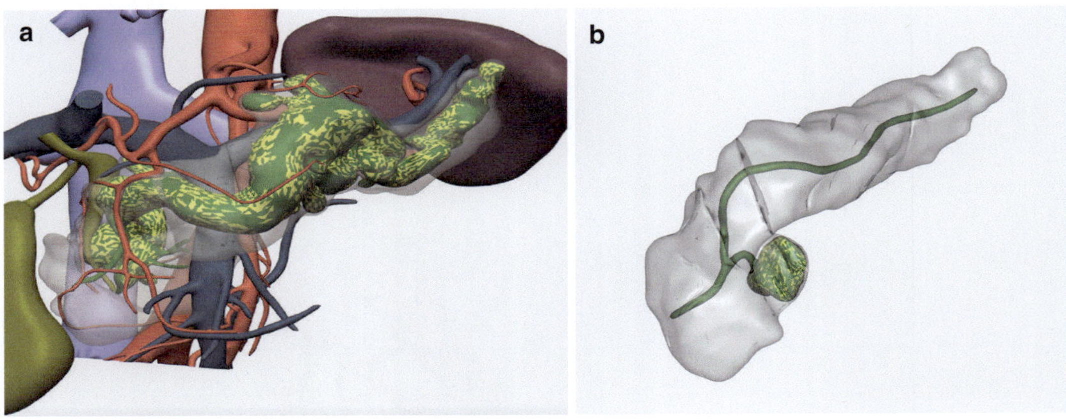

Fig. 14.7 (**a**) Malignant main branch IPMN (**b**) Malignant secondary branch IPMN

14.4 Evaluation of the Benefits of Information Obtained with 3DM

14.4.1 Achieving a Precise Anatomical Definition of the Surgical and Tumor Areas

Tumor staging is a crucial step in establishing an appropriate therapeutic strategy, a concept that remains widely accepted. However, longstanding limitations in diagnostic methodologies have resulted in a lack of rigor in this area. 3DM enables a detailed understanding of both the patient's anatomy and the characteristics of lesions within the pancreas (T1–T2) or with extraglandular extension (T3–T4), accurately defining the size of such extensions in the latter case.

14.4.2 Improved Therapeutic Planning

3DM enables the establishment of accurate criteria for operability and resectability. It helps determine the extent of treatment needed in the pancreas, including the necessity for multivisceral and/or vascular resections, as well as the characteristics, length, diameter, and condition of the affected vessels. Its primary value lies in managing locally advanced lesions, where this information serves as a strong rationale for neoadjuvant treatment. Additionally, it provides insights into collateral flow in patients with significant venous involvement, which is essential for evaluating and ensuring the patency of any subsequent venous resections.

14.4.3 Oncological Evaluation of the Surgical Procedure

3DM assesses the likelihood of achieving an R0 resection (including radial margin), the urgency of the procedure, the potential morbidities and mortalities associated with it, and the capacity to establish an appropriate risk/benefit ratio for the proposed surgery.

14.4.4 Effect of Neoadjuvant Therapy

Neoadjuvant treatment is a significant therapeutic strategy in the management of pancreatic cancer [16–18]. Assessing the morphological changes that occur after preparatory chemoradiotherapy is challenging, as it is difficult to distinguish between neoplastic and fibrotic tissue without evaluating tumor viability. Currently, 3DM offers indirect information regarding the response to neoadjuvant treatment, Fig. 14.8.

14.4.5 Personal Experience with 3DM in Pancreatic Cancer

The existing literature on 3DM in pancreatic cancer patients is limited [19–22]. From September 2019 to September 2024, our service completed a total of 980 3D reconstructions, primarily for various oncological processes (92%). Of the 379 reconstructions for pancreatic conditions, 324 (85%) were diagnosed as pancreatic cancer. At our center, 3D modeling is routinely conducted prior to pancreatic surgery, aiding in intraoperative surgical navigation. As this is a preliminary study, we focused on analyzing the most complex cases involving vascular resection.

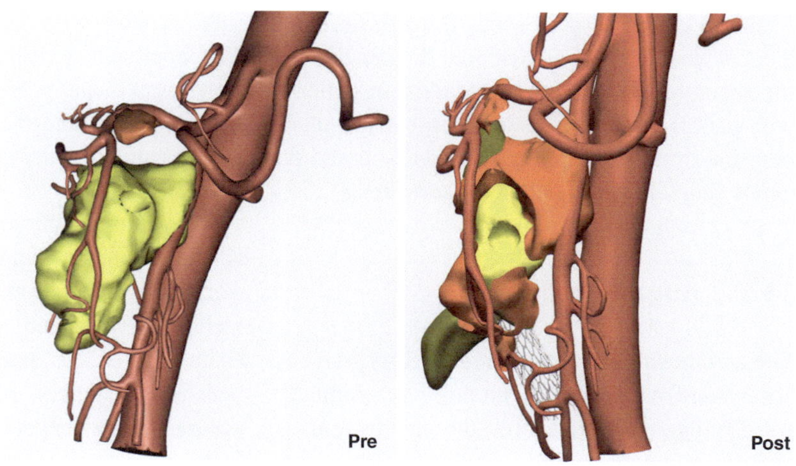

Fig. 14.8 Response to neoadjuvant treatment (chemotherapy/radiotherapy)

During the first of our observational study (2019), 10 patients underwent either cephalic or distal pancreatectomy with associated vascular resection. A celiac trunk resection was performed in five patients, and in one of these cases, a circumferential resection of the superior mesenteric vein was also completed, followed by end-to-end handsewn reconstruction. Additionally, seven patients underwent tangential resection of the portal mesenteric axis, which included tangential reconstruction. Vascular infiltration was confirmed in six cases, and tumor infiltration at the resected margins was observed in 30% of patients. 3D reconstruction models demonstrated 100% sensitivity and 100% specificity in identifying celiac trunk involvement, outperforming traditional imaging methods (CT scan, MRI, and endoscopic ultrasound), which showed sensitivity rates of 60%, 40%, and 80%, respectively. Moreover, the 3D technique accurately detected all cases requiring vascular resection due to portal mesenteric trunk involvement, achieving 100% accuracy compared to 25%, 50%, and 30% for CT scan, MRI, and endoscopic ultrasound, respectively. Regarding tumor diameter, 3D imaging reconstruction tended to overestimate tumor sizes, showing a mean difference of 0.8 cm compared to pathological measurements. In contrast, CT and MRI demonstrated larger mean differences of 1.1 cm and 1.2 cm, respectively.

Based on our experience, 3D reconstruction models have become an essential diagnostic tool for accurate preoperative evaluation in patients with pancreatic cancer, aiding surgeons in planning the optimal therapeutic approach based on tumor characteristics and vascular invasion.

14.5 Augmented Reality

The advancement of augmented reality (AR) as a new and promising technology is gradually solidifying. AR allows for the integration of real environments with virtual objects by overlaying 3D images onto the affected organ in the surgical field in real time. This enhances the visual information available to the surgeon during minimally invasive procedures. AR can project the patient's radiological tests, reconstructing their pathology and the previously developed surgical plan. With AR, "image-guided surgery" can be performed, merging the real and virtual worlds by adding a virtual component to the existing reality.

The advantages of AR for patients are clear, as it increases the precision and safety of surgical procedures. This illustrates that technological innovation often leads to enhanced accuracy while minimizing intervention risks without compromising safety and efficacy.

Predicting the future of pancreatic cancer surgery is challenging. However, recent advancements in techniques and technology, such as 3D modeling, suggest that the next generation of surgeries, supported by artificial intelligence and AR, may enable us to perform hepatopancreatobiliary (HPB) procedures previously beyond our imagination.

14.6 Conclusion

3D virtual surgical planning using images from PET, CT, or MRI can aid surgeons in accurately locating tumors and assessing their local extent, while also providing enhanced visualization of surgical sites with improved depth perception. This approach reinforces the concept of "precision surgery" and personalized surgical treatment for patients. Additionally, 3D technology serves an educational purpose for both students and surgeons.

3D reconstruction, utilizing mathematical algorithms and artificial intelligence, represents a significant innovation in pancreatic surgery. It facilitates advanced image segmentation and evaluation of the extent, pathophysiology, and benefits of surgery, offering greater diagnostic accuracy than conventional imaging techniques. 3DM is a valuable tool in HPB centers for both open and minimally invasive pancreatic surgeries.

References

1. Tempero MA, Malafa MP, Al-Hawary M, Asbun H, Bain A, Behrman SW, et al. Pancreatic adenocarcinoma, Version 2.2017. NCCN clinical practice guidelines in oncology. J Natl Compr Cancer Netw. 2017;15:1028–61.
2. Clanton J, Oh S, Kaplan SJ, Johnson E, Ross A, Kozarek R. Does mesenteric venous imaging assessment accurately predict pathologic invasion in localized pancreatic ductal adenocarcinoma? HPB (Oxford). 2018;20:925–31.
3. Quijano Y, Vicente E, Duran H, Diaz E, Fabra I, Caruso R, et al. Carcinoma de cabeza de pancreas. ¿Cómo y cuándo realizar la resección vascular? Monografia de la AEC. Controversias en el tratamiento quirúrgico del cáncer de páncreas. Arán Ediciones SL. 2019:22–5.
4. Wall J, Krummel T. The digital surgeon: how big data, automation, and artificial intelligence will change surgical practice. J Pediatr Surg. 2020;55:47–50.
5. Uchida M. Recent advances in 3D computed tomography techniques for simulation and navigation in hepatobiliary pancreatic surgery. J Hepatobiliary Pancreat Sci. 2014;21:239–45.
6. Marconi S, Pugliese L, Del Chiaro M, Pozzi Mucelli R, Auricchio F, Pietrabissa A. An innovative strategy for the identification and 3d reconstruction of pancreatic cancer from CT images. Updat Surg. 2016;68:273–8.
7. Pizzuti G, Quijano Y, Vicente E, Caruso R. First-reported case of vaginal late recurrence of Wilms tumor treated with complete pelvic exenteration. Int J Surg Case Rep. 2024;123:110136.
8. Vicente E, Quijano Y, Ferri V, Caruso R. The use of 3D virtual surgical planning springer nature Switzerland Ag Glissonean pedicles approach in minimally invasive liver surgery, 2023. Ch 23, 161–164.
9. García-Picazo A, Sánchez-Velázquez P, Burdio F, et al. Anatomical variations of the hepatic artery in duodenopancreatectomy: tips and tricks in the minimally invasive surgical approach. Updates Surg. 2025. https://doi.org/10.1007/s13304-025-02307-w. Epub ahead of print. PMID: 40593390.
10. Xu Y-C, Yang F, Fu D-L. Clinical significance of variant hepatic artery in pancreatic resection: a comprehensive review. World J Gastroenterol. 2022;28:2057–75.
11. Petrova E, Mazzella E, Eichler K, Gruber-Rouh T, Schulze F, Bechstein WO, et al. Influence of aberrant right hepatic artery on survival after pancreatic resection for ductal adenocarcinoma of the pancreatic head. Langenbeck's Arch Surg. 2024;409:111.
12. Rammohan A. Implications of the presence of an aberrant right hepatic artery in patients undergoing pancreaticoduodenectomy. World J Gastrointest Surg. 2014;6:9.
13. Pyras C, Lukas C, Janot-Mattuschek M, Herzog T, Tannapfel A, Uhl W, et al. Preservation of aberrant right hepatic arteries does not affect safety and oncological radicality of pancreaticoduodenectomy. Own results and a systematic review of the literature. Hepato biliary Surg Nutr. 2022;11:25–37.
14. Arslan A, Buanes T, Geitung JT. Pancreatic carcinoma: MR, MR angiography and dynamic helical CT in the evaluation of vascular invasion. Eur J Radiol. 2001;38:151–9.
15. Giovinazzo F, Turri G, Katz MH, Heaton N, Ahmed I. Meta-analysis of benefits of portal- superior mesenteric vein resection in pancreatic resection for ductal adenocarcinoma. Br J Surg. 2016;103:179–91.
16. Alvarez R, Musteanu M, Garcia-Garcia E, Lopez-Casas PP, Megias D, Guerra C, et al. Stromal disrupting effects of nab-paclitaxel in pancreatic cancer. Br J Cancer. 2013;109:926–33.
17. Ielpo B, Duran H, Diaz E, Fabra I, Caruso R, Ferri V, et al. Preoperative treatment with gemcitabine plus nab-paclitaxel is a safe and effective chemotherapy for pancreatic adenocarcinoma. Eur J Surg Oncol. 2016;42:1394–400.
18. Ielpo B, Caruso R, Duran H, Diaz E, Fabra I, Malavé L, et al. A comparative study of neoadjuvant treatment with gemcitabine plus nab-paclitaxel versus surgery first for pancreatic adenocarcinoma. Surg Oncol. 2017;26:402–10.
19. Mahmoud A, Bennett M. Introducing 3-dimensional printing of a human anatomic pathology specimen: potential benefits for undergraduate and postgraduate education and anatomic pathology practice. Arch Pathol Lab Med. 2015;139:1048–51.
20. Sampogna G, Pugliese R, Elli M, Vanzulli A, Forgione A. Routine clinical application of virtual reality in abdominal surgery. Minim Invasive Ther Allied Technol. 2017;26:135–43.
21. Vicente E, Quijano Y, Duran H, Diaz E, Fabra I, Malave L, Ruiz P, Pizzuti G, Naldini C, De Nobili G, Caruso R, Ferri V. Can 3D imaging modeling recognize functional tissue and predict liver failure? A retrospective study based on 3D modelling of the major hepatectomies after hepatic modulation. BMC Surg. 2023;23(1):316. https://doi.org/10.1186/s12893-023-02196-z. PMID: 37853412; PMCID: PMC10583474.
22. Shi W, Wang J, Gao J, Zou X, Dong Q, Huang Z, et al. Utilization of 3D printing technology in hepatopancreatobiliary surgery. J Zhejiang Univ Sci B. 2024;25:123–34.

Bleeding Control During Minimally Invasive Pancreaticoduodenectomy

15

Alessia Fassari, Edoardo Rosso, and Vito De Blasi

15.1 Introduction

Minimizing intraoperative bleeding is the goal in almost all surgical procedures. In medium-high complexity surgery, this also represents a quality index as well as an important prognostic factor for postoperative outcomes. Pancreatic surgery acts as an excellent example in this regard due to the technical challenge of demolitive-reconstructive surgical maneuvers and the anatomical complexity of pancreas and surrounding vascular structures.

According to the most recent evidence, intraoperative bleeding during pancreaticoduodenectomy (PD) is widely considered as an independent predictive element of postoperative clinically significant pancreatic fistula (CR-POPF) on par with other well recognized factors like small duct, soft pancreas, and high-risk pathology [1–3]. In 2021, Casciani et al. elaborated a propensity score model including 966 patients undergoing PD with high estimated blood loss and 966 patients with lower estimated blood loss. In the first group, there was a significantly higher rate of POPF, transfusions, reoperations, intensive care unit transfers, and 90-day mortality [2].

High blood loss could contribute to the onset of pancreatic fistula and postoperative complications by triggering mechanisms that interfere with the anastomosis healing process. These include subsequent relative local ischemia due to hypoperfusion of residual pancreatic parenchyma, the immunosuppressive effect of transfusions, and the reperfusion edema of pancreatic and intestinal tissues.

With the advent of minimally invasive approaches, bleeding control has become one of the most important criteria for establishing not only the safety and feasibility of the technique but also the surgeon's proficiency and represents the most frequent reason for conversion to laparotomy.

Supplementary Information The online version contains supplementary material available at https://doi.org/10.1007/978-3-031-99695-5_15. The videos can be accessed individually by clicking the DOI link in the accompanying figure caption or by scanning this link with the SN More Media App.

A. Fassari (✉) · E. Rosso · V. De Blasi
General Surgery Unit, Centre Hospitalier de Luxembourg, Luxembourg City, Luxembourg
e-mail: alessia.fassari@gmail.com; edoardo_rosso@hotmail.com; DeBlasi.Vito@chl.lu

B. Ielpo et al. (eds.), *Minimally Invasive Pancreatoduodenectomy in Cancer*,
https://doi.org/10.1007/978-3-031-99695-5_15

15.2 All You Need to Know Before You Go: Prevention Is Better Than Cure

Ignoranti quem portum petat nullus suus ventus est (For the sailor who does not know which port he is headed for, no wind will be favorable), Seneca, Ep. ad Luc 71. Preoperative study plays an essential role in knowing what you will face and predicting a possible complication is certainly the best way to treat it. Therefore, the experience of a surgeon is measured first and foremost in the ability to plan the operation and select patients, adapting the surgical approach on a case-by-case basis.

In minimally invasive PD, the two most important variables to evaluate before surgery are the presence of anatomical variants and the neoplastic involvement of vessels.

It is widely known that the normal vascular anatomy for the resected area occurs in only 55–79% of cases, while in the rest of patients vascular variations are found making the procedure even more challenging [4]. According to the literature, the most common vascular anomaly encountered is a replaced right hepatic artery (rRHA) originating in most of cases from the superior mesenteric artery (SMA) or in other cases from gastroduodenal artery (GDA) and celiac trunk. The second most common anatomical vascular variant is represented by a replaced left hepatic artery (rLHA) originating from left gastric artery (LGA), followed by replaced gastroduodenal artery (rGDA) and accessory hepatic artery (AHA).

These arterial variants could cause iatrogenic hemorrhagic and ischemic damage if not recognized [5] (Fig. 15.1).

Awareness of the relationship between the GDA and the hepatic artery is important in order to avoid accidental ligation of the hepatic artery. Moreover, due to frequent tumor involvement of the uncinate process, documentation of aberrant vessels in this area is crucial for preventing unexpected bleeding.

Finally, knowing in advance the need for a vascular resection and reconstruction following neoplastic involvement could lead in some cases, based on the skills of the individual surgeon, to prefer from the beginning a laparotomy approach rather than a minimally invasive one.

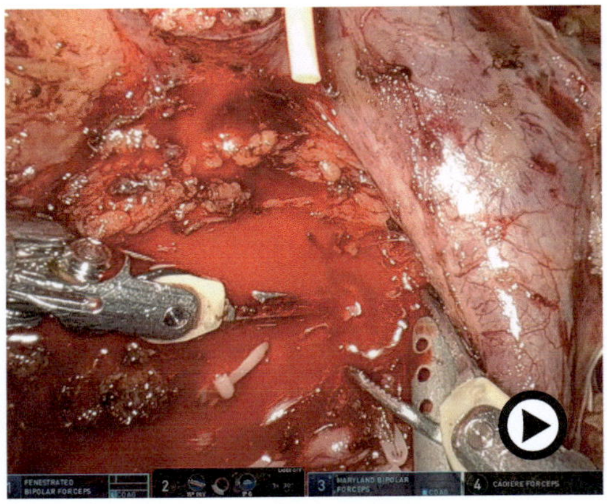

Fig. 15.1 Bleeding from superior mesenteric artery (Intraoperative bleeding control techniques (▶ https://doi.org/10.1007/000-hez))

Although sonography, magnetic resonance, and endoscopic sonography are used to assess local resectability, the most accurate and accessible imaging technique for vascular anatomy is the 3-phase computed tomographic angiography (CTA). As extensively explained in the previous chapter the use of 3D virtual surgical planning can now be made commercially. With this new technology, surgeons can simulate their planned surgical intervention improving their procedure choices.

15.3 Intraoperative Bleeding Control: Tips and Tricks

As shown in the video, the artery-first represents our preferred approach not only for reasons of oncological radicality but also for the safety it guarantees us on bleeding control. Firstly described in 1993 in order to verify the possible involvement of SMA margin before reaching the point of no return, the artery-first approach to PD has demonstrated in a recent meta-analysis to be associated with both reduced estimated blood loss, intraoperative transfusions, and CR-POPF rates compared with the standard approach [6]. Currently, at least six artery-first approaches are described in literature and for all the details you can refer to the dedicated chapter. Here, we focus on the advantages coming from this technique in vascular control. As shown in the video, the first is represented by an easier identification and ligation of the inferior pancreaticoduodenal arteries before the afferent veins, reducing congestion and bleeding from the pancreatic head. Secondly, it enables simpler recognition and preservation of aberrant RHA or CHA originating from SMA. In this case, we identify the SMA origin at the upper edge of the left renal vein and we continue with a periadventitial dissection from the aorta to the mesentery until reaching the point of emergence of the RHA or CHA. The aberrant vessel is encircled at its distal margin and then released from the surrounding tissue posteriorly to the pancreatic head. This allows to safely tie and divide the superior pancreatic artery and the GDA in case of CHA at their origins.

Finally, in the case of venous neoplastic involvement, once the extension and the precise point (at portal or mesenteric vein or at the porto-mesenteric confluence) have been preoperatively established, an enormous advantage comes from the suspension of the specimen on the venous axis, including the mesopancreas, now completely detached from everything else. This allows for great freedom in surgical maneuvers which are easier and safer, resulting in shorter venous clamping and reconstruction times.

Beyond the technical details, one last tip for managing intraoperative blood loss in minimally invasive setting is to keep calm, clean and identify as soon as possible the source of bleeding, take time to reflect by swabbing with a hemostatic gauze (SURGICEL™ Absorbable Hemostat), and don't hesitate to convert when the procedure is no longer safe.

15.4 Conclusions

Minimally invasive PD requires significant expertise and resources which may not be within the reach of all surgeons. Among the variables associated with increased blood loss, the relative impact of those that could be modified by the surgeon was approximately 40% [3, 7–9]. This means that the ability to reduce bleeding is the result of a combination of techniques and decision-making skills that together make what we call *surgical experience*.

Statements and Declarations No funding sources were received specific to this paper.

References

1. Trudeau MT, Casciani F, Maggino L. Et al; pancreas fistula study group. The influence of intraoperative blood loss on fistula development following Pancreatoduodenectomy. Ann Surg. 2022;276(5):e527–35. https://doi.org/10.1097/SLA.0000000000004549. Epub 2020 Nov 12. PMID: 33201132.
2. Casciani F, Trudeau MT, Asbun HJ, et al. Pancreas Fistula Study Group. The effect of high intraoperative blood loss on pancreatic fistula development after pancreatoduodenectomy: an international, multi-institutional propensity score matched analysis. Surgery. 2021;170(4):1195–204. https://doi.org/10.1016/j.surg.2021.03.044. Epub 2021 Apr 28. PMID: 33931208.
3. Seykora TF, Ecker BL, McMillan MT, et al. Pancreas fistula study group. The beneficial effects of minimizing blood loss in pancreatoduodenectomy. Ann Surg. 2019;270(1):147–57. https://doi.org/10.1097/SLA.0000000000002714. PMID: 29489483.
4. Mansour S, Damouny M, Obeid M, Farah A, Halloun K, Marjiyeh R, Ghalia J, Kluger Y, Khuri S. Impact of vascular anomalies on pancreatoduodenectomy procedure. J Clin Med Res. 2021;13(3):158–63. https://doi.org/10.14740/jocmr4455. Epub 2021 Mar 19. PMID: 33854655; PMCID: PMC8016524.
5. Zimmitti G, Manzoni A, Codignola C, Postiglione V, Garatti M, Rosso E. How to deal with replaced common hepatic artery during laparoscopic pancreaticoduodenectomy. Dig Med Res. 2019;2:4. https://doi.org/10.21037/dmr.2019.03.03.
6. Jiang X, Yu Z, Ma Z, et al. Superior mesenteric artery first approach can improve the clinical outcomes of pancreaticoduodenectomy: a meta-analysis. Int J Surg. 2020;73:14–24. https://doi.org/10.1016/j.ijsu.2019.11.007. Epub 2019 Nov 18. PMID: 31751791.
7. Casciani F, Trudeau MT, Asbun HJ, et al. Pancreas Fistula Study Group. Surgeon experience contributes to improved outcomes in pancreatoduodenectomies at high risk for fistula development. Surgery. 2021;169(4):708–20. https://doi.org/10.1016/j.

surg.2020.11.022. Epub 2020 Dec 30. PMID: 33386129.
8. Ielpo B, Anselmo A, Koh Y, Burdio F, De Blasi V, Sanchez-Velazquez P, Azagra JS, Huscher C, Giuliani A, Pellino G, Rosso E. Minimally invasive pancreatic anastomosis after pancreaticoduodenectomy: multi-institutional step by step video description of the technique. Updat Surg. 2023;75(1):255–9. https://doi.org/10.1007/s13304-022-01389-0. Epub 2022 Nov 12. PMID: 36371550.
9. Ielpo B, Anselmo A, Masuda Y, Xuan MYH, Burdio F, De Blasi V, Sanchez-Velazquez P, Giuliani A, Azagra JS, Viola GM, Podda M, Pellino G, Rosso E. Superior mesenteric artery first approach for minimally invasive pancreaticoduodenectomy: a step-by-step surgical technique video. Ann Surg Oncol. 2023;30(3):1500–3. https://doi.org/10.1245/s10434-022-12743-2. Epub 2022 Nov 5. PMID: 36335270.

How to Achieve a Total Mesopancreas Excision During Minimally Invasive Pancreaticoduodenectomy

16

Manuel Barberio, Barbara Leone, and Massimo Giuseppe Viola

16.1 Introduction

Pancreatic cancer (PC) is one of the deadliest cancer types in the Western world (9.3% of 5-year survival among all cases) [1]. Future projections envisage a consistent incidence increase and PC should become the second tumor-related cause of death by 2030 [2]. Early diagnosis remains difficult, mainly because the disease progresses silently and symptoms (e.g., jaundice, pain, gastric outlet impairment, etc.) mostly occur at an advanced stage. This results in only 15% of patients with PC eligible to undergo surgery by the time of diagnosis [3]. Currently, R0 surgical resection, combined with perioperative chemotherapy protocols, represents the only potential curative option for these patients. Since PC arises more frequently within the head of the pancreas (60–70% of cases) [4], pancreaticoduodenectomy (PD), one of the most challenging abdominal surgical procedures, represents often the operation of choice. In fact, given its complexity, PD is associated with high rates of postoperative morbidity along with a mortality rate reaching up to 9% in modern series [5].

However, major technical advances have been made in the field of oncological pancreatic surgery over the last decades. First, surgical anatomical studies have improved the knowledge of the architecture of lymphatic and perineural tissue around the pancreas, introducing the concept of mesopancreas [6]. As a result, mesopancreas excision (ME) has been proposed [7, 8] concomitantly to PD, and this approach appears to consistently increase the rate of R0 resections and the number of harvested lymph nodes, decreasing the local recurrence rate [9, 10]. Secondly, "artery-first" approaches (AFA) have been implemented into operative standards by many pancreatic surgery centers worldwide. AFA strategies implicate the dissection around the superior mesenteric artery as an initial procedural step. On one hand, AFA allows to verify tumor resectability at an early procedural stage, and on the other hand, it facilitates "en bloc" resection of the mesopancreas together with the pancreatic head [11].

Concurrently, the constant technological and technical evolution is progressively lowering the minimally invasive feasibility threshold in favor of more complex gastrointestinal procedures. As a result, laparoscopic pancreaticoduodenectomy (LPD) has been increasingly performed worldwide

Supplementary Information The online version contains supplementary material available at https://doi.org/10.1007/978-3-031-99695-5_16. The videos can be accessed individually by clicking the DOI link in the accompanying figure caption or by scanning this link with the SN More Media App.

M. Barberio (✉) · B. Leone · M. G. Viola
General Surgery Department, Ospedale Card. G. Panico, Tricase (LE), Italy
e-mail: mbarberio17@gmail.com; barbara.leone508@gmail.com; masgiuviola@yahoo.it

B. Ielpo et al. (eds.), *Minimally Invasive Pancreatoduodenectomy in Cancer*,
https://doi.org/10.1007/978-3-031-99695-5_16

since its first description in the 90 s [12]. Although LPD offers better results in terms of reduced intra-operative blood loss, reduced hospital stay, and faster overall recovery as compared to the open approach [3, 13–18], periampullary malignancies have been regarded as a contraindication for LPD, for many years [19]. In fact, only recently LPD has been advocated as a valid alternative to open surgery [3] and new evidence suggested at least its non-inferiority in terms of oncological safety as compared to open PD [16–18, 20].

Nevertheless, LPD has a steep learning curve [3, 21], requiring a high degree of proficiency in both advanced laparoscopy and hepatobiliary surgeries. For such reasons, its diffusion is currently limited to a few centers, and it is mostly restricted either to benign conditions or to early-stage malignancies [19, 22, 23].

16.2 Laparoscopic PD: Setup

In our standardized surgical procedure, the patient is placed in a slight reverse Trendelenburg position, with the operating surgeon between the patient's legs and one assistant surgeon on each side. The trocars are positioned as follows: one in the right pararectal region 10–/12-mm optic trocar (right postero-lateral control of AFA), one 10–/12-mm trocar in the right region 4 cm to the optic one, and one 5-mm trocar in right subcostal region. One optic trocar 10–/12-mm is placed in the left pararectal region (left postero-lateral control of AFA), one 10–/12-mm trocar in the left region 4 cm to the optic one, one 5-mm trocar in the left subcostal region. The pneumoperitoneum is maintained at 12 mmHg and an energy device, either bipolar or radiofrequency (according to the surgeon's preference and availability) is used (Fig. 16.1).

16.3 Robotic PD: Setup

In robotic procedure, the trocars are placed as follows: four supraumbilical 10–12-mm trocars and an assistant trocar (5 mm) on the right region, between optic trocar and the operative one 10–12-mm and another assistant 5-mm trocar in the left subcostal region (Fig. 16.2).

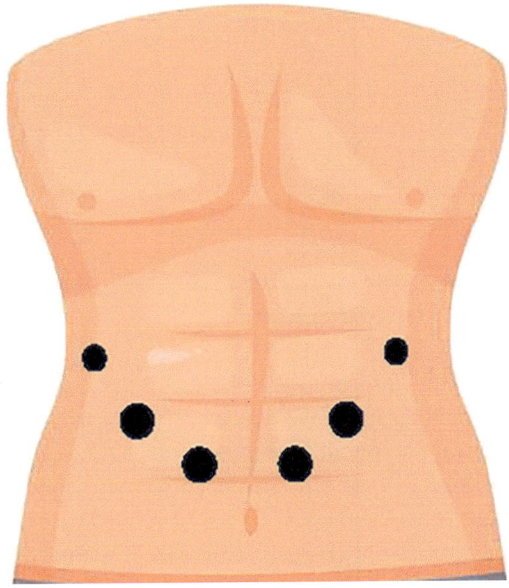

Fig. 16.1 Laparoscopic PD setup

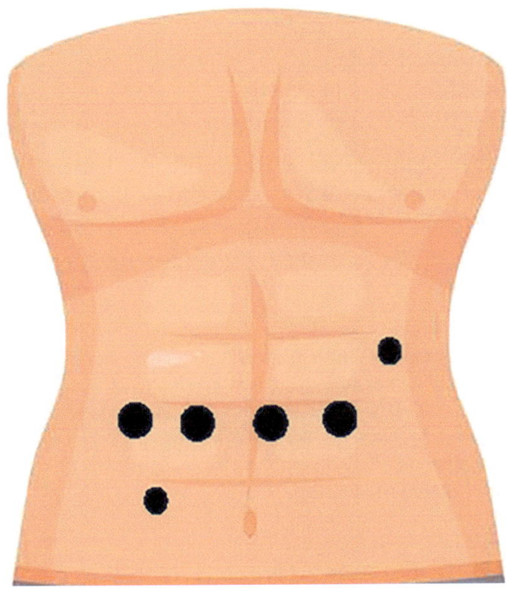

Fig. 16.2 Robotic PD setup

16.4 Surgical Procedure Step-by-Step

Step 1 As shown in the video, the gastrocolic ligament is opened, and a Cattell-Braasch maneuver is then performed (takedown of the hepatic flexure, mobilization of the right colon, and division of the mesentery root from the ileocecal junction to the left side of the mesenteric artery up to the Treitz ligament) [24].

Step 2 An extended Kocher maneuver is performed, and the right gastroepiploic vessels are identified and divided at their origin. This strategy, called right posterior AFA [25], allows to widely expose the origin of the SMA, thereby assessing tumor resectability before initiating any irreversible step (i.e., pancreas or stomach division). Additionally, the right posterior AFA provides an excellent control over the aortic plane at the level of the origin of the SMA and of the celiac artery (CA). Since this is the area where the mesopancreatic root is located, this unique view facilitates ME during minimally invasive DP. In fact, while the pancreatic isthmus is dissected from the SMA, if a cleavage plane is achieved, the ME is started around the origin of the SMA and carried on up to the CA's origin (Fig. 16.3).

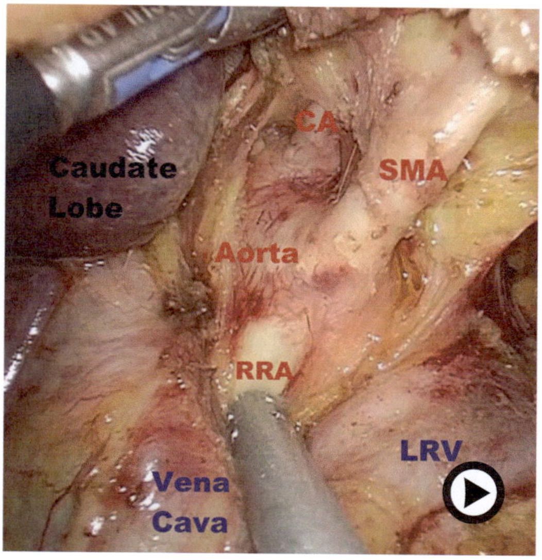

Fig. 16.3 Artery-first approach (AFA) view. The surgical plane achieved during the right posterior AFA is visible. The confluence of the left renal vein (LRV) into the vena cava represents the surgical landmark to identify the origin of the superior mesenteric artery (SMA) from the aorta. The origin of the celiac artery (CA) lies cranially, and the origin of the right renal artery (RRA) from the aorta is also visible. As displayed in the picture, the mesopancreas root has been dissected from the right side of the aorta and from the CA and SMA origins. Approaching the mesopancreas root during AFA facilitates the execution of a radical ME (Artery first approaches (▶ https://doi.org/10.1007/000-hf0))

Step 3 Division of the small omentum and lymphadenectomy of the retroportal area, common, and proper hepatic artery is performed. The origin of the gastroduodenal artery is identified, and the vessel is divided between clips.

Step 4 Division of the pancreas at the isthmus (video), hence further access to the SMA is achieved, then the inferior pancreaticoduodenal artery can be identified and ligated. The ME is then completed by further detachment of the mesopancreas from the right aspect of the SMA (Fig. 16.4). The resection is completed with the division of the hepatic duct above the cystic duct insertion and concomitant cholecystectomy.

Step 5 The ligament of Treitz is dissected, intestinal derotation is performed, the second jejunal loop is isolated and divided, and the first jejunal vein and artery are sectioned. This allows dissection of the duodenal and proximal jejunal mesentery together with the mesopancreas. At this stage, the "en bloc" specimen consisting of pancreatic head, duodenum, first jejunal loop (with the corresponding mesentery), and mesopancreas (Fig. 16.4b) is retrieved from a Pfannenstiel mini-laparotomy.

16.5 Postoperative Management

Patients are mobilized on the 1 postoperative day (POD) and gradually resume oral diet. Drain fluid amylase level is measured on 1 POD,

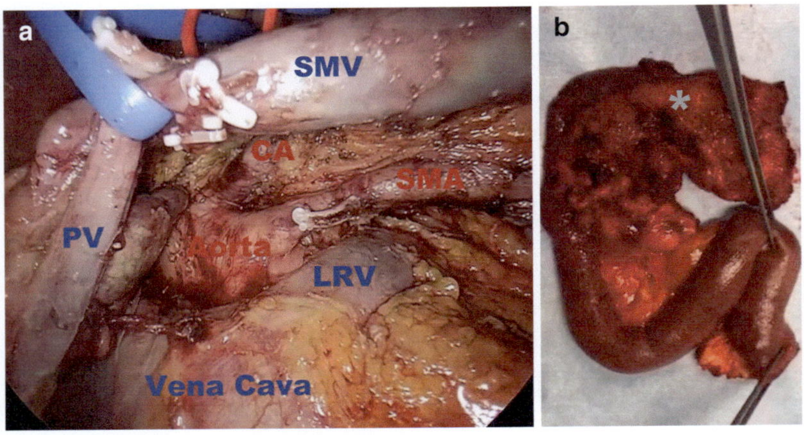

Fig. 16.4 Mesopancreas excision (ME). (**a**) shows the surgical plane achieved after completing ME. LRV, left renal vein; SMA, superior mesenteric artery; CA, celiac artery; PV, portal vein; SMV, superior mesenteric vein. The mesopancreas detached from the right side of the aorta and from the CA's and SMA's origins, during AFA, has now been detached from the right aspect of the SMA. In (**b**), the surgical specimen consisting of the pancreatic head with mesopancreas, duodenum with the mesoduodenum, and of the first jejunal loop with its mesentery, is shown

and drains with low amylase level and output are removed following the protocol of early drain removal management [26]. However, before pancreatic drains removal, a CT scan is always performed, to exclude possible intraabdominal fluid collections due to drains dislocation, even in case of low amylase level and low fluid output.

16.6 Tips and Tricks

- In our operative technique for pancreatic head's cancer, one of the first steps is represented by the right posterior AFA, which allows to promptly assess cancer resectability. Additionally, right posterior AFA provides an optimal view of the origins of the SMA and CA from the inframesocolic level. This unique view both provides an excellent control over the origins of the major arterial vessels (SMA and CA) and facilitates the dissection of the mesopancreatic root from those two vessels and the right aspect of the aorta.
- Cattell-Braasch maneuver allows the derotation of the entire intestine with en bloc resection of the mesoduodenum, mesojejunum, and pancreas, dominating the decrose of the superior mesenteric vessels which are in vertical axis during all the maneuvers.

References

1. Gromisch C, Qadan M, Machado MA, et al. Pancreatic adenocarcinoma: unconventional approaches for an unconventional disease. Cancer Res. 2020;80:3179–92.
2. Strobel O, Neoptolemos J, Jäger D, et al. Optimizing the outcomes of pancreatic cancer surgery. Nat Rev Clin Oncol. 2019;16:11–26.
3. Kang CM, Lee WJ. Is laparoscopic pancreaticoduodenectomy feasible for pancreatic ductal adenocarcinoma? Cancer. 2020;12:3430.
4. Artinyan A, Soriano PA, Prendergast C, et al. The anatomic location of pancreatic cancer is a prognostic factor for survival. HPB. 2008;10:371–6.
5. Farges O, Bendersky N, Truant S, et al. The theory and practice of pancreatic surgery in France. Ann Surg. 2017;266:797–804.
6. Gockel I, Domeyer M, Wolloscheck T, et al. Resection of the mesopancreas (RMP): a new surgical classification of a known anatomical space. World J Surg Oncol. 2007;5:1–8.
7. Hackert T, Strobel O, Michalski CW, et al. The TRIANGLE operation–radical surgery after neoadjuvant treatment for advanced pancreatic

cancer: a single arm observational study. HPB. 2017;19:1001–7.

8. Inoue Y, Saiura A, Oba A, et al. Optimal extent of superior mesenteric artery dissection during pancreaticoduodenectomy for pancreatic cancer: balancing surgical and oncological safety. J Gastrointest Surg. 2019;23:1373–83.
9. Quero G, Fiorillo C, Menghi R, et al. Total mesopancreas excision for periampullary malignancy: a single-center propensity score-matched comparison of long-term outcomes. Langenbeck's Arch Surg. 2020;405:303–12.
10. Fernandes ESM, Strobel O, Girão C, et al. What do surgeons need to know about the mesopancreas. Langenbeck's Arch Surg. 2021:1–12.
11. Sanjay P, Takaori K, Govil S, et al. 'Artery-first' approaches to pancreatoduodenectomy. J Br Surg. 2012;99:1027–35.
12. Gagner M, Pomp A. Laparoscopic pylorus-preserving pancreatoduodenectomy. Surg Endosc. 1994;8:408–10.
13. Asbun HJ, Stauffer JA. Laparoscopic vs open pancreaticoduodenectomy: overall outcomes and severity of complications using the accordion severity grading system. J Am Coll Surg. 2012;215:810–9.
14. Kim H, Song KB, Hwang DW, et al. Laparoscopic versus open pancreaticoduodenectomy for pancreatic neuroendocrine tumors: a single-center experience. Surg Endosc. 2019;33:4177–85.
15. Han SH, Kang CM, Hwang HK, et al. The Yonsei experience of 104 laparoscopic pancreaticoduodenectomies: a propensity score-matched analysis with open pancreaticoduodenectomy. Surg Endosc. 2020;34:1658–64.
16. Feng Q, Liao W, Xin Z, et al. Laparoscopic pancreaticoduodenectomy versus conventional open approach for patients with pancreatic duct adenocarcinoma: an up-to-date systematic review and meta-analysis. Front Oncol. 2021;11:4266.
17. Jiang Y-L, Zhang R-C, Zhou Y-C. Comparison of overall survival and perioperative outcomes of laparoscopic pancreaticoduodenectomy and open pancreaticoduodenectomy for pancreatic ductal adenocarcinoma: a systematic review and meta-analysis. BMC Cancer. 2019;19:1–9.
18. Yin Z, Jian Z, Hou B, et al. Surgical and oncological outcomes of laparoscopic versus open pancreaticoduodenectomy in patients with pancreatic duct adenocarcinoma. Pancreas. 2019;48:861–7.
19. van Hilst J, de Rooij T, Hilal MA, et al. Worldwide survey on opinions and use of minimally invasive pancreatic resection. HPB. 2017;19:190–204.
20. Sun R, Yu J, Zhang Y, et al. Perioperative and oncological outcomes following minimally invasive versus open pancreaticoduodenectomy for pancreatic duct adenocarcinoma. Surg Endosc. 2021;35:2273–85.
21. Choi M, Hwang HK, Lee WJ, et al. Total laparoscopic pancreaticoduodenectomy in patients with periampullary tumors: a learning curve analysis. Surg Endosc. 2021;35:2636–44.
22. Nickel F, Haney CM, Kowalewski KF, et al. Laparoscopic versus open pancreaticoduodenectomy: a systematic review and meta-analysis of randomized controlled trials. Ann Surg. 2020;271:54–66.
23. van Hilst J, de Graaf N, Abu Hilal M, et al. The landmark series: minimally invasive pancreatic resection. Ann Surg Oncol. 2021;28:1447–56.
24. Muttillo EM, Felli E, Pessaux P. Cattell-Braasch maneuver in pancreatic surgery. No need of venous graft for vascular resection. J Surg Oncol. 2020;122:1612–5.
25. Ielpo B, Anselmo A, Masuda Y, et al. Superior mesenteric artery first approach for minimally invasive pancreaticoduodenectomy: a step-by-step surgical technique video. Ann Surg Oncol. 2022:1–4.
26. Bassi C, Molinari E, Malleo G, et al. Early versus late drain removal after standard pancreatic resections: results of a prospective randomized trial. Ann Surg. 2010;252:207–14.

17 When and How to Convert During Robotic Pancreaticoduodenectomy

Maria Christodoulou, Tara M. Pattilachan, and Sharona B. Ross

17.1 Introduction

Pancreatic cancer presents a formidable challenge in the medical community, being the fourth leading cause of cancer-related deaths worldwide [1]. The mortality rates for pancreatic cancer are alarmingly close to its incidence rates, and as the prevalence of this disease continues to increase, it is anticipated that pancreatic cancer-related deaths may surpass those of other major cancers [2]. Surgical intervention, particularly pancreaticoduodenectomy, remains the only treatment for tumors located in the pancreatic head, periampullary region, and distal bile duct [3]. Pancreaticoduodenectomy is considered one of the most intricate and challenging operations in surgical practice, with a significant risk of perioperative morbidity and mortality. Despite the widespread adoption of laparoscopic techniques due to their positive impact on patient perioperative outcomes, pancreaticoduodenectomy predominantly is undertaken in an open approach in most centers [4]. This is largely due to the technical complexities and steep learning curve associated with these operations [5, 6]. Recently, robotic-assisted pancreaticoduodenectomy is increasingly recognized as a highly promising minimally invasive alternative to the traditional open approach, providing enhanced stability, dexterity, and three-dimensional (3D) high-resolution visualization [7, 8]. The advanced capabilities of the robotic platform enable precise intracorporeal suturing and greater control in difficult anatomical regions, thereby improving oncological outcomes and reducing postoperative complications [9].

Despite the advancements and benefits of robotic pancreaticoduodenectomy, certain intraoperative challenges may necessitate conversion to an open operation [10]. Conversions, though often perceived as a setback, are sometimes necessary decisions to ensure patient safety and optimal outcomes. Understanding the circumstances that lead to conversion and how to manage them effectively is essential for surgeons undertaking such complex operations. Based on existing literature, the rates of unplanned conversions often reflect a surgeon's ability to manage complex intraoperative challenges or unexpected disease presentations [11]. Patients requiring conversion tend to have poorer short-term and long-term outcomes, including higher mortality rates [12]. Previous studies in other surgical fields

Supplementary Information The online version contains supplementary material available at https://doi.org/10.1007/978-3-031-99695-5_17. The videos can be accessed individually by clicking the DOI link in the accompanying figure caption or by scanning this link with the SN More Media App.

M. Christodoulou · T. M. Pattilachan · S. B. Ross (✉)
Digestive Health Institute, AdventHealth Tampa, Tampa, FL, USA
e-mail: christodouloum20@gmail.com; tarapattilachan@gmail.com; mysharonaross@gmail.com

B. Ielpo et al. (eds.), *Minimally Invasive Pancreatoduodenectomy in Cancer*,
https://doi.org/10.1007/978-3-031-99695-5_17

have indicated that unplanned conversions are associated with worse outcomes compared to both minimally invasive and traditionally open operations [13].

This chapter aims to provide a detailed analysis of the circumstances necessitating a conversion from a robotic to an open approach during pancreaticoduodenectomy. Additionally, the chapter will discuss the strategic decision-making process and technical considerations crucial for undertaking a safe and effective conversion. By understanding these elements, surgeons will be better equipped to manage intraoperative challenges and optimize patient outcomes, even when conversion becomes necessary.

17.2 Indications for Conversions

The likelihood of unplanned conversions is influenced by various factors, including the surgeon's experience, patient characteristics, and intraoperative events. Conversion rates are higher at the beginning of the learning curve but decrease as surgeons gain more experience and as preoperative planning and patient selection improve. The reduction in conversion rates over time underscores the importance of meticulous patient selection and growing surgical expertise. Surgeons should carefully consider factors such as the extent of disease, tumor size, and patient obesity when evaluating candidates for robotic pancreaticoduodenectomy. Additionally, they should account for their level of expertise and where they stand on the learning curve. The increasing effectiveness of neoadjuvant chemotherapy for borderline resectable pancreatic adenocarcinoma is also crucial in enhancing surgical outcomes [14]. Studies utilizing the American College of Surgeons National Surgical Quality Improvement Program (ACS-NSQIP) database indicate unplanned conversion rates of 15% for robotic and 25% for laparoscopic pancreaticoduodenectomy [7, 11]. Our tertiary institution observed a lower conversion rate of 10.5%, likely due to a consistently high volume of cases and standardized operations from a single institution, unlike the varied settings in the ACS-NSQIP data [15]. These rates are typically higher for surgeons early in their learning curve but improve with increased experience [7]. Enhanced preoperative imaging and the growing use of neoadjuvant chemotherapy have also aided in better patient selection, contributing to reduced conversion rates [16].

Unplanned conversion can occur due to several intraoperative challenges. One significant reason is unexpected vascular involvement [15]. When operating on more extensive or locally advanced tumors, unforeseen engagement with major blood vessels may necessitate conversion. This is particularly relevant when manual palpation is required in cases of pancreatitis and fibrosis, which often obscure clear dissection planes commonly seen in pancreaticoduodenectomies. Another scenario necessitating conversion is uncontrolled intraoperative bleeding [15]. The inability to secure effective hemostasis or the necessity for extensive vascular repair presents a considerable challenge, particularly when the lead surgeon is operating from the console. While temporary bleeding control can be managed with local pressure, definitive hemostasis around critical vessels like the superior mesenteric artery and vein often requires open access for effective management. Visceral obesity is another factor that can lead to conversion. High BMI and central obesity complicate surgical exposure and make dissection more challenging. Although obesity has been identified as a risk factor for postoperative complications, it has not emerged as an independent risk factor in studies [17, 18]. The difficulty in achieving adequate exposure and navigating through the excess fatty tissue often necessitates conversion.

Patients who undergo unplanned conversion to open pancreaticoduodenectomy typically have worse outcomes compared to those whose operations are undertaken in a completely robotic fashion [19]. These patients tend to experience higher estimated blood loss (EBL), greater need for blood transfusions, increased complication rates, higher rates of clinically relevant postoperative pancreatic fistula (CR-POPF), prolonged ICU and hospital stays, and higher mortality rates. These adverse outcomes are consistent with findings in other surgical disciplines, where unplanned conversions from minimally invasive to an open operation are associated with poorer results [11, 12, 20, 21].

17.3 Preoperative Planning

17.3.1 Patient Selection and Assessment

Thorough preoperative planning is essential for the successful execution of robotic pancreaticoduodenectomy. Patient selection should be carefully considered, taking into account the individual's overall health, comorbidities, and anatomical characteristics. Individuals without significant vascular involvement or visceral obesity may be optimal candidates for robotic pancreaticoduodenectomy, as these factors can significantly increase the risk of conversion to an open operation [16]. Previous investigations at our high-volume tertiary center have demonstrated that robotic pancreaticoduodenectomy can yield positive outcomes even in octogenarians, indicating that advanced age alone should not disqualify patients from this surgical approach [22]. Conversely, a study conducted at our institution revealed an association between elevated BMI and longer operative durations in robotic pancreaticoduodenectomy [23]. This emphasizes the importance of strategic planning in these patients, as increased BMI can pose surgical challenges and prolong operative times. However, other perioperative outcomes, including estimated blood loss, intraoperative complications, conversion to an open operation, and length of stay, were not significantly impacted by BMI [25].

In addition to these considerations, our institution has developed the Tampa Difficulty Score, an online, open-source novel scoring system designed to predict the difficulty of robotic pancreaticoduodenectomy based on preoperative variables. This tool incorporates factors such as history of alcoholism, tumor size, preoperative endoscopic intervention, pancreatic duct dilation, and nodal disease on preoperative imaging. The Tampa Difficulty Score helps surgeons in preoperative planning by matching the complexity of the case to the surgeon's skill level and ensuring appropriate resource allocation. We believe the incorporation of this tool into routine preoperative assessment for robotic pancreaticoduodenectomy could improve surgical decision-making and patient outcomes.

17.3.2 Preoperative Imaging and Planning

Preoperative imaging is critical for planning the surgical approach and anticipating potential challenges. Triple-phase IV contrast abdominal CT scans with 1-mm cuts with reconstructions are widely used for diagnosis and staging and are standard at our institution. These imaging techniques help assess tumor size, location, and vascular involvement, which are key factors in determining the feasibility of robotic pancreaticoduodenectomy. In addition to detecting metastatic disease, triple-phase CT enables assessment of tumor characteristics (location, size, and extension), vascular involvement, and dilation of the biliary and pancreatic ducts [24, 25] (Fig. 17.1a, b). Additionally, MRI/MRCP can offer supplementary information for equivocal CT findings, particularly regarding hepatic lesions presumed to be metastatic, though CT remains more efficient in defining vascular involvement [26] (Fig. 17.1c, d). Endoscopic ultrasound (EUS) allows for histologic sampling via fine needle aspiration (FNA) to obtain a definitive pathological diagnosis prior to treatment initiation [27]. EUS may provide additional value in tumor staging and vessel involvement assessment. Routine endoscopic retrograde cholangiopancreatography (ERCP) with stenting for obstructing disease may increase postoperative complications and should be reserved for specific indications, such as neoadjuvant therapy, cholangitis, or biliary obstruction with a long interval to resection [28] (Fig. 17.1e). PET/CT's role in staging pancreatic ductal adenocarcinoma is debated due to variability in tumor PET avidity [29]. Our recommendation is a thorough review

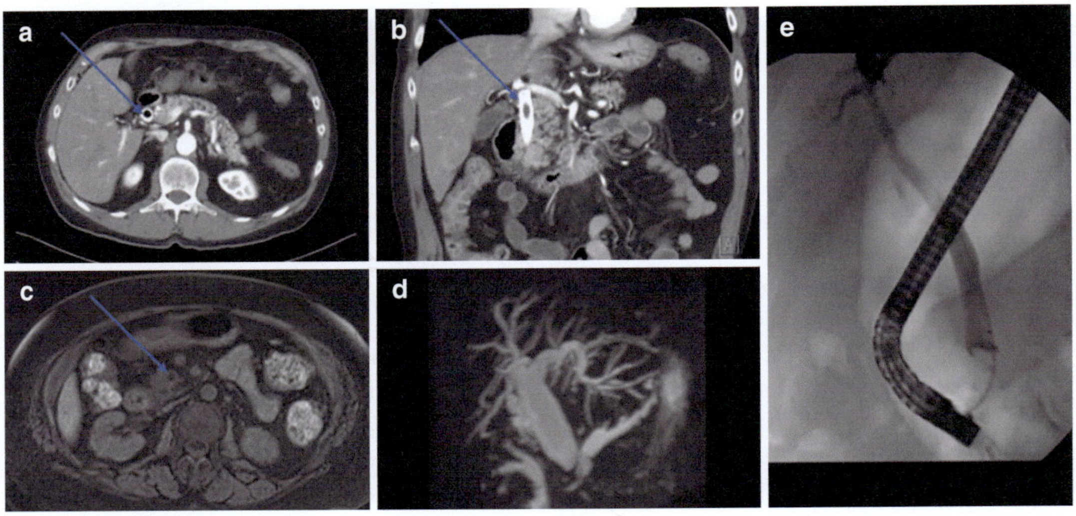

Fig. 17.1 Imaging modalities in evaluating robotic pancreaticoduodenectomy candidates. Triple-phase abdominal CT scan with 1 mm cuts shows cross-sectional (**a**) and coronal (**b**) views. Abdominal MRI (**c**) and MRCP (**d**) highlight common bile duct (CBD) dilation in the head of the pancreas (arrow). Endoscopic retrograde cholangiopancreatography (**e**) also demonstrates CBD

of all preoperative imaging to plan a reconstructive strategy, considering any vascular aberrations that may influence the decision for a robotic approach [30].

17.3.3 Multidisciplinary Team Approach and Optimization

A multidisciplinary team approach is necessary for the comprehensive management of patients undergoing robotic pancreaticoduodenectomy. This team should include surgeons, radiologists, gastroenterologists, oncologists, and anesthesiologists [30, 31]. Regular tumor board meetings can facilitate collaborative decision-making, ensuring that each patient's treatment plan is tailored to their specific needs [26]. This multidisciplinary approach should also be customized based on the stage of the disease, which is crucial to distinguish between early resectable, borderline resectable, and locally advanced disease [32, 33]. Moreover, thorough systemic assessments must also be conducted. For instance, upon diagnosis of pancreatic ductal adenocarcinoma, a majority of patients present with advanced disease not suitable for immediate surgical resection [34]. These patients are typically referred to an oncologist for neoadjuvant therapy (e.g., FOLFIRINOX) to potentially improve the chances of successful resection later on. Glycemic control is essential, as over 20% of pancreatic cancer patients present with hyperglycemia, ranging from impaired fasting glucose to new-onset diabetes mellitus, which should be managed preoperatively [32]. Cardiac assessment is recommended for patients at high risk for perioperative cardiac events [35, 36]. Although age does not preclude the robotic approach, age and frailty should still be considered preoperatively, as they may be associated with dismal postoperative outcomes [37, 38].

17.4 Managing Intraoperative Complications

Managing intraoperative complications during robotic pancreaticoduodenectomy is critical for ensuring patient safety and improving surgical outcomes, as intraoperative bleeding is one of the most challenging complications that can arise, and its early identification and prompt management are essential to prevent significant morbidity and mortality [16]. Continuous monitoring of the surgical field and hemodynamic parameters can help detect bleeding early. Visualization tools, such as the robotic system's 3D high-resolution imaging capacities, can also aid in identifying the source of bleeding more precisely [39].

17.4.1 Identification of Intraoperative Bleeding

As shown in the video, early identification of intraoperative bleeding is fundamental (Fig. 17.2). Surgeons must continuously monitor the surgical field and the patient's hemodynamic status. Immediate application of pressure to control the hemorrhage is essential. The use of robotic instruments (e.g., arm #1—fenestrated bipolar) to apply direct pressure or pack the bleeding area with gauze can also provide temporary control, such as the use of bipolar forceps, clip appliers, and suction/irrigation devices for effective hemostasis [16, 40].

17.4.2 Techniques for Temporary Control

Temporary control of bleeding is critical to stabilize the patient and allow for situational assessment (Fig. 17.3). Techniques such as direct pressure, packing, and the application of hemostatic agents are commonly used. Hemostatic agents, including fibrin glue (e.g., Tisseel™), oxidized regenerated cellulose (e.g., Surgicel™), and thrombin-based products (e.g., Floseal™), are effective in controlling bleeding and should be readily available in the operating room [41]. These agents must be applied meticulously to ensure adequate coverage of the bleeding site without compromising surrounding structures. It's important to note that although temporary hemostasis can often be achieved through simple measures such as direct pressure, definitive control of bleeding, particularly around the dorsal aspect of the superior mesenteric vessels, can be challenging before specimen removal [16].

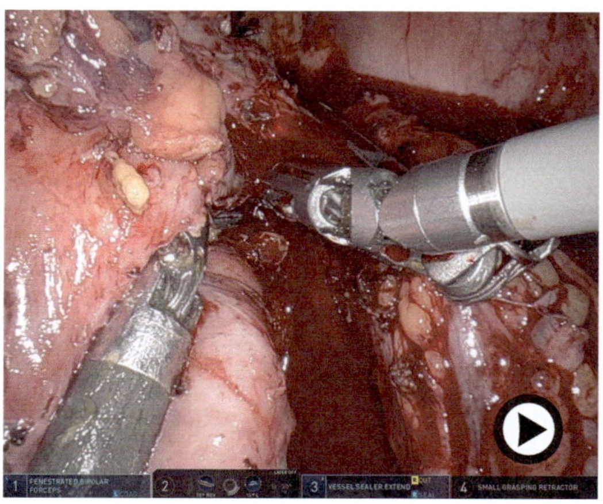

Fig. 17.2 Intraoperative bleeding encountered during robotic pancreaticoduodenectomy (▶ https://doi.org/10.1007/000-hf1)

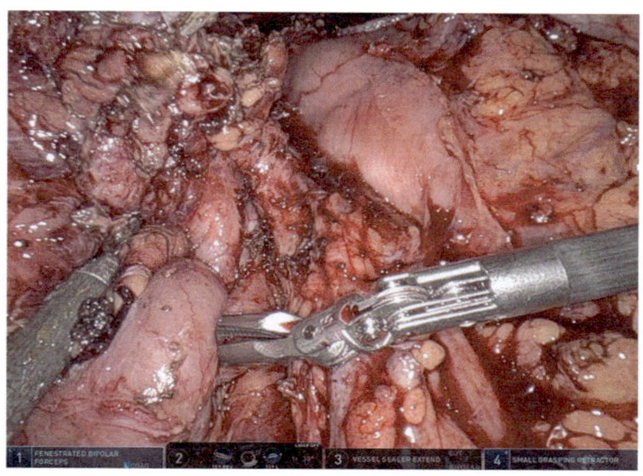

Fig. 17.3 Temporary control of intraoperative bleeding achieved

17.4.3 Vascular Structures Prone to Bleeding

Certain anatomical areas are particularly prone to bleeding during robotic pancreaticoduodenectomy. Just deep to the gastroduodenal artery (GDA) is the portal vein, which should be visible during dissection. On the right side is the common bile duct (CBD) [41, 42]. Careful dissection of the gastroduodenal vein, typically found on the right side of the GDA, is essential, as its injury can cause significant bleeding. The "first jejunal trunk" (FJT) in the region of the uncinate process is notorious for causing bleeding due to its U-shaped loop through the process [42]. The FJT is present in 58–88% of cases, and the proximal jejunal vein (PJV) located ventral to the superior mesenteric artery (SMA) is found in 13–37% of cases; both are associated with increased intraoperative bleeding and higher transfusion rates compared to those without these anatomical variations [43]. Thus, ensuring proper dissection and securing these veins are imperative to control bleeding in this area. Additionally, the gastrocolic trunk of Henle and the SMA are critical structures that, if injured, can lead to significant hemorrhage [44]. Proper identification and careful dissection of these vessels are essential to avoid uncontrolled bleeding (Fig. 17.4).

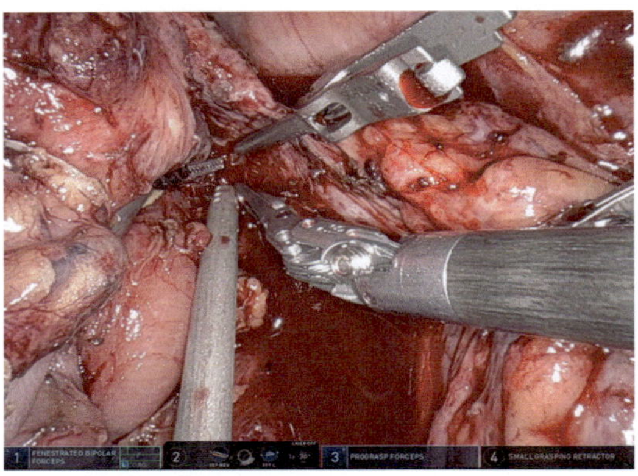

Fig. 17.4 Unsuccessful attempts to control bleeding robotically

17.4.4 Preparedness

"Disaster training" should occur frequently, with clearly delineated roles for everyone involved. It is recommended to remind the team of the steps for a safe unplanned conversion at the start of every operation during the briefing [16]. Once bleeding is identified, the first step is to obtain temporary control by grasping the bleeding vessel or applying pressure to the area. At this point, it is critical to call for the assistance of another experienced surgeon, even if the decision to convert has not yet been made. Effective communication with the bedside assistant, scrub tech, anesthesiologist, and the rest of the OR staff is imperative to update them on the situation. The surgeon should allow time for the OR team to optimize resources, obtain necessary blood products, and prepare the equipment required for conversion, if necessary. An experienced program coordinator can be helpful in orchestrating these efforts.

17.5 Stepwise Algorithm for Safe Conversion

Robotic pancreaticoduodenectomy involves several meticulously coordinated steps to ensure a successful outcome. The operation begins with precise port placement under direct videoscopic visualization and is followed by confirmation of the absence of metastatic disease (Fig. 17.5). Key dissection steps include undertaking the Kocher maneuver to mobilize the duodenum, dividing the jejunum, the gastrohepatic ligament, the duodenum, and the pancreatic neck. Meticulous dissection along the SMV, SMA, and portal vein is also essential to minimize bleeding risk during the operation. Reconstruction involves creating three anastomoses, hepaticojejunostomy, pancreatojejunostomy, and duodenojejunostomy, using advanced suturing techniques to ensure secure connections. Each operation phase has been thoroughly detailed in previously published chapters,

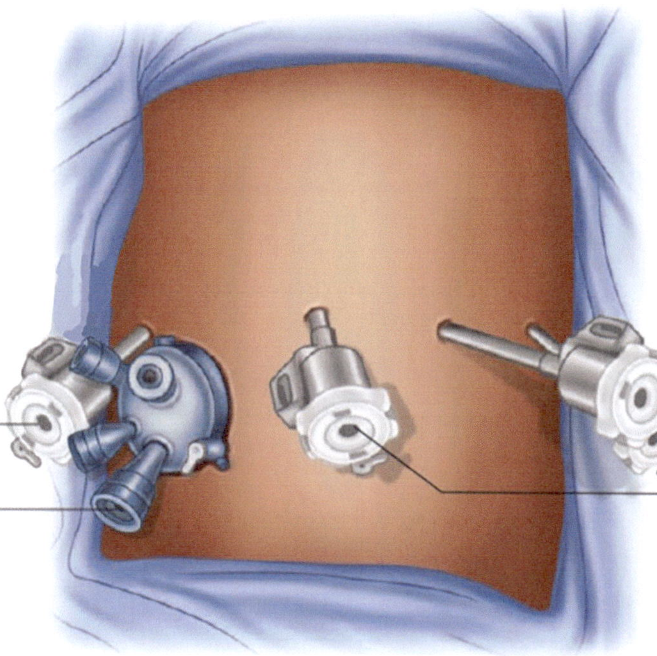

Fig. 17.5 Port placement for robotic pancreaticoduodenectomy

providing comprehensive guidance on the technical and critical maneuvers essential for minimizing complications and enhancing patient outcomes in undertaking robotic pancreaticoduodenectomy [30, 45–47].

Given the complexity of this operation, the decision to convert from a robotic to an open operation should be made promptly when it becomes evident that bleeding cannot be controlled robotically (Fig. 17.4). Factors influencing this decision include the surgeon's experience, the location and severity of bleeding, and the patient's hemodynamic stability. An organized stepwise approach ensures patient safety and minimizes complications during conversion. To achieve this, we suggest the following structured algorithm for managing unplanned conversions due to uncontrollable intraoperative bleeding (Fig. 17.6). It is recommended that at the beginning of each operation, a brief reminder of the steps for a safe unplanned conversion should be included in the team briefing. When significant bleeding occurs, the first step is to achieve temporary control. This can be done by grasping the bleeding vessel or applying pressure to the bleeding site. It is critical to call for the assistance of another experienced surgeon immediately, even if the decision to convert has not yet been finalized. Effective communication with the assistant at the bedside, the scrub tech, the anesthesiologist, and the rest of the OR staff is essential to keep them informed about the current situation. Allow adequate time for the OR team to optimize resources, including obtaining necessary blood products and opening conversion-specific equipment. Calling for additional experienced personnel, such as other surgeons or the anesthesia care team, is strongly recommended. Having an experienced program coordinator to manage this process is crucial.

When all else seems to have failed, it's time to ask for help, and if that fails, it's now time to convert to open. If the decision to convert is made, avoid removing the robotic instruments and scope immediately. The scope (arm 2) and the instrument providing hemostasis (typically arm 1) should remain in place to maintain the stability of the temporary control while the incision is made (Fig. 17.7). The scope should remain in place to ensure continued visualization and con-

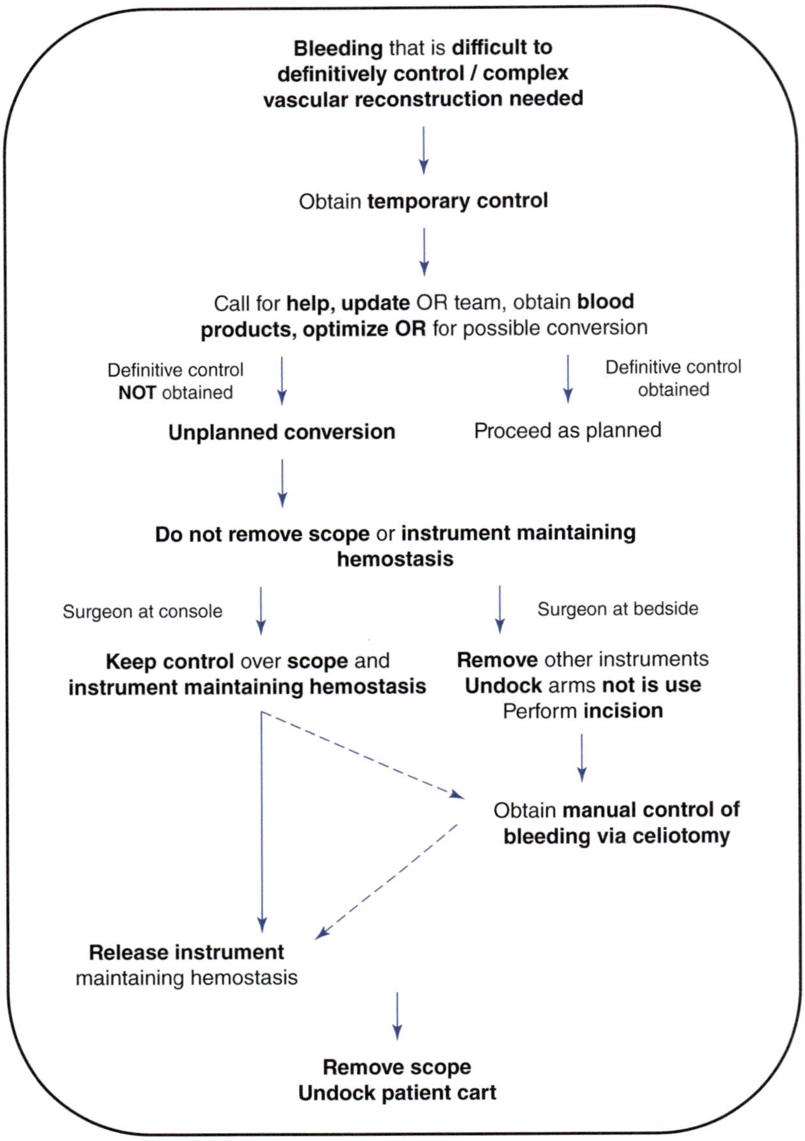

Fig. 17.6 Stepwise algorithm for safe conversion to open operation in robotic pancreaticoduodenectomy

trol. Removing the scope could lead to manual and blind control of the instrument, which is not advisable.

Incising the peritoneal membrane should not be undertaken until everything is ready for rapid vascular control. One experienced surgeon must remain at the robotic console while another scrubs in to undertake the remaining of the operation in an open approach. At this stage, robotic instruments in arms 3 and 4 can be removed, their arms undocked, and the trocars taken out. A right subcostal incision (Kocher incision) is recommended for better access around arms 1 and 2. Once the incision is made and the bedside surgeon has manual control of the bleeding, the console surgeon can release the instrument in arm 1 (Fig. 17.8). The scope (arm 2) can then be removed, and the robot undocked. After undocking, continue to manage the patient according to the principles of an open operation. Stabilize the patient, complete necessary hemostatic maneuvers, and address

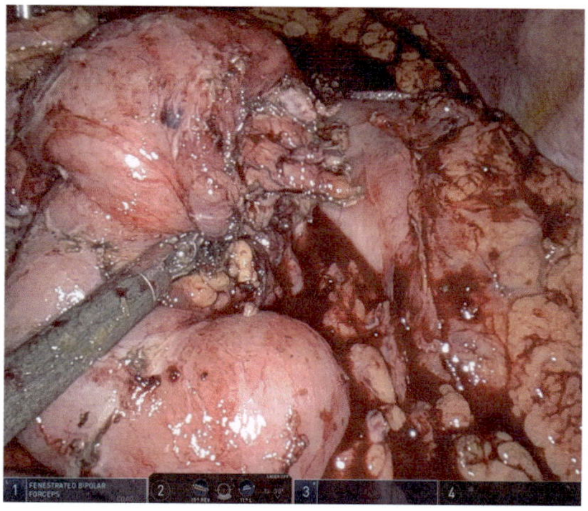

Fig. 17.7 Temporary control of bleeding prior to the decision to convert to "Open"

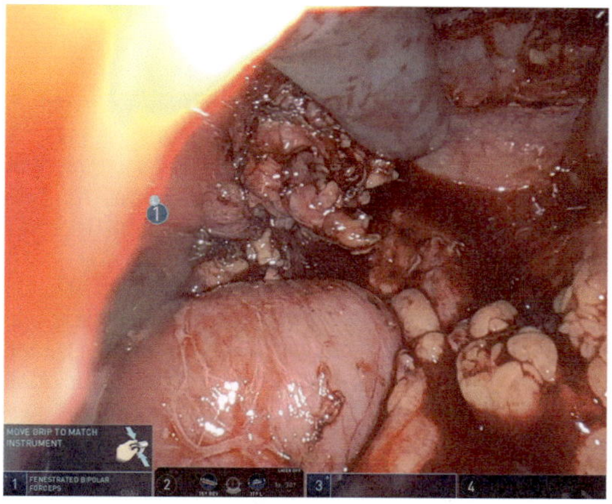

Fig. 17.8 Conversion to "Open:" removal of robotic instruments and manual control of bleeding

any additional complications. An example of a safe unplanned conversion is presented in Supplemental Material Video 1.

17.6 Practical Tips and Tricks

17.6.1 Practical Tips from Experienced Surgeons

- *Preoperative planning:* Conduct a thorough imaging review and brief the team on potential challenges and conversion steps. Utilize tools such as our Tampa Difficulty Score to assess case complexity and plan accordingly. Ensure all necessary equipment and hemostatic agents are available.
- *Experience and mastery:* Recognize that unplanned conversions significantly impair short-term outcomes and increase mortality. However, their occurrence decreases with growing surgeon and team experience. Achieving mastery on the steep learning curve is critical to reducing unplanned conversions and improving patient outcomes [1].
- *Regular "Disaster" training:* Conduct "disaster training" frequently to prepare the team for potential complications, intraoperative hemorrhages, and unplanned conversions [1].
- *Psychological preparedness:* Mental preparedness is key. Encourage mindfulness and stress-management techniques among the surgical team to maintain focus and composure during high-pressure situations.
- *Time management in conversion:* Prompt decision-making and quick action are essential during conversion. Delaying the decision to convert can increase the risk of complications. Once the decision is made, follow the structured, stepwise algorithm to ensure a safe and efficient conversion process.

17.6.2 Key Decision Points

- *Assessing bleeding severity:* Evaluate if bleeding can be controlled robotically based on its location, severity, and the patient's stability.
- *Calling for assistance:* Promptly seek help from an experienced surgeon if initial measures fail. Clear communication with the OR team is essential to ensure readiness for conversion if needed.
- *Implementing the stepwise algorithm for conversion:* Obtain temporary control of bleeding, take a deep breath, communicate the need for help, and prepare for conversion by optimizing resources and maintaining stability until manual control is achieved.

17.7 Conclusions

Robotic pancreaticoduodenectomy signifies a substantial advancement in minimally invasive surgery, offering increased precision, visualization, and the potential for improved patient outcomes. However, the possibility of unplanned conversion to an open operation demonstrates the importance of thorough preoperative planning, strategic intraoperative decision-making, and effective communication among the surgical team. Ensuring patient safety during such conversions requires comprehensive preparation and seamless coordination. Future research should focus on refining robotic techniques, developing robust predictive tools for conversion, and improving training programs to better navigate the steep learning curve, minimizing conversion rates in itself. Continued innovation and collaboration within the surgical community will be paramount in advancing the efficacy and safety of robotic pancreaticoduodenectomy.

Statements and Declarations No funding sources was received specific to this paper.

References

1. American Society of Clinical Oncology. Pancreatic Cancer Statistics. Cancer Net; 2023. https://www.cancer.net/cancer-types/pancreatic-cancer/statistics#:~:text=It%20is%20the%20fourth%20leading,worldwide%20died%20from%20pancreatic%20cancer
2. GBD 2017 Pancreatic Cancer Collaborators. The global, regional, and national burden of pancreatic cancer and its attributable risk factors in 195 countries and territories, 1990–2017: a systematic analysis for the Global Burden of Disease Study 2017 [published correction appears in Lancet Gastroenterol Hepatol. 2020 Mar;5(3):e2]. Lancet Gastroenterol Hepatol. 2019;4(12):934–947.
3. Zureikat AH, Beane JD, Zenati MS, Al Abbas AI, Boone BA, Moser AJ, Bartlett DL, Hogg ME, Zeh HJ 3rd. 500 minimally invasive robotic pancreatoduodenectomies: one decade of optimizing performance. Ann Surg. 2021;273(5):966–72. https://doi.org/10.1097/SLA.0000000000003550.
4. Wei Q, Fan Y, Wang C. Surgical procedures and experience sharing of robotic pancreaticoduodenectomy. Int Surg. 2023;6:34–9. https://doi.org/10.1016/j.isurg.2023.06.001.
5. Shyr BU, Chen SC, Shyr YM, Wang SE. Learning curves for robotic pancreatic surgery-from distal pancreatectomy to pancreaticoduodenectomy. Medicine. 2018;97(45):e13000. https://doi.org/10.1097/MD.0000000000013000.
6. Haney CM, Karadza E, Limen EF, de Santibanes M, Kinny-Koester B, Müller PC, Bintintan VV, Kulu Y, Hackert T, Müller-Stich BP, Nickel F. Training and learningcurves in minimally invasive pancreatic surgery: from simulationto mastery. J Pancreatol. 2020;2020(3):101–10. https://doi.org/10.1097/JP9.0000000000000050.
7. Davis CH, Grandhi MS, Gazivoda VP, Greenbaum A, Kennedy TJ, Langan RC, Alexander HR, Pitt HA, August DA. Robotic pancreatoduodenectomy: trends in technique and training challenges. Surg Endosc. 2023;37(1):266–73. https://doi.org/10.1007/s00464-022-09469-3.
8. Rosemurgy A, Ross S, Bourdeau T, Jacob K, Thomas J, Przetocki V, Luberice K, Sucandy I. Cost analysis of pancreaticoduodenectomy at a high-volume robotic hepatopancreaticobiliary surgery program. J Am Coll Surg. 2021;232(4):461–9. https://doi.org/10.1016/j.jamcollsurg.2020.12.062.
9. Rosemurgy AS, Ross SB, Espeut A, Nguyen D, Crespo K, Syblis C, Vasanthakumar P, Sucandy I. Survival and robotic approach for pancreaticoduodenectomy: a propensity score-match study. J Am Coll Surg. 2022;234(4):677–84. https://doi.org/10.1097/XCS.0000000000000137.
10. Abd El Aziz MA, Grass F, Behm KT, D'Angelo AL, Mathis KL, Dozois EJ, Larson DW. Trends and consequences of surgical conversion in the United States. Surg Endosc. 2022;36(1):82–90. https://doi.org/10.1007/s00464-020-08240-w.
11. Stiles ZE, Dickson PV, Deneve JL, Glazer ES, Dong L, Wan JY, Behrman SW. The impact of unplanned conversion to an open procedure during minimally invasive pancreatectomy. J Surg Res. 2018;227:168–77. https://doi.org/10.1016/j.jss.2018.02.028.
12. Halpern AL, Friedman C, Torphy RJ, Al-Musawi MH, Mitchell JD, Scott CD, Meguid RA, McCarter MD, Weyant MJ, Gleisner AL. Conversion to open surgery during minimally invasive esophagectomy portends worse short-term outcomes: an analysis of the National Cancer Database. Surg Endosc. 2020;34(8):3470–8. https://doi.org/10.1007/s00464-019-07124-y.
13. Lee YF, Albright J, Akram WM, Wu J, Ferraro J, Cleary RK. Unplanned robotic-assisted conversion-to-open colorectal surgery is associated with adverse outcomes. J Gastrointest Surg. 2018;22(6):1059–67. https://doi.org/10.1007/s11605-018-3706-0.
14. van Veldhuisen E, Klompmaker S, Janssen QP, Hilal MA, Alseidi A, Balduzzi A, Balzano G, Bassi C, Berrevoet F, Bonds M, Busch OR, Butturini G, Conlon KC, Frigerio IM, Fusai GK, Gagnière J, Griffin O, Hackert T, Halimi A, Keck T, Scientific Committee of the European-African Hepato-Pancreato-Biliary Association. Surgical and oncological outcomes after preoperative FOLFIRINOX chemotherapy in resected

pancreatic cancer: an international multicenter cohort study. Ann Surg Oncol. 2023;30(3):1463–73. https://doi.org/10.1245/s10434-022-12387-2.
15. Slavin M, Ross SB, Sucandy I, Saravanan S, Crespo KL, Syblis CC, Trotto MS, Rosemurgy AS. Unplanned conversions of robotic pancreaticoduodenectomy: short-term outcomes and suggested stepwise approach for a safe conversion. Surg Endosc. 2024;38(2):964–74. https://doi.org/10.1007/s00464-023-10527-7.
16. de Geus SWL, Sachs TE. A paradigm shifts: neoadjuvant therapy for clearly resectable pancreatic cancer. Ann Surg Oncol. 2023;30(6):3427–36. https://doi.org/10.1245/s10434-023-13281-1.
17. Tanaka K, Yamada S, Sonohara F, Takami H, Hayashi M, Kanda M, Kobayashi D, Tanaka C, Nakayama G, Koike M, Fujiwara M, Kodera Y. Pancreatic fat and body composition measurements by computed tomography are associated with pancreatic fistula after pancreatectomy. Ann Surg Oncol. 2021;28(1):530–8. https://doi.org/10.1245/s10434-020-08581-9.
18. Greenblatt DY, Kelly KJ, Rajamanickam V, Wan Y, Hanson T, Rettammel R, Winslow ER, Cho CS, Weber SM. Preoperative factors predict perioperative morbidity and mortality after pancreaticoduodenectomy. Ann Surg Oncol. 2011;18(8):2126–35. https://doi.org/10.1245/s10434-011-1594-6.
19. Villano AM, Ruth K, Castellanos J, Farma JM, Reddy SS. Discrepancies in survival after conversion to open in minimally invasive pancreatoduodenectomy. Am J Surg. 2023;225(4):728–34. https://doi.org/10.1016/j.amjsurg.2022.10.056.
20. Stiles ZE, Behrman SW, Glazer ES, Deneve JL, Dong L, Wan JY, Dickson PV. Predictors and implications of unplanned conversion during minimally invasive hepatectomy: an analysis of the ACS-NSQIP database. HPB (Oxford). 2017;19(11):957–65. https://doi.org/10.1016/j.hpb.2017.06.012.
21. Nassour I, Wang SC, Porembka MR, Augustine MM, Yopp AC, Mansour JC, Minter RM, Choti MA, Polanco PM. Conversion of minimally invasive distal pancreatectomy: predictors and outcomes. Ann Surg Oncol. 2017;24(12):3725–31. https://doi.org/10.1245/s10434-017-6062-5.
22. Ross S, Sucandy I, Vasanthakumar P, Christodoulou M, Pattilachan T, Rosemurgy A. A comparative analysis of robotic versus open pancreaticoduodenectomy in octogenarians. J Robot Surg. 2024;18(1):183.
23. Rayman S, Ross SB, Sucandy I, et al. Weighing the outcomes: the role of BMI in complex robotic esophageal and hepatobiliary operations. Updat Surg. 2024;76(3):1031–9.
24. Elbanna KY, Jang HJ, Kim TK. Imaging diagnosis and staging of pancreatic ductal adenocarcinoma: a comprehensive review. Insights Imaging. 2020;11(1):58.
25. Tamm EP, Balachandran A, Bhosale PR, et al. Imaging of pancreatic adenocarcinoma: update on staging/resectability. Radiol Clin North Am. 2012;50(3):407–28.
26. Fogel EL, Shahda S, Sandrasegaran K, et al. A multidisciplinary approach to pancreas cancer in 2016: a review. Am J Gastroenterol. 2017;112(4):537–54.
27. He MJ, Chen TY, Liu XY, Xu XY, Zhou PH, Zhang YQ. Utility of endoscopic ultrasound-guided fine-needle aspiration in pancreatic cancer patients who failed to obtain a pathological diagnosis in surgical exploration. Gland Surg. 2022;11(2):426–31.
28. van der Gaag NA, Rauws EA, van Eijck CH, et al. Preoperative biliary drainage for cancer of the head of the pancreas. N Engl J Med. 2010;362(2):129–37.
29. Ghanta B, Thambi-Pillai TC, Timmerman G, Fischer C, Nelson A, Bleeker JS. Role of FDG PET/CT scan in preoperative pancreatic cancer staging. J Clin Oncol. 2018;36(4_suppl):511.
30. Ross SRS, Sucandy I, Syblis C, Rosemurgy A. Whipple's operation and distal pancreatectomy. Costello's Principles and Practice of Robotic Surgery. 2023; In press
31. Taberna M, Gil Moncayo F, Jané-Salas E, et al. The multidisciplinary team (MDT) approach and quality of care. Front Oncol. 2020;10:85.
32. Singhi AD, Koay EJ, Chari ST, Maitra A. Early detection of pancreatic cancer: opportunities and challenges. Gastroenterology. 2019;156(7):2024–40.
33. Tempero MA. NCCN guidelines updates: pancreatic cancer. J Natl Compr Cancer Netw. 2019;17(5.5):603–5.
34. Ansari D, Gustafsson A, Andersson R. Update on the management of pancreatic cancer: surgery is not enough. World J Gastroenterol. 2015;21(11):3157–65.
35. Wiltberger G, Muhl B, Benzing C, et al. Preoperative risk stratification for major complications following pancreaticoduodenectomy: identification of high-risk patients. Int J Surg. 2016;31:33–9.
36. Smilowitz NR, Berger JS. Perioperative cardiovascular risk assessment and management for noncardiac surgery: a review. JAMA. 2020;324(3):279–90.
37. Mogal H, Vermilion SA, Dodson R, et al. Modified frailty index predicts morbidity and mortality after pancreaticoduodenectomy. Ann Surg Oncol. 2017;24(6):1714–21.
38. Liang Y, Zhao L, Jiang C, et al. Laparoscopic pancreaticoduodenectomy in elderly patients. Surg Endosc. 2020;34(5):2028–34.
39. Wang Y, Cao D, Chen SL, Li YM, Zheng YW, Ohkohchi N. Current trends in three-dimensional visualization and real-time navigation as well as robot-assisted technologies in hepatobiliary surgery. World J Gastrointest Surg. 2021;13(9):904–22.
40. Brown KGM, Solomon MJ. Topical haemostatic agents in surgery. Br J Surg 2024; 111(1).
41. Ielpo B, Anselmo A, Koh Y, Burdio F, De Blasi V, Sanchez-Velazquez P, Azagra JS, Huscher C, Giuliani A, Pellino G, Rosso E. Minimally invasive pancreatic anastomosis after pancreaticoduodenectomy: multi-institutional step by step video description of the technique. Updat Surg. 2023;75(1):255–9. https://doi.org/10.1007/s13304-022-01389-0. Epub 2022 Nov 12. PMID: 36371550

42. Agarwal BB, Dhamija N. Robotic assisted pancreaticoduodenectomy. In: Sharma D, Hazrah P, editors. Recent concepts in minimal access surgery, vol. 1. Singapore: Springer Singapore; 2022. p. 111–32.
43. Kang MJ, Han SS, Park SJ, Park HM, Kim SW. Do jejunal veins matter during pancreaticoduodenectomy? Ann Hepatobiliary Pancreat Surg. 2022;26(3):229–34.
44. AlMasri S, Kraftician J, Zureikat A, Paniccia A. Management of intra-operative hemorrhage and safe venous resection in robotic-assisted pancreaticoduodenectomy: techniques to avoid open conversion. J Gastrointest Surg. 2023;27(8):1753–6.
45. Ross SB, Downs D, Sucandy I, Rosemurgy AS. Robotic pylorus-preserving pancreaticoduodenectomy. In: Fong Y, Woo Y, Hyung W, Lau C, Strong V, editors. The SAGES atlas of robotic surgery. Cham.: 319-334 Online 9/9/2018.: Springer; 2018. https://doi.org/10.1007/978-3-319-91045-1_28.
46. Rosemurgy A, Ross S, Luberice K, Browning H, Sucandy I. In: Martin R, editor. Robotic pancreatic surgery for solid, cystic, and mixed lesions, vol. 100. Surgical Clinics of North America: Robotic Surgery; 2020. p. 303–36.
47. Ross SB, Bourdeau T, Sucandy I, Rosemurgy AS. Robotic pancreaticoduodenectomy. Robotic General Surgery. Atlas of Robotic General Surgery E-Book.

Complex Pancreatic Anastomosis After Pancreaticoduodenectomy: A Comprehensive Guide

18

Gemma Vellalta Muxi, Benedetto Ielpo, and Edoardo Rosso

18.1 Introduction

Pancreaticoduodenectomy (PD) is a critical surgical procedure for treating pancreatic and periampullary disorders, whether malignant or benign. Traditionally, it has been associated with high morbidity and mortality, especially due to the complexity of pancreatic anastomosis (PA). In parallel, the advent of minimally invasive surgery, including both laparoscopic and robotic techniques, has significantly demonstrated improved patient outcomes. However, these advancements bring new challenges, particularly in mastering PA in a minimally invasive setting.

Complex PA, even following minimally invasive pancreaticoduodenectomy (MIPD), remains a challenging situation, often associated with a high risk of postoperative pancreatic fistula and its consequences. Factors determining whether a PA might be considered a high-complexity case involve invisible pancreatic ducts, bulky and fatty pancreatic stumps, ongoing acute pancreatitis, or the need for reintervention [1]. In addition, any patient presenting general risk factors such as high comorbidity is also considered complex PA.

In recent years, several new techniques have been introduced, each offering specific advantages [2–6]. However, the choice of PA technique still largely depends on the surgeon's experience. Additionally, while many complications can be predicted, unexpected situations may arise during surgery, requiring quick, in-the-moment decisions in the operating room.

This chapter provides a comprehensive guide to managing complex PAs, offering strategies for preoperative, intraoperative, and reintervention scenarios. It aims to equip surgeons with the knowledge and techniques necessary to handle the complexities of PA in the context of MIPD, ultimately improving patient outcomes and reducing complications.

Supplementary Information The online version contains supplementary material available at https://doi.org/10.1007/978-3-031-99695-5_18. The videos can be accessed individually by clicking the DOI link in the accompanying figure caption or by scanning this link with the SN More Media App.

G. Vellalta Muxi (✉)
General Surgery and Laparoscopic Surgery, Clínica Corachan, Barcelona, Spain
e-mail: vellalta.muxi@gmail.com

B. Ielpo
Hepato-Biliary and Pancreatic Surgery Unit, Department of Surgery, Hospital del Mar, Pompeu Fabra University, Barcelona, Spain

E. Rosso
Centre de Chirurgie Digestive – Pole Santé Sud, Le Mans, France

B. Ielpo et al. (eds.), *Minimally Invasive Pancreatoduodenectomy in Cancer*,
https://doi.org/10.1007/978-3-031-99695-5_18

18.2 Management of Complex Pancreatic Anastomosis Patients

Managing complex PA patients requires a structured and thorough approach. This involves careful preoperative planning, choosing the appropriate intraoperative techniques, and proper postoperative management, including rare special cases that need reintervention. Here, we provide detailed guidance on each stage of the process, aiming to optimize patient outcomes and reduce complications. By addressing the specific challenges of PA, including but not limited to those specific to minimally invasive pancreaticoduodenectomy, surgeons can improve their proficiency and patient care.

Figure 18.1 provides a schematic with the main recommended approaches for each given scenario covered in this manuscript for managing complex PAs, providing surgeons with a quick reference.

18.2.1 Preoperative Management

Effective preoperative management is crucial for optimizing outcomes in complex pancreatic anastomosis (PA) patients. This includes thorough assessment and preparation of the intervention, including the necessary patient prehabilitation and detailed planning of the intervention. As is well known, prehabilitation strategies, which include nutritional support and physical conditioning, can improve patient resilience and readiness for surgery [7, 8].

Notwithstanding, preoperative preparation is particularly important for those patients with high-risk factors. These are more susceptible to severe postoperative complications, such as Grade C postoperative pancreatic fistula (POPF), postoperative biliary fistula, postoperative hemorrhage, or infected fluid collections. Metrics such as "failure to rescue" (FTR) which describes the mortality following a major complication can help understand how high-risk patients can benefit from well-executed preoperative management.

For these high-risk patients with significant comorbidities, a preoperative evaluation might lead to considering a total pancreatectomy. This preoperative decision often allows for a planned spleen-preserving pancreatectomy. Video 1. shows a totalization procedure with spleen preservation in an 86-year-old patient with pancreatic adenocarcinoma.

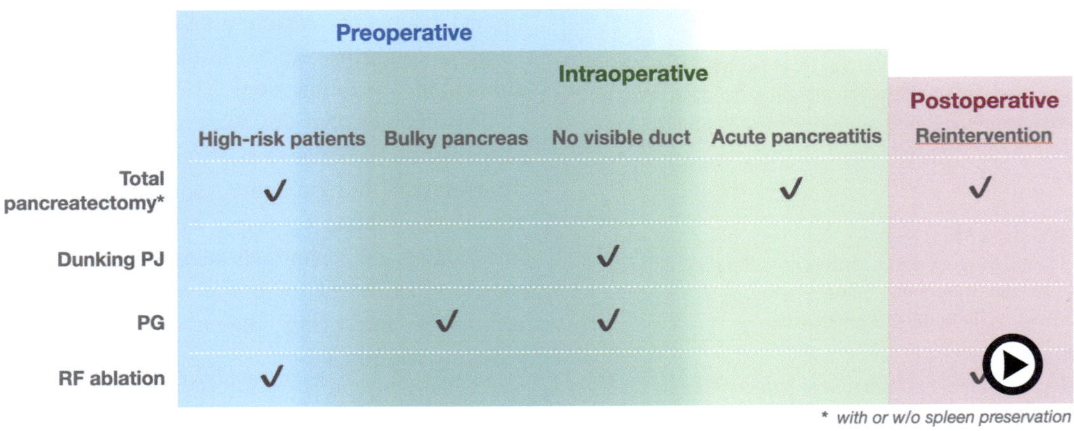

Fig. 18.1 Schematic showing the main recommended approaches for each of the complex PA situations tackled in this chapter (Footage of a totalization procedure with spleen preservation in an 86-year-old patient with pancreatic adenocarcinoma (▶ https://doi.org/10.1007/000-hf4))

18.2.2 Intraoperative Management

Intraoperative management of complex pancreatic anastomosis (PA) often involves adapting techniques to unexpected challenges encountered during surgery. Here are key considerations for managing such complexities:

18.2.2.1 Absence of a Visible Main Pancreatic Duct

The absence of a visible main pancreatic duct (MPD) can complicate the creation of a secure anastomosis. Lack of MPD visibility is quite often associated with premalignant pathologies, benign pathologies, or borderline tumors with low malignant potential. Less frequent are anatomical variations or developmental anomalies, such as ansa pancreatica and meandering main pancreatic duct, pancreas divisum, or accessory pancreatic duct, that may obscure the duct [9, 10]. In these cases, traditional duct-to-mucosa pancreaticojejunostomy (PJ) is not feasible. Alternatives like dunking PJ [2] or pancreaticogastrostomy (PG), which involve invaginating the pancreas into the small intestine or stomach, respectively, can be employed to bypass the need for formal anastomosis on the Wirsung duct.

18.2.2.2 Fatty-Bulky Pancreatic Stump

A bulky and fatty pancreatic stump presents another intraoperative challenge (Fig. 18.2). While these conditions are frequently identified intraoperatively, they can sometimes be detected preoperatively through MRI and CT scans [11, 12] (Fig. 18.2c, d), often associated with obesity and older age. High body mass index and stump morphology are predictors of an increased risk of clinically relevant POPF [1, 13, 14]. The diameter of the pancreatic stump often exceeds the height of the small bowel, complicating the anastomosis and suturing process.

In these cases, PG is preferred over PJ, as the size of the stump might prevent PJ's such as Blumgart or Peng. Key technical steps to attaining a safe PG include mobilizing the pancreatic stump from both the splenic vein and artery to avoid tension on the anastomosis in the so-called Pisa Tower effect [15], making an incision on the stomach wall that matches the stump's length in order to prevent intussusception, and adopting a purse-string technique, avoiding stitches that could easily tear the pancreatic wall.

In video 2, we present a case involving a fatty, bulky pancreas and describe several technical details related to the procedure. The footage demonstrates the surgeons' decision to perform a pancreaticogastrostomy, which was an appropriate choice given the circumstances.

18.2.2.3 Ongoing Acute Pancreatitis

Inflammation, swelling, and steatonecrosis are rare findings but can sometimes be noticed during PD, usually when inspecting the remaining pancreas after the resection phase. Pancreatitis in the pancreatic stump introduces additional risks. The inflamed and fragile nature of the tissue makes it difficult to achieve stable and leak-proof anastomosis. Surgeons need to adapt their techniques to manage these delicate tissues effectively.

In cases of acute pancreatitis with significant inflammation and necrosis, total pancreatectomy may be considered to avoid the complications associated with PA.

Footage of a cephalic duodenopancreatectomy (CDP) is shown in video 3, where, after portal vein resection, the surgeons opted for a totalization after findings of pancreatitis in the pancreatic stump.

18.2.2.4 Patients with Overall High Risk—Estimating Risk (Risk Calculators)

Identifying high-risk patients intraoperatively is crucial to deciding between performing a PA or opting for a near-total or total pancreatectomy [16, 17].

Besides preoperative risk factors such as underlying conditions, sarcopenia, or obesity, the main intraoperative factors that drive the surgeon's decision include the consistency of the pancreas, the duct's diameter, and intraoperative bleeding.

To help the surgeon in this decision, statistical risk scoring models [18–20] and their online risk

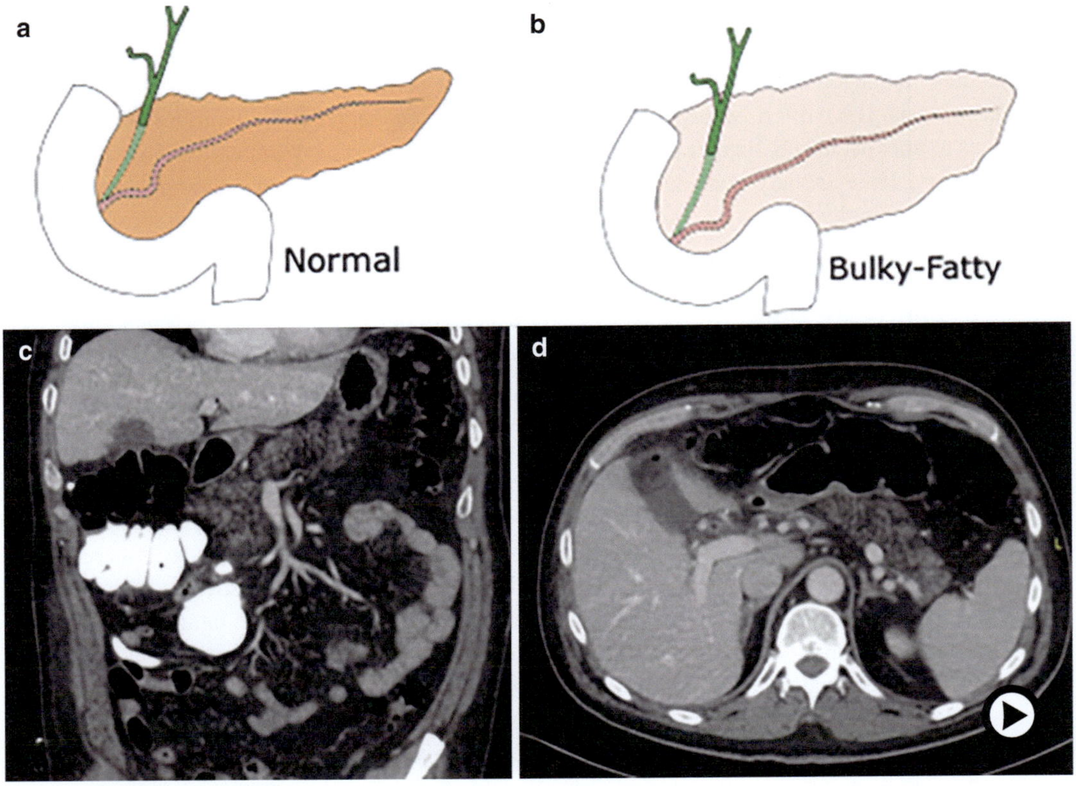

Fig. 18.2 Anatomy of the bulky-fatty pancreas. In contrast to a normal pancreas (**a**) vs. bulk-fatty pancreas (**b**) is larger in size and contains a larger proportion of fat tissue, providing it a pale tone of color. (**c**, **d**) CT-scan imaging of a bulky-fatty pancreas (This video presents a case of fatty, bulky pancreas. The footage describes a few technical details pivotal to achieving a safe PG: (I) mobilization of the pancreatic stump from both the splenic vein and artery should be enough to avoid the so-called "Pisa Tower Effect" (when the angle between the pancreatic surface and splenic vessels is smaller than 90 degrees, case in which the PG anastomosis is subject to excessively imbalanced tensions); (II) the incision on the posterior wall of the stomach should be of the same length of the stump to facilitate the intussusception; (III) a purse-string technique should be adopted avoiding stitches which can easily tear the pancreatic stump, as shown in the video. Reproduced here with the permission of the authors (▶ https://doi.org/10.1007/000-hf3))

calculator counterparts have been made available. These come in extremely handy in informing the decision in these cases. For instance, the Pancreatic Fistula Risk Score (FRS) calculator available through MDCalc's website (https://www.mdcalc.com/calc/10194/pancreatic-fistula-risk-score) is based on the FRS system proposed by Callery et al. [18]. The tool uses information about the gland texture (firm or soft), pathology (whether adenocarcinoma or pancreatitis, or any other), duct diameter, and intraoperative blood loss and uses an easy-to-understand scoring system to assign patients a risk group and a rate of clinically relevant POPF.

18.2.2.5 Radiofrequency Ablation of the Pancreatic Duct

An alternative technique, still under active research, is that of radiofrequency ablation of the MPD.

It has been shown that duct obstruction induces acinar atrophy and exocrine pancreatic insufficiency without pancreatitis signs while preserving the endocrine function through unaltered Langerhans islets [21, 22]. Ligation of the duct or its sealing with glue are procedures that have arisen to decimate pancreatic exocrine activity and reduce the risks associated with POPF. While ligation and sealing have been successfully applied in animal models and proven safe, these techniques have not been widely accepted as human treatments, either due to the high risk of fistula in humans in the ligation case or due to re-permeabilization in the case of glue.

Preoperative pancreatic intraductal ablation is also an interesting emerging management technique currently in research that might reduce the risk of POPF. Initial results in animal models indicate that endoluminal radiofrequency ablation of the pancreatic duct might be a safer and more effective alternative to inducing acinar atrophy preoperatively [23]. In addition to the results in animals, RFA has been successfully applied to six high-risk patients (Figs. 18.3 and 18.4). In those cases, RFA was chosen after careful consideration of the pre- and intraoperative findings [24, 25]. From this group of high-risk patients, all patients presented fistula, but none of them presented clinically relevant grade C fistula, and the mortality was 0%. While further research is definitely needed to confirm the readiness of this treatment in humans, these early results bear great promise.

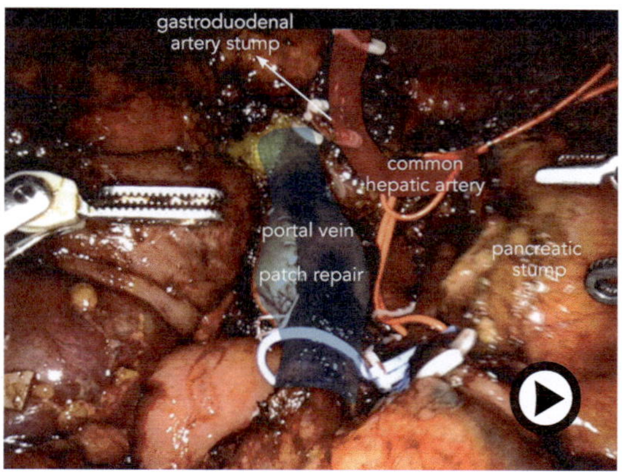

Fig. 18.3 Bulky, fatty pancreas stump with signs of acute pancreatitis (Footage of a patient with a bulky, fatty pancreas stump with signs of acute pancreatitis. In this case, a total pancreatectomy is performed. Reproduced here with the permission of the authors (▶ https://doi.org/10.1007/000-hf2))

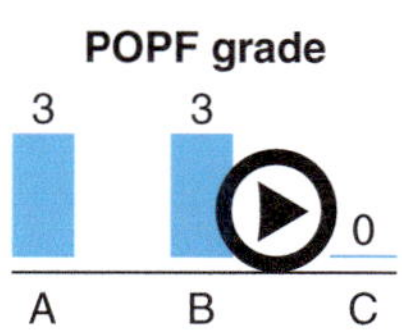

Fig. 18.4 Summary of the POPF grade fistula in six high-risk patients from the study [24, 25] who underwent endoluminal RFA intraoperatively during elective pancreaticoduodenectomy (data shared by the authors) (This video shows a radiofrequency ablation procedure in a patient with a high risk of fistula. The decision was made intraoperatively (▶ https://doi.org/10.1007/000-hf5))

Video 4 shows one such radiofrequency ablation procedure in a patient with a high risk of postoperative pancreatic fistula. The decision was made intraoperatively, taking into account preoperative factors as well as intraoperative findings.

18.2.3 Postoperative Management and Special Reintervention Cases

Cases requiring surgical reintervention due to failed initial anastomosis and subsequent development of POPF are particularly complex. These situations often involve navigating through altered anatomy, managing inflammation, and overcoming tissue fibrosis, all of which demand high levels of surgical expertise and adaptability.

Redoing the PA is sometimes possible if the pancreatic stump can be adequately mobilized. Yet, total or sub-total pancreatectomy may be the preferred intervention if the PA appears unsafe. In these cases, while performing a totalization often, the preservation of the spleen is not possible.

Again, innovative techniques such as radiofrequency ablation are emerging as a promising alternative for managing failed PAs by preserving endocrine function and reducing the need for total pancreatectomy.

18.3 Conclusions and Final Remarks

The management of complex pancreatic anastomosis after pancreaticoduodenectomy requires a tailored approach, considering the unique challenges of each patient's pancreatic anatomy and comorbidities.

In this chapter, we offer a guide to managing complex PA, offering tips and tricks focused on preoperative, intraoperative, as well as special postoperative situations.

Surgeons must be prepared to adapt their techniques and consider alternative strategies to ensure the best possible outcomes. Advances in preoperative imaging, intraoperative decision-making, and innovative techniques like radiofrequency ablation offer new avenues for improving the safety and efficacy of these procedures. This comprehensive guide aims to provide a framework for addressing the complexities of PA, encouraging the adoption of minimally invasive approaches even in the most challenging cases.

References

1. Sugimoto M, Takahashi S, Kojima M, Kobayashi T, Gotohda N, Konishi M. In patients with a soft pancreas, a thick parenchyma, a small duct, and fatty infiltration are significant risks for pancreatic fistula after pancreaticoduodenectomy. Gastrointest Surg. 2017;21:846–54. https://doi.org/10.1007/s11605-017-3356-7.
2. Kim EY, You YK, Kim DG, Hong TH. A simple pancreaticojejunostomy technique for hard pancreases using only two transpancreatic sutures with buttresses: a comparison with the previous pancreaticogastrostomy and dunking methods. Surg Treat Res. 2016;90:64–71. https://doi.org/10.4174/astr.2016.90.2.64.
3. Kawaida H, Kono H, Hosomura N, et al. Surgical techniques and postoperative management to prevent postoperative pancreatic fistula after pancreatic surgery. J Gastroenterol. 2019;28(25):3722–37. https://doi.org/10.3748/wjg.v25.i28.3722.
4. Marcucci F, Carillo G, Sánchez-Velázquez P, et al. Practical Approaches to High-Risk Anastomoses in Robotic Pancreatoduodenectomy. Ann Surg Oncol. 2025;32(8):5717–19. https://doi.org/10.1245/s10434-025-17402-w. Epub 2025 May 6.
5. Fiorentini G, Tamburrino D, Belfiori G, Crippa S, Partelli S, Falconi M. Which is the best pancreatic anastomosis? Minerva Chir. 2019;74:241–52. https://doi.org/10.23736/S0026-4733.19.07997-5.
6. Wang W, Zhang Z, Gu C, Liu Q, Liang Z, He W, Chen J, Lai J. The optimal choice for pancreatic anastomosis after pancreaticoduodenectomy: a network meta-analysis of randomized control trials. J Surg. 2018;57:111–6. https://doi.org/10.1016/j.ijsu.2018.04.005.
7. De Luca R, Gianotti L, Pedrazzoli P, Brunetti O, Rizzo A, Sandini M, Paiella S, Pecorelli N, Pugliese L, Pietrabissa A, Zerbi A, Salvia R, Boggi U, Casirati A, Falconi M, Caccialanza R. Immunonutrition and prehabilitation in pancreatic cancer surgery: a new concept in the era of ERAS® and neoadjuvant treatment. Eur J Surg Oncol. 2023;49(3):542–9. https://doi.org/10.1016/j.ejso.2022.12.006. PMID: 36577556
8. Zhang QH, Ma JD, Lu YM, Zhang RN, Zhao ZH, Li YT, Chen QP. Sarcopenia adversely impacts clinical outcomes in patients undergoing pancreaticoduodenectomy: a systematic review and meta-analysis. World J Gastrointest Surg. 2024;16(6):1857–70. https://doi.org/10.4240/wjgs.v16.i6.1857. PMID: 38983342
9. Adibelli ZH, Adatepe M, Imamoglu C, Esen OS, Erkan N, Yildirim M. Anatomic variations of the pancreatic duct and their relevance with the Cambridge classification system: MRCP findings of 1158 consecutive patients. Radiol Oncol. 2016;50(4):370–7. https://doi.org/10.1515/raon-2016-0041.
10. Türkvatan A, Erden A, Türkoğlu MA, Yener Ö. Congenital variants and anomalies of the pancreas and pancreatic duct: imaging by magnetic resonance cholangiopancreaticography and multidetector computed tomography. Korean J Radiol. 2013;14(6):905–13. https://doi.org/10.3348/kjr.2013.14.6.905.
11. Hanaki T, Uejima C, Amisaki M, et al. The attenuation value of preoperative computed tomography as a novel predictor for pancreatic fistula after pancreaticoduodenectomy. Surg Today. 2018;48:598–608. https://doi.org/10.1007/s00595-018-1626-y.
12. Tranchart H, Gaujoux S, Rebours V, et al. Preoperative CT scan helps to predict the occurrence of severe pancreatic fistula after pancreaticoduodenectomy. Ann Surg. 2012;256:139–45. https://doi.org/10.1097/SLA.0b013e318256c32.
13. Rosso E, Casnedi S, Pessaux P, et al. The role of "fatty pancreas" and of BMI in the occurrence of pancreatic fistula after pancreaticoduodenectomy. Gastrointest Surg. 2009;13:1845–51. https://doi.org/10.1007/s11605-009-0974-8.
14. Gaujoux S, Cortes A, Couvelard A, et al. Fatty pancreas and increased body mass index are risk factors of pancreatic fistula after pancreaticoduodenectomy. Surgery. 2010;148:15–23. https://doi.org/10.1016/j.surg.2009.12.005.
15. Vellalta Muxí G, Ielpo B, Anselmo A, de Blasi V, Rosso E. Managing complex pancreatic anastomoses after minimally invasive pancreaticoduodenectomy. Laparosc Surg. 2024;8 https://doi.org/10.21037/ls-23-15.
16. Salvia R, Lionetto G, Perri G, Malleo G, Marchegiani G. Total pancreatectomy and pancreatic fistula: friend or foe? Updat Surg. 2021;73:1231–6. https://doi.org/10.1007/s13304-021-01130-3.
17. Luu AM, Olchanetski B, Herzog T, Tannapfel A, Uhl W, Belyaev O. Is primary total pancreatectomy

in patients with high-risk pancreatic remnant justified and preferable to pancreaticoduodenectomy? -a matched-pairs analysis of 200 patients. Gland Surg. 2021;10:618–28. https://doi.org/10.21037/gs-20-670.

18. Callery MP, Pratt WB, Kent TS, Chaikof EL, Vollmer CM Jr. A prospectively validated clinical risk score accurately predicts pancreatic fistula after pancreatoduodenectomy. J Am Coll Surg. 2013;216(1):1–14. https://doi.org/10.1016/j.jamcollsurg.2012.09.002. PMID: 23122535
19. Miller BC, Christein JD, Behrman SW, Drebin JA, Pratt WB, Callery MP, Vollmer CM Jr. A multi-institutional external validation of the fistula risk score for pancreatoduodenectomy. J Gastrointest Surg. 2014;18(1):172–9; discussion 179–80. https://doi.org/10.1007/s11605-013-2337-8. PMID: 24002771
20. Perri G, Marchegiani G, Partelli S, Crippa S, Bianchi B, Cinelli L, Esposito A, Pecorelli N, Falconi M, Bassi C, Salvia R. Preoperative risk stratification of postoperative pancreatic fistula: a risk-tree predictive model for pancreatoduodenectomy. Surgery. 2021;170(6):1596–601. https://doi.org/10.1016/j.surg.2021.06.046. PMID: 34315629
21. Quesada R, Burdío F, Iglesias M, Dorcaralo D, Cáceres M, Andaluz A, Poves I, Castiella T, Sánchez P, Berjano E, Grande L. Radiofrequency pancrea5c ablation and sec5on of the main pancreatic duct does not lead to necrotizing pancreatitis. Pancreas. 2014;43(6):931–7. https://doi.org/10.1097/MPA.0000000000000156. PMID: 24977335
22. Quesada R, Andaluz A, Cáceres M, Moll X, Iglesias M, Dorcaralo D, Poves I, Berjano E, Grande L, Burdío F. Long-term evolution of acinar-to-ductal metaplasia and β-cell mass a>er radiofrequency-assisted transection of the pancreas in a controlled large animal model. Pancreatology. 2016;16(1):38–43. https://doi.org/10.1016/j.pan.2015.10.014. PMID: 26639388
23. Andaluz A, Ewertowska E, Moll X, Aguilar A, García F, Fondevila D, Quesada R, Berjano E, Grande L, Burdío F. Endoluminal radiofrequency ablation of the main pancreatic duct is a secure and effective method to produce pancreatic atrophy and to achieve stump closure. Sci Rep. 2019;9(1):5928. https://doi.org/10.1038/s41598-019-42411-7. PMID: 30976043
24. Ielpo B, Pueyo-Périz EM, Radosevic A, Andaluz A, Berjano E, Grande L, Sánchez-Velázquez P, Burdío F. Clinical case report: endoluminal thermal ablation of main pancreatic duct for patients at high risk of postoperative pancreatic fistula after pancreaticoduodenectomy. Int J Hyperth. 2021;38(1):755–9. https://doi.org/10.1080/02656736.2021.1917703. PMID: 33941013
25. Moll X, Fondevila D, García-Arnas F, Pérez JJ, Ielpo B, Sánchez-Velázquez P, Grande L, Jaume S, Radosevic A, Barranco L, Berjano E, Burdio F, Andaluz A. Is occlusion of the main pancreatic duct by thermal ablation really safe? A surgical innovation assessed according to IDEAL recommendations. Int J Hyperth. 2023;40(1):2203888. https://doi.org/10.1080/02656736.2023.2203888. PMID: 37126121

19 How and When to Drain

Domenico Bassi, Giampaolo Perri, Umberto Cillo, and Giovanni Marchegiani

19.1 Introduction

The positioning of one or more intraoperative drains during pancreatic surgery is a long-debated, ever-evolving practice. Historically, drains were routinely placed after every open pancreatic resection, aiming at reduction or mitigation of surgical complications such as postoperative pancreatic fistula (POPF) [1], biliary leak, intra-abdominal abscesses, and bleeding. By facilitating the removal of blood, clots, and possible pancreatic/biliary/enteric secretions, drains help prevent the accumulation of fluids that could otherwise lead to the formation of intra-abdominal collections and infections. Therefore, drains are traditionally accepted a standard of care, theoretically reducing the risk of severe postoperative complications or allowing for early therapeutic intervention whenever they occur. However, the routine use of intraoperative drains does not come without risks. Infections related to prolonged use, physical or psychological discomfort, and delayed recovery are recognized downsides of surgical drains that may contribute to extended hospital stays and increased healthcare costs. Moreover, the question of whether drains truly prevent severe complications such as clinically relevant POPF, or merely provide a window into the development of such complications, is still open. Recent studies have challenged the routine placement of drains in selected patients during pancreatoduodenectomy (PD), especially in low-risk cases [2], or even supported routine omission during distal pancreatectomy [3], suggesting that drainless policies in certain circumstances can lead to similar or better outcomes. In addition to "when," "how" to drain is also a hot topic in pancreatic surgery, as many open questions remain, such as superiority of closed over open systems or suction over gravity drainage.

Furthermore, with the advent of minimally invasive pancreatoduodenectomy (MIPD), surgical drains have come under renewed scrutiny. Both robotic and laparoscopic approaches have introduced new challenges in drain placement, positioning, and management, compared to open procedures. Although potentially offering significant advantages such as reduced blood loss, shorter recovery times, and decreased postoperative pain, MIPD requires careful reconsideration of traditional drain practices to optimize outcomes, as in this context drain placement presents unique challenges. The minimally invasive nature of robotic and laparoscopic techniques offers reduced surgical trauma, but also alters the

D. Bassi · G. Perri · U. Cillo · G. Marchegiani (✉)
Hepato-Pancreato-Biliary and Liver Transplant Surgery Unit, Department of Surgical, Oncological and Gastroenterological Sciences (DiSCOG), University of Padua, Padua, Italy
e-mail: domenico.basssi@aopd.veneto.it; giampaolo.perri@unipd.it; cillo@unipd.it; giovanni.marchegiani@unipd.it

B. Ielpo et al. (eds.), *Minimally Invasive Pancreatoduodenectomy in Cancer*,
https://doi.org/10.1007/978-3-031-99695-5_19

anatomy and dissection planes, potentially influencing the dynamics of fluid collection and drainage. Additionally, MIPD typically involves a smaller surgical field with limited access, making the precise positioning of drains more technically demanding.

This chapter explores the role of intraoperative drains in MIPD, both robotic and laparoscopic, focusing on when and how to place drains effectively and outlining current evidence and surgical techniques.

19.2 When to Drain?

19.2.1 Risk Stratification and Drain Omission

Deciding to place one or more drains during PD is a critical step of the intraoperative management and should be guided by intraoperative risk factors and patient-specific considerations. The most important determinant in this decision-making process remains the risk of developing POPF, the most frequent and potentially life-threatening complication after PD, characterized by leakage of pancreatic secretions from the pancreatic anastomosis. One of the first and most validated tool to assess POPF risk is the Fistula Risk Score (FRS), developed by Callery et al. in 2013 [4]. The FRS is calculated based on several intraoperative variables, including pancreatic gland texture, pancreatic duct size, pathology type, and intraoperative blood loss. These factors are assigned weighted scores and combined to generate the overall FRS, which stratifies patients into negligible (FRS 0), low (FRS 1–2), moderate (FRS 3–6), and high risk (FRS 7–10) of developing POPF. Soft glands are associated with a significantly higher risk of POPF due to the friable nature of the tissue, which makes anastomoses less secure, and a "functional" pancreatic remnant (as opposed to obstructive chronic pancreatitis), which is more likely to produce higher quantities of amylase-rich pancreatic secretion. A small duct diameter (≤3 mm) is also more likely to develop a fistula for both technical (narrow ducts limit the ability to form a secure anastomosis with the jejunal mucosa) and biological reasons (absence of long-lasting obstruction). Pancreatic gland texture (soft vs. firm) and duct diameter (> or ≤ 3 mm) are the most important and can be sufficient to accurately predict POPF risk, as recently demonstrated by the ISGPS A-B-C-D class system [5]. Conversely, the presence of non-malignant diseases (e.g., benign or premalignant lesions, like intraductal papillary mucinous neoplasms) and increased blood loss (≥1000 mL) during surgery represent surrogate metrics, as the first is often associated with softer pancreatic tissue, while the latter may be a marker of a technically demanding surgery leading to compromised anastomotic healing.

Several other scores and calculators have been developed after the FRS [6], but regardless of the preferred method, POPF risk stratification has become an essential tool in guiding surgical decision-making around drain placement. The concept of tailored drain management, based on intraoperative FRS and patient-specific factors, is gaining support as surgeons move away from a "one-size-fits-all" approach. Selective drain placement allows surgeons to balance the need for early detection of complications against the risks of drain-related issues such as infection, prolonged drainage, and increased hospital stays.

In high-risk patients, surgical drains have several fundamental functions: (1) early POPF detection, by measuring amylase levels in the drain fluid; (2) controlled drainage of pancreatic secretions, preventing the formation of collections and abscesses, leading to clinically relevant POPF (grade B or C); and (3) serve as a route for therapeutic interventions, should a clinically relevant POPF develop. Conversely, for patients with a negligible or low POPF risk—those with a firm pancreatic gland and a large duct diameter—the omission of drains is increasingly considered safe and may even improve outcomes. Several studies have challenged the routine use of drains in low-risk patients, suggesting that avoiding drains in such individuals can (1) reduce the risk of retrograde infections, which can occur if bacteria from the skin or external environment migrate along the drain track into the abdominal cavity; (2) decrease the duration of hospital stay, by eliminating the need for prolonged monitoring and care associated with drain management; and (3) improve patient comfort and mobility, as drains can limit postoperative activity and contribute to discomfort.

Interestingly, the first randomized multicenter trial [7] to ever evaluate the outcome of PD without routine intraperitoneal drainage seemed to exclude the possibility of safe drain omission. Elimination of intraperitoneal drainage in all cases of PD increased the frequency and severity of complications, requiring the safety monitoring board to stop the study early because of an increase in mortality from 3% to 12%. However, in this trial, participants were not stratified according to POPF risk. In 2017, McMillan and colleagues [8] provided the first risk-adjusted trial for drain omission after PD, demonstrating that drain omission was not only safe, but also beneficial in patients with negligible POPF risk, reducing POPF rate from 3.6% to 0.

For patients with moderate FRS scores, the decision to place a drain is less clear-cut and often relies on additional intraoperative findings and the surgeon's judgment. Factors that may influence the decision include (1) the complexity of the anastomosis: a technically challenging pancreatico-jejunostomy or hepatico-jejunostomy, particularly in cases where tension is present or vascularity is questionable, may warrant drain placement even in patients with moderate risk scores; (2) patient comorbidities: patients with significant comorbidities, such as obesity, diabetes, or cardiovascular disease, may have impaired wound healing and an increased risk of infection, justifying more conservative management with drains; and (3) surgeon experience: surgeons with extensive experience in open PD or MIPD may feel more comfortable omitting drains in select patients, while less experienced surgeons may prefer to place drains as a precautionary measure in moderate-risk cases.

19.2.2 Considerations and Challenges Specific to MIPD

As already mentioned, to stratify POPF risk is mandatory before deciding whether to drain or not. However, the FRS was developed for open PD, with no validation in MIPD cohorts. Recently, an updated alternative-FRS (ua-FRS) [9] was validated and optimized for POPF risk prediction in MIPD, by including sex and adjusting based on anastomotic technique. The ua-FRS (consisting of body mass index, pancreatic texture, duct size, and male sex) can be used for perioperative risk prediction and post-hoc risk adjustment, in both open PD and all subgroups of MIPD (laparoscopic, robot-assisted, and hybrid).

It is important to notice that drainless policies for PD have also been developed in patients undergoing open surgery. Moreover, reports on POPF rates after MIPD have been discordant, with some series reporting similar outcomes compared to open PD [10] and other reporting higher rates of POPF (up to 10%) after MIPD [11]. These results should be interpreted considering two main confounding factors: (1) patient selection, as typically (especially for less experienced programs) MIPD is reserved to resectable pancreatic cancers or benign and premalignant lesions—by definition technically less demanding resections, but with higher POPF risk and (2) surgeon experience: MIPD is a technically complex procedure, where the surgeon's objective technical skills are strictly connected to outcomes (including POPF) [12], and centers with lower MIPD volume may experience worse outcomes especially earlier in the learning curve [13]. Nevertheless, the first randomized controlled trial (EUROPA trial) [14] comparing robotic PD to open PD, performed by surgeons with sufficient experience (≥40 procedures), was recently published. Despite the primary outcome (overall 90-day morbidity) was similar, patient who underwent robotic PD had a higher rate of pancreas-specific complications (58.6% vs. 33.3%). For this reason, a word of caution should be spent over drainless policies after MIPD, to be considered only in very low-risk patients and after adequate learning curve. In all the other cases, drain placement with early drain removal policies is to be preferred.

19.3 How to Drain?

19.3.1 Drain Types

Surgical drains used in MIPD can be broadly categorized into two types, similarly to open surgery: (1) open drains and (2) closed drains. Each type offers distinct advantages and limitations depending on the clinical situation. Open drains rely on passive capillary action to evacuate fluid from the abdominal cavity. Examples of open drains include Penrose drain (soft, flexible, and flat drain, often used for passive drainage in superficial wound sites) and corrugated drain (a variation of the Penrose drain, with a corrugated surface to increase capillary action and encourage fluid flow). Open drains are simple, inexpensive, and effective for passive drainage. However, they carry a higher risk of contamination and infection, as the exposed fluid can become in contact with the external environment. Closed system drains collect fluid in a closed reservoir, reducing the risk of external contamination. These further include (1) active closed drains, which use suction to actively remove fluid, such as the Jackson-Pratt drain (a flexible silicone drain connected to a bulb, creating negative pressure to suction fluids) and (2) passive closed drains, such as the round drain (which rely on gravity or intra-abdominal pressure to evacuate fluids). Closed drains, particularly active systems, offer the advantage of controlled, continuous evacuation of fluid, while reducing the risk of infection. Passive closed drains, however, may not provide sufficient evacuation in cases of large fluid collections or high output. In open PD, studies have shown no significant differences in terms of morbidity and mortality using open or closed drainage systems [15]. In many practices, including Author's own, open drains are routinely used in MIPD. Open drains, like Penrose drains, are easier to position and manipulate in the confined operative field of laparoscopic or robotic surgery, and they are less prone to occlusion compared to closed drains with active suction systems. This is particularly important in the pancreatic bed, where debris and clotted blood can obstruct drains.

19.3.2 Drain Positioning

In MIPD, as in open surgery, two drains are usually placed in the peritoneal cavity. The positioning of these drains is strategically designed to cover the critical anastomotic sites, namely the pancreatico-jejunostomy (PJ) and the hepatico-jejunostomy (HJ) (Fig. 19.1). In MIPD, as in other minimally invasive procedures in the abdomen, adhesion formation is typically low. This could reduce collections compartmentation and drainage, especially in patients that tend to produce ascites o chylous fluids. Such double-drain configuration ensures that the critical areas where leaks are most likely to occur are adequately covered, providing early detection of pancreatic, biliary, or gastric leaks. The first drain is inserted from the right flank, directed posteriorly to the HJ, and from there routed to reach the superior margin of the PJ, ensuring effective drainage of fluids accumulating near both sites. The second drain is inserted from the left flank and positioned to run posteriorly toward the gastro-jejunostomy (G-J) and from there inserted anteriorly (or, if possible, posteriorly) to the PJ. It could be further advanced to drain the area posterior to the lesser sac, where fluid collections are common. Drains in MIPD are routinely placed before completing the anastomoses, for two key reasons: to avoid mechanical trauma and to ensure proper positioning. In laparoscopic and robotic PD, placing drains after the completion of the anastomoses can be challenging, and the posterior anastomotic aspects are especially vulnerable due to the limited dexterity and reduced tactile feedback. Placing the drain before the anastomoses are performed ensures appropriate positioning, mitigating the need for complex maneuvers after the anastomotic suturing is complete. Once the anastomoses are completed, the distal end of the pre-

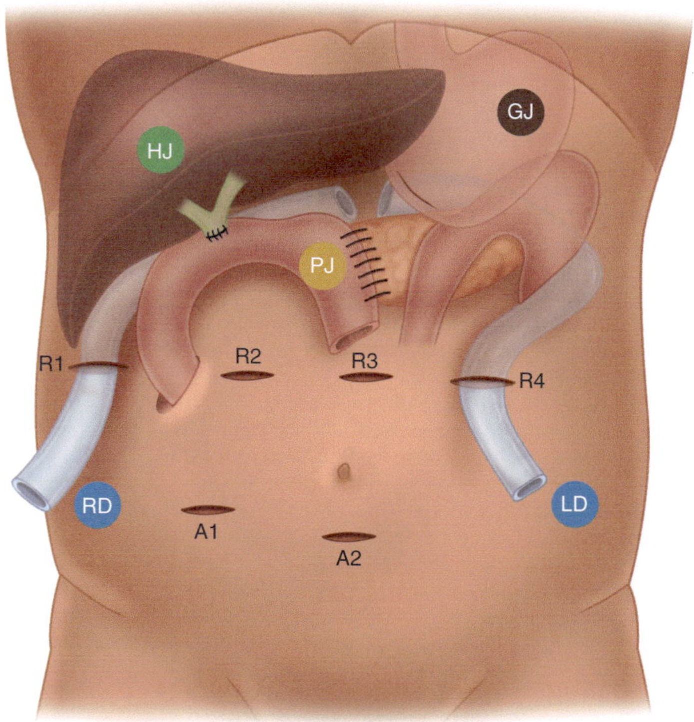

Fig. 19.1 Drain positioning after robotic pancreatoduodenectomy. Legend: *R* robotic trocar access, *A* laparoscopic assistant trocar access, *RD* right drain, *LD* left drain, *HJ* hepatico-jejunostomy, *PJ* pancreatico-jejunostomy, *GJ* gastro-jejunostomy

viously positioned drains can be extracted from the trocar incisions, without the need for further incisions.

19.4 Conclusions

The role of intraoperative drainage in pancreatic surgery, particularly in MIPD, remains critical and requires careful consideration. While historically routine, the use of drains is evolving, with increasing emphasis on individualized approaches based on patient-specific and intraoperative risk factors. For MIPD, the technical challenges of drain placement, including limited access and altered adhesions formation, demand heightened precision. The placement of two drains is commonly recommended to effectively cover critical anastomotic sites, such as the PJ and HJ, ensuring early detection of leaks. Although emerging evidence suggests that selective drain omission can be safe in selected low-risk patients, caution is advised, particularly in MIPD. Drainless strategies should be considered only after surgeons have completed an adequate learning curve and in very low/negligible-risk patients. In all other cases, the placement of surgical drains remains a critical tool to mitigate the risks of serious postoperative complications in MIPD.

References

1. Bassi C, Dervenis C, Butturini G, Fingerhut A, Yeo C, Izbicki J, et al. Postoperative pancreatic fistula: an international study group (ISGPF) definition. Surgery [Internet]. 2005;138(1):8–13. Available from: http://www.ncbi.nlm.nih.gov/pubmed/16003309
2. McMillan MT, Malleo G, Bassi C, Butturini G, Salvia R, Roses RE, et al. Drain management after pancreatoduodenectomy: reappraisal of a prospective randomized trial using risk stratification. J Am Coll Surg [Internet]. 2015;221(4):798–809. Available from: http://www.ncbi.nlm.nih.gov/pubmed/26278037
3. van Bodegraven EA, Balduzzi A, van Ramshorst TME, Malleo G, Vissers FL, van Hilst J, et al. Prophylactic abdominal drainage after distal pancreatectomy (PANDORINA): an international, multicentre, open-label, randomised controlled, non-inferiority trial. lancet Gastroenterol Hepatol

[Internet]. 2024;9(5):438–47. Available from: http://www.ncbi.nlm.nih.gov/pubmed/38499019
4. Callery MP, Pratt WB, Kent TS, Chaikof EL, Vollmer CM. A prospectively validated clinical risk score accurately predicts pancreatic fistula after pancreatoduodenectomy. J Am Coll Surg [Internet]. 2013;216(1):1–14. Available from: http://www.ncbi.nlm.nih.gov/pubmed/23122535
5. Schuh F, Yildirim B, Klotz R, Pianka F, Boskovic A, Werba A, et al. Prospective Validation of the Pancreatic Fistula Risk Classification by the International Study Group for Pancreatic Surgery (PARIS trial). Ann Surg [Internet]. 2024 Aug 8.; Available from: http://www.ncbi.nlm.nih.gov/pubmed/39114920
6. Mungroop TH, van Rijssen LB, van Klaveren D, Smits FJ, van Woerden V, Linnemann RJ, et al. Alternative fistula risk score for pancreatoduodenectomy (a-FRS): design and international external validation. Ann Surg [Internet]. 2019;269(5):937–43. Available from: http://www.ncbi.nlm.nih.gov/pubmed/29240007
7. Van Buren G, Bloomston M, Hughes SJ, Winter J, Behrman SW, Zyromski NJ, et al. A randomized prospective multicenter trial of pancreaticoduodenectomy with and without routine intraperitoneal drainage. Ann Surg. 2014;259(4):605–12.
8. McMillan MT, Malleo G, Bassi C, Allegrini V, Casetti L, Drebin JA, et al. Multicenter, prospective trial of selective drain management for pancreatoduodenectomy using risk stratification. Ann Surg [Internet]. 2017;265(6):1209–18. Available from: https://journals.lww.com/00000658-201706000-00028
9. Mungroop TH, Klompmaker S, Wellner UF, Steyerberg EW, Coratti A, D'Hondt M, et al. Updated alternative fistula risk score (ua-FRS) to include minimally invasive pancreatoduodenectomy. Ann Surg [Internet]. 2021;273(2):334–40. Available from: https://journals.lww.com/10.1097/SLA.0000000000003234
10. McMillan MT, Zureikat AH, Hogg ME, Kowalsky SJ, Zeh HJ, Sprys MH, et al. A propensity score–matched analysis of robotic vs open pancreatoduodenectomy on incidence of pancreatic fistula. JAMA Surg [Internet] 2017;152(4):327. Available from: http://archsurg.jamanetwork.com/article.aspx?doi=10.1001/jamasurg.2016.4755
11. Klompmaker S, van Hilst J, Wellner UF, Busch OR, Coratti A, D'Hondt M, et al. Outcomes after minimally-invasive versus open pancreatoduodenectomy. Ann Surg [Internet]. 2020;271(2):356–63. Available from: https://journals.lww.com/10.1097/SLA.0000000000002850
12. van den Broek BLJ, Zwart MJW, Bonsing BA, Busch OR, van Dam JL, de Hingh IHJT, et al. Video grading of pancreatic anastomoses during robotic pancreatoduodenectomy to assess both learning curve and the risk of pancreatic fistula. Ann Surg [Internet]. 2023;278(5):e1048–54. Available from: https://journals.lww.com/10.1097/SLA.0000000000005796
13. Zwart MJW, van den Broek B, de Graaf N, Suurmeijer JA, Augustinus S, Te Riele WW, et al. The feasibility, proficiency, and mastery learning curves in 635 robotic pancreatoduodenectomies following a multicenter training program: "standing on the shoulders of giants". Ann Surg [Internet]. 2023;278(6):e1232–41. Available from: http://www.ncbi.nlm.nih.gov/pubmed/37288547
14. Klotz R, Mihaljevic AL, Kulu Y, Sander A, Klose C, Behnisch R, et al. Robotic versus open partial pancreatoduodenectomy (EUROPA): a randomised controlled stage 2b trial. Lancet Reg Heal Eur [Internet]. 2024;39:100864. Available from: http://www.ncbi.nlm.nih.gov/pubmed/38420108
15. Marchegiani G, Perri G, Pulvirenti A, Sereni E, Azzini AM, Malleo G, et al. Non-inferiority of open passive drains compared with closed suction drains in pancreatic surgery outcomes: a prospective observational study. Surg (United States) [Internet]. 2018;164(3):443–9. https://doi.org/10.1016/j.surg.2018.04.025.

20 Safe Venous Dissection

Alessia Fassari, Vito De Blasi, and Edoardo Rosso

20.1 Introduction

Dissection of the head of the pancreas from the porto-mesenteric vein (PMV) axis is one of critical steps during pancreaticoduodenectomy (PD). In up to 45% of the cases [1] of pancreatic head cancer, a certain degree of attachment to the PMV is identified during the intervention. Iatrogenic PMV injuries can occur during PD for cancer and are associated with high morbidity and mortality as a result of massive bleeding, such events are more frequent in case of tumoral or inflammatory adhesions to the venous axis [2–4]. Emergency repair of PMV injuries is particularly complex and are associated with a high incidence of severe postoperative immediate and long-term complications (stenosis, thrombosis, liver failure, etc.) [2]. Prevention of intraoperative PMV injuries during PD requires an adjustment of the surgical technique which we named safe venous dissection strategy (SVDs) [5–9].

20.2 Indications

SVDs is required in the following cases:

1. The presence of inflammatory adhesions between the head of the pancreas and the PMV axis precluding an easy and straightforward mobilization of the head of the pancreas from vein (Figs. 20.1 and 20.2). Such plane in most of the cases is clearly visible by combing a gentle traction of the duodenum toward the right side combined and by pushing the PMV toward the left.
2. The presence of cancer abutment of the PMV on the preoperative abdominal CT scan which in most of the cases cannot be distinguished by a formal cancer invasion.
3. The presence of a large tumoral mass of the head of the pancreas (ex. degenerated IPMN), in those cases mobilizations are particularly challenging and are associated with a high risk of PMV injury.

Supplementary Information The online version contains supplementary material available at https://doi.org/10.1007/978-3-031-99695-5_20. The videos can be accessed individually by clicking the DOI link in the accompanying figure caption or by scanning this link with the SN More Media App.

A. Fassari · V. De Blasi · E. Rosso (✉)
Service de Chirurgie Générale et Viscérale—Centre Hospitalier de Luxembourg,
Rollingergrund-North Belair, Luxembourg
e-mail: alessia.fassari@gmail.com; DeBlasi.Vito@chl.lu; edoardo_rosso@hotmail.com

B. Ielpo et al. (eds.), *Minimally Invasive Pancreatoduodenectomy in Cancer*,
https://doi.org/10.1007/978-3-031-99695-5_20

20.3 Surgical Technique

As shown in the video, SVDs include two main steps: (1) venous vascular control and (2) clearance of the superior mesenteric margin (SMA) before venous dissection; the purpose of this approach is to leave the area of venous attachment "suspended" on the vein having completed all the other steps of the resection phase. In this way, it is possible to clamp the venous axis to proceed to a safe dissection of the vein attachment (Figs. 20.1 and 20.2, Videos).

20.3.1 Venous Vascular Control

Once the major mobilization has been completed including the section of the first jejunal loop and of the stomach/duodenum, the pancreas is divided, then the portal vein (PV), the superior mesenteric vein (SMV), and the splenic vein (SpV) are surrounded with vessel loop. In case of the presence of accessory colic veins at the angle between the SMV and the SpV, those branches are ligated, not clipped (to avoid to the blockage of the bulldog clamps), and sectioned. If the inferior mesenteric vein originated from the SMV or at the insertion with SpV in the superior mesenteric vein, it should be controlled separately with a vessel loop.

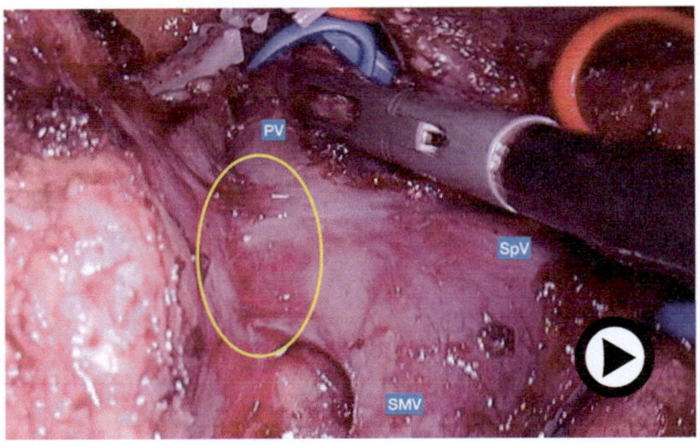

Fig. 20.1 Site of portale vein attachment. *PV* portal vein, *SMV* superior mesenteric vein, *SpV* splenic vein. Yellow mark: site of portal vein attachment (▶ https://doi.org/10.1007/000-hf7)

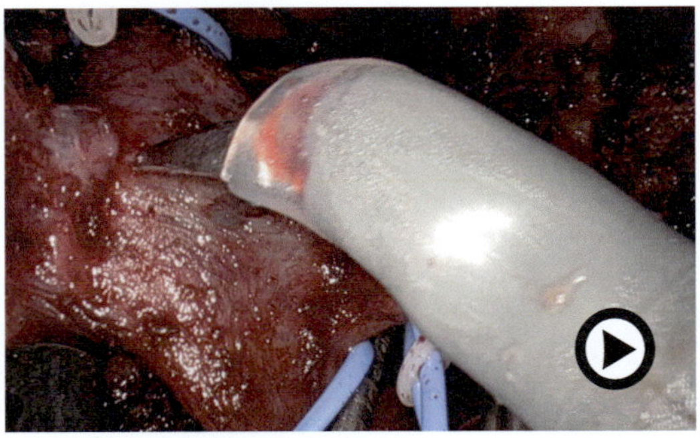

Fig. 20.2 An intraoperative robotic view of portal vein attachment (▶ https://doi.org/10.1007/000-hf6)

As shown in the video, particular attention should be paid to the insertion of right gastric vein (RgV), if it originates from the left border of the PV, the vessel loop below the insertion of the RgV should be controlled separately with a vessel loop (or ligated and divided). Similarly, in case the RgV originates from the superior border of the SpV at its insertion with the PV, after having mobilized the pancreatic stump from the SpV for 2–3, the RgV should be controlled separately or ligated.

In case of difficulty in surrounding the PV to place the vessel loop, a helpful trick is to divide the biliary duct; such maneuver facilitates the isolation of PV.

20.3.2 Clearence of the Superior Mesenteric Artery Margin

Once venous vascular control is achieved, to "suspend" the specimen at the venous attachment site, it is necessary to divide the SMA margin. Two main approaches are possible: (1) tilting completely the specimen toward the left and following the SMA till the origin, dividing between clips the inferior pancreatic duodenal arteries, such approach is ideal in cases of small specimen, and (2) using an anterior approach by identification of SMA on the right of SMV and then proceeding to the gradual division of the SMA margin toward the aorta.

20.4 Safety Tips and Trips

To perform a SVDs, apart from having achieved a venous vascular control and having divided the SMA margin, it is important to be ready for a vascular resection or a bail out procedure (planned conversion to open laparotomy). Therefore, before clamping and proceeding to SVDs:

- Bring into the operating room the necessary materials for a vascular reconstruction (bovine patch, or peritoneal patch, synthetic vascular prothesis or cryopreserved veins, etc.)
- Install on the table the surgical retractor to be ready for a conversion to open surgery.
- Ask for extra assistance if necessary.
- Get a short break.

Once everything is ready, then you can clamp the venous axis and proceed to the venous dissection.

20.5 Conclusion

SVDs should be adopted each time the dissection of the head of the pancreas from the venous axis is not clearly simple, to reduce the risk of major bleeding or being surprised by an unexpected venous resection.

References

1. Li J, Liu Z, Xu X, Chen J. The role of vascular resection and reconstruction in pancreaticoduodenectomy. Asian J Surg. 2024;47(1):63–71. https://doi.org/10.1016/j.asjsur.2023.09.039. Epub 2023 Sep 16
2. Mandolfino T, Canciglia A, Taranto F, et al. Outcome of iatrogenic injuries to the abdominal and pelvic veins. Surg Today. 2008;38:1009–12. https://doi.org/10.1007/s00595-008-3793-8.
3. Herrero A, Souche R, Panaro F, et al. Endovascular balloon occlusion during reconstruction of portal vein injury. Langenbeck's Arch Surg. 2020;405:391–5. https://doi.org/10.1007/s00423-020-01886-z.
4. Kawaguchi Y, Velayutham V, Fuks D, Mal F, Kokudo N, Gayet B. Operative techniques to avoid near misses during laparoscopic hepatectomy. Surgery. 2017;161(2):341–6. https://doi.org/10.1016/j.surg.2016.07.023. Epub 2016 Aug 25
5. Ielpo B, Anselmo A, Masuda Y, Xuan MYH, Burdio F, De Blasi V, Sanchez-Velazquez P, Giuliani A, Azagra JS, Viola GM, Podda M, Pellino G, Rosso E. Superior mesenteric artery first approach for minimally invasive pancreaticoduodenectomy: a step-by-step surgical technique video. Ann Surg Oncol. 2023;30(3):1500–3. https://doi.org/10.1245/s10434-022-12743-2. Epub 2022 Nov 5
6. Morales E, Zimmitti G, Codignola C, Manzoni A, Garatti M, Sega V, Rosso E. Follow "the superior mesenteric artery": laparoscopic approach for total mesopancreas excision during pancreaticoduodenectomy. Surg Endosc. 2019;33(12):4186–91. https://doi.org/10.1007/s00464-019-06994-6. Epub 2019 Jul 22
7. Ielpo B, d'Addetta MV, Anselmo A, Rosso E, de Blasi V, Sanchez-Velazquez P, Vellalta G, Podda M, Burdio F. Levels of robotic mesopancreas dissection according to malignancy and vascular anatomy: what surgeons need to know. Ann Surg Oncol. 2024;31(3):1916–8. https://doi.org/10.1245/s10434-023-14686-8. Epub 2023 Dec 10
8. Rosso E, Frey S, Zimmitti G, Manzoni A, Garatti M, Iannelli A. Laparoscopic radical antegrade modular pancreatosplenectomy with vascular resection for pancreatic cancer: tips and tricks. J Gastrointest Surg. 2020;24(12):2896–902. https://doi.org/10.1007/s11605-020-04695-3. Epub 2020 Jul 14
9. Rosso E, Zimmitti G, Iannelli A, Garatti M. The 'TRIANGLE Operation' by laparoscopy: radical pancreaticoduodenectomy with major vascular resection for borderline resectable pancreatic head cancer. Ann Surg Oncol. 2020;27(5):1613–4. https://doi.org/10.1245/s10434-019-08101-4. Epub 2019 Dec 4

ERAS® in MI PD

21

Raffaele De Luca, Isabella Frigerio, and Luca Gianotti

21.1 Enhanced Recovery After Surgery (ERAS®)

The Enhanced Recovery After Surgery (ERAS®) protocol was developed by a group of academic surgeons in Europe in 2001 when they founded the ERAS® Study group.

Although the term fast-track surgery had been described for the first time in 1994 by Kehlet [1], the group wanted to emphasize that the key surgical end point is the quality, rather than speed, of recovery. The concept rested on several components [2]: a multidisciplinary team working together around the patient, a multimodal approach to undertaking issues that delay recovery and cause complications, a scientific, evidence-based approach to care protocols, and a change in management using interactive and continuous audit. The trimodal approach including nutrition, physical exercise, and stress-reducing psychological component is summarized in Table 21.1.

A key challenge in surgical patient care is the journey through various hospital components: outpatient clinics, preoperative units, the operating room, postoperative recovery facility, and the ward. Each unit has unique focuses, personnel, and specialists that impact subsequent steps based on treatment decisions. For example, if a surgeon prescribes oral bowel preparation, and the patient is unable to replace fluid loss, the anesthetist may encounter a dehydrated patient during anesthesia induction.

Few stakeholders in the surgical pathway can grasp and participate in the entire perioperative patient journey. Hospital staff frequently concentrate on immediate clinical management, limiting strategic thinking. Numerous essential elements of ERAS® care have robust scientific backing. These components are integrated throughout the patient journey and administered by various hospital departments and professionals. Therefore, the surgeon, as the clinician with ultimate responsibility for the patient, is in the best position to provide a comprehensive perspective to guide the process. Consensus on management endpoints is

Created by authors using the available data from the literature including ERAS website.

R. De Luca
Department of Surgical Oncology, I.R.C.C.S Istituto Tumori "Giovanni Paolo II", Bari, Italy
e-mail: dr.raffaele.deluca@gmail.com

I. Frigerio (✉)
HPB Surgery, Pederzoli Hospital, Peschiera del Garda, Italy

Collegium Medicum, University of Social Sciences, Łodz, Poland
e-mail: isifrigerio@yahoo.com

L. Gianotti
School of Medicine and Surgery, University of Milano-Bicocca Foundation IRCCS San Gerardo Hospital, Monza, Italy
e-mail: luca.gianotti@unimib.it

B. Ielpo et al. (eds.), *Minimally Invasive Pancreatoduodenectomy in Cancer*,
https://doi.org/10.1007/978-3-031-99695-5_21

Table 21.1 ERAS® flowchart

	Preadmission	Preoperative	Intraoperative	Postoperative
Surgery	Nutritional support Cessation of smoking Control alcohol intake		Minimally invasive surgery Minimize drains and tubes	Early drain removal Stop IV fluids
Anesthesia	Medical optimization	Preop carbohydrates No NPO PONV prophylaxis	Regional analgesia Opioids-sparing anesthesia Fluids balance Temperature control	Multimodal opioid-sparing pain control
Nursing	Preoperative information			Early mobilization Early oral intake Post-discharge follow-up

crucial for cohesive action, such as the patient being fit for discharge when meeting criteria like adequate oral intake, bowel function, pain management, and self-care mobility, without complications requiring continued hospital care. Enhancing surgical outcomes necessitates a multimodal approach to perioperative care that leverages all available strategies for recovery improvement. The goal is to establish synergy between successive care elements.

A large body of evidence suggest that ERAS® program should be considered the gold standard for perioperative care as it minimizes surgery-induced stress, maintains a homeostatic balance, and reduces catabolism leading thus to cell and organ dysfunction control.

21.2 ERAS® in Pancreatic Surgery

Despite that colon resection was the basis for the development of ERAS® and still dominates the field, it has been shown that ERAS® can be implemented, with improved outcomes, in many other surgical domains, including hepato-biliary and pancreatic, upper GI, cardio-thoracic, urology, gynecology, orthopedic, and emergency surgery.

Among pancreatic surgeries, pancreatoduodenectomy (PD) is the most challenging operation because of the magnitude of dissection and resection, the resultant global stress, and the high morbidity rate [3].

PD reconstruction consists in three anastomoses (pancreatic, biliary, and digestive) leading to a change in physiology of early phases of digestion and slow gain of dietary autonomy [4]. Any postoperative complication easily involves one of these anastomoses therefore impairing the ability to oral food intake, prolonging maintenance of abdominal drains or nasogastric tube. Given the benefit of both MIS and ERAS® in the postoperative outcome, it could be that, once standardized, they would enhance each other beneficial effects.

Implementation of the ERAS® program in such demanding field may be difficult for several reasons, some depending on patient characteristics and underlying disease and some others depending on postoperative events (Table 21.2).

Nevertheless, already more than 10 years ago, large studies [5] and data pooled in meta-analyses consistently showed that patients treated with ERAS® after pancreatic resection have better outcomes as reported by Kagedan et al. in his review [6]. Among ten analyzed studies investigating ERAS protocols in pancreatic surgery, equivalent or better outcomes were reported specifically in morbidity, length of hospital stay, mortality, and readmission rates without evidence of harm.

Additionally, Coolsen et al. [7] reported a systematic review and meta-analysis that revealed that implementation of ERAS® program in pancreatic resections may contribute to a shorter hospital stay and does not seem to compromise

Table 21.2 Factors affecting ERAS® adoption in pancreatic surgery patients

Patient related	Surgery related
Cachexia Fatigue Hypomobility Taste changes Hyporexia Steatorrhea Early satiety Weight loss Abdominal pain Low mood Prolonged opioids use Poor compliance Chemotherapy side effects	Pancreatic fistula Biliary fistula Digestive fistula Chile leak Postoperative pancreatitis Postoperative hemorrhage Ileus Surgical site infection Abdominal collection Need for contact isolation

outcome measures, such as delayed gastric emptying, pancreatic fistula, mortality, and readmission.

More recent publications reported even more favorable results. A meta-analysis of individual patient data [8], from 17 trials and comprising 3108 patients, showed a significant benefit of ERAS® in time to functional recovery, overall postoperative morbidity, and postoperative length of stay. However, benefits were lost when looking at pancreatic specific morbidity such as POPF, PPH, reoperation rate, and mortality.

Further studies have indicated that ERAS remains safe and its advantages are maintained in the treatment of high-risk patients, including those aged over 70 years [9]. Despite limited reports, ERAS® protocols application seems to achieve similar benefits both in open and minimally invasive pancreatectomy [10].

The global trust to ERAS® among pancreatic surgeons has recently been investigated: regardless known specific benefits, surgeons' adherence was 38%, which is very low. When looking at relevant challenges to the application of individual ERAS® components, MIS technique is not considered as a relevant obstacle if applied to PD [11].

In view of the advantages of ERAS®, the implementation of such programs is possible both in open and in MIS and should be encouraged in all centers performing pancreatic surgery [12].

21.3 Minimally Invasive Pancreatoduodenectomy (MIPD) and ERAS®

Minimally Invasive Pancreatic Surgery (MIPS) and ERAS® share common goals but direct impact of ERAS® protocols on MIPS patients, particularly MIPD, is still in its early study phase.

An impactful benefit of ERAS® is the shorter time to return to intended oncological therapy (RIOT) initially conceived for colorectal cancer patients scheduled to adjuvant chemotherapy: institutional ERAS® with almost 70% adherence to the items was associated to shorter RIOT [13], and so to better oncological outcome. These findings could be considered when evaluating benefits of MIS and ERAS® applied to pancreatic head resection given the survival benefit when access to adjuvant therapy is possible within 8 weeks from surgery. As published by the MD Anderson Cancer Center surgical team in a retrospective series, they compared patients undergone robotic or open surgery for PC (distal pancreatectomy or pancreatoduodenectomy) during the first 3 years of their robotic pancreatectomy experience. Rate of early RIOT in the robotic group was significantly better than that in the open group. Moreover, in multivariable analysis, a robotic approach was associated with earlier RIOT which support the oncological safety of robotic pancreatectomy program even during its implementation [14].

The latest version of ERAS® guidelines published in 2019 did not include the MI approach among surgical items in patients undergoing pancreatoduodenectomy [20], indeed the higher level of evidence-based results about MIPS [15–19] has been achieved very recently. Due to worldwide implementation of MIPD programs only in recent years, there is a knowledge gap of the real benefit expected by the application of ERAS® protocols in this specific group of patients.

21.4 How to Implement ERAS® Protocols in MIPS

As identified by Karunakaran [10], key for success and improvement of ERAS® protocols in MIPD are similar to open surgery: ERAS® dedicated team and nurse, patient's empowerment, regular audit and continuous improvement, clear discharge criteria, and commitment of the Hospital Board. All these should work in accordance and coordination. Nurses play a crucial role in the adoption, dissemination, and sustainment of an ERAS® clinical pathway, such as described by Brown and co-workers [21] within a health care organization context.

All of these are crucial to establish a working group focused not only into Guidelines and/or Recommendations, but also on quality of evidence of literature [15, 16, 18, 19] and local facilities and resources. A common objective and strategy are needed. A monthly audit to assess adherence to ERAS® items, conversion rate and reason for conversion in MIS, 30-day and 90-day morbidity-mortality rate, and hospital readmission rate are crucial to define data and improve them.

A Deming Cycle, based on the four steps: plan, do, check, and act could be a methodological strategy for continuous improvement.

Anesthesiologist and surgeon are key figures for specific intraoperative items: Grant and coworkers [22] have showed how a dedicated operating room and team are related to improvement of adherence to intraoperative ERAS® items and clinical outcomes. This could become critical considering also technical aspects (positioning, abdominal pressure and insufflation, fluid balance) in MIPD.

Implementing educational resources (booklet, checklist, educational videos) and communication allows to improve achievement of ERAS® items among patients, reducing also errors and intraoperative adverse events.

In conclusion, ERAS® is proven to provide benefits in specific surgical domains while pancreatic surgery has specific challenges to face. Adoption of MIS approach for PD may enhance ERAS® benefits already documented in open pancreatic surgery; however, the continuing learning process of MIPD among units may still have an impact on potential ERAS® benefits.

All pancreas units have to adopt ERAS® protocols, but it should be acknowledged that not all patients undergoing pancreatic resection are suitable for ERAS®.

References

1. Bardram L, Funch-Jensen P, Jensen P, Crawford ME, Kehlet H. Recovery after laparoscopic colonic surgery with epidural analgesia, and early oral nutrition and mobilisation. Lancet. 1995;345(8952):763–4.
2. Gianotti L, Sandini M, Romagnoli S, Carli F, Ljungqvist O. Enhanced recovery programs in gastrointestinal surgery: actions to promote optimal perioperative nutritional and metabolic care. Clin Nutr. 2020;39(7):2014–24.
3. Bassi C, Marchegiani G, Giuliani T, Di Gioia A, Andrianello S, Zingaretti CC, Brentegani G, De Pastena M, Fontana M, Pea A, Paiella S, Malleo G, Tuveri M, Landoni L, Esposito A, Casetti L, Butturini G, Falconi M, Salvia R. Pancreatoduodenectomy at the verona pancreas institute: the evolution of indications, surgical techniques, and outcomes: a retrospective analysis of 3000 consecutive cases. Ann Surg. 2022;276(6):1029–38. https://doi.org/10.1097/SLA.0000000000004753. Epub 2021 Jan 15. PMID: 33630454
4. Gianotti L, Besselink MG, Sandini M, Hackert T, Conlon K, Gerritsen A, Griffin O, Fingerhut A, Probst P, Abu Hilal M, Marchegiani G, Nappo G, Zerbi A, Amodio A, Perinel J, Adham M, Raimondo M, Asbun HJ, Sato A, Takaori K, Shrikhande SV, Del Chiaro M, Bockhorn M, Izbicki JR, Dervenis C, Charnley RM, Martignoni ME, Friess H, de Pretis N, Radenkovic D, Montorsi M, Sarr MG, Vollmer CM, Frulloni L, Büchler MW, Bassi C. Nutritional support and therapy in pancreatic surgery: a position paper of the International Study Group on Pancreatic Surgery (ISGPS). Surgery. 2018;164(5):1035–48. https://doi.org/10.1016/j.surg.2018.05.040. Epub 2018 Jul 17. PMID: 30029989
5. Braga M, Pecorelli N, Ariotti R, Capretti G, Greco M, Balzano G, Castoldi R, Beretta L. Enhanced recovery after surgery pathway in patients undergoing pancreaticoduodenectomy. World J Surg. 2014;38(11):2960–6.

6. Kagedan DJ, Ahmed M, Devitt KS, Wei AC. Enhanced recovery after pancreatic surgery: a systematic review of the evidence. HPB. 2015;17(1):11–6.
7. Coolsen M, Van Dam R, Van Der Wilt A, Slim K, Lassen K, Dejong C. Systematic review and meta-analysis of enhanced recovery after pancreatic surgery with particular emphasis on pancreaticoduodenectomies. World J Surg. 2013;37(8):1909–18.
8. Kuemmerli C, Tschuor C, Kasai M, Alseidi AA, Balzano G, Bouwense S, et al. Impact of enhanced recovery protocols after pancreatoduodenectomy: meta-analysis. Br J Surg. 2022;109(3):256–66.
9. Kuemmerli C, Balzano G, Bouwense SA, Braga M, Coolsen M, Daniel SK, et al. Are enhanced recovery protocols after pancreatoduodenectomy still efficient when applied in elderly patients? A systematic review and individual patient data meta-analysis. J Hepatobiliary Pancreat Sci. 2024;31(5):308–17.
10. Pagano D, Li Petri S, di Francesco F, Calamia S, Accardo C, Vella I, Barbàra M, Gruttadauria S. Which factors are associated with distal pancreatectomy outcomes' optimization with the application of an enhanced recovery after surgery program? J Laparoendosc Adv Surg Tech A. 2024;34(2):106–12. https://doi.org/10.1089/lap.2023.0445. Epub 2023 Nov 29. PMID: 38029364
11. Karunakaran M, Roulin D, Ullah S, Shrikhande SV, De Boer HD, Demartines N, Barreto SG. Global Perceptions on ERAS® in Pancreatoduodenectomy. World J Surg. 2023;47(12):2977–89. https://doi.org/10.1007/s00268-023-07198-9. Epub 2023 Oct 3. PMID: 37787776; PMCID: PMC10694106
12. Robertson N, Gallacher PJ, Peel N, Garden OJ, Duxbury M, Lassen K, Parks RW. Implementation of an enhanced recovery programme following pancreaticoduodenectomy. HPB (Oxford). 2012;14(10):700–8. https://doi.org/10.1111/j.1477-2574.2012.00521.x. PMID: 22954007; PMCID: PMC3461377
13. The Italian ColoRectal Anastomotic Leakage (iCral3) Study Group. Patient-reported outcomes and return to intended oncologic therapy after colorectal enhanced recovery pathway. The iCral3 prospective study. Ann Surg Open. 2023;4(1):e267. https://doi.org/10.1097/AS9.0000000000000267. PMCID: PMC10431437
14. Lu PW, Lyu HG, Prakash LR, Chiang YS, Maxwell JE, Snyder RA, Kim MP, Tzeng CWD, Katz MHG, Ikoma N. Effect of surgical approach on early return to intended oncologic therapy after resection for pancreatic ductal adenocarcinoma. Surg Endosc. 2024;38(9):4986–95. https://doi.org/10.1007/s00464-024-11022-3. PMID: 38987482
15. Reis PCA, Bittar V, Almirón G, Schramm AJ, Oliveira JP, Cagnacci R. Camandaroba MPG laparoscopic versus open pancreatoduodenectomy for periampullary tumors: a systematic review and meta-analysis of randomized controlled trial J Gastrointest. Cancer. 2024;55(3):1058–68. PMID: 39028397
16. Sattari SA, Sattari AR, Makary MA, Hu C, He J. Laparoscopic versus open pancreatoduodenectomy in patients with periampullary tumors: a systematic review and meta-analysis. Ann Surg. 2023;277(5):742–55. https://doi.org/10.1097/SLA.0000000000005785. PMID: 36519444
17. de Graaf N, Hilal MA. Besselink MG robotic pancreatoduodenectomy: an ongoing exploration. Lancet Reg Health Eur. 2024;39:100880. https://doi.org/10.1016/j.lanepe.2024.100880. PMID: 38464481
18. Uijterwijk BA, Wei K, Kasai M, Ielpo B, van Hilst J, Chinnusamy P, Lemmers DHL, Burdio F, Senthilnathan P, Besselink MG, Hilal MA, Qin RM. Inimally invasive versus open pancreatoduodenectomy for pancreatic ductal adenocarcinoma: individual patient data meta-analysis of randomized trials. Surg Endosc. 2024;38(9):4986–95. https://doi.org/10.1007/s00464-024-11022-3. PMID: 37076411
19. Valle V, Pakataridis P, Marchese T, Ferrari C, Chelmis F, Sorotou IN, Gianniou MA, Dimova A, Tcholakov O, Ielpo B. Comparative analysis of open, laparoscopic, and robotic pancreaticoduodenectomy: a systematic review of randomized controlled trials. Medicina (Kaunas). 2025;61(7):1121. https://doi.org/10.3390/medicina61071121. PMID: 40731751; PMCID: PMC12298437.
20. Melloul E, Lassen K, Roulin D, Grass F, Perinel J, Adham M, Wellge EB, Kunzler F, Besselink MG, Asbun H, Scott MJ, Dejong CHC, Vrochides D, Aloia T, Izbicki JR, Demartines N. Guidelines for perioperative care for pancreatoduodenectomy: Enhanced Recovery After Surgery (ERAS®) recommendations 2019. World J Surg. 2020;44(7):2056–84. https://doi.org/10.1007/s00268-020-05462-w. PMID: 32161987
21. Brown D, Xhaja A. Nursing perspectives on enhanced recovery after surgery. Surg Clin North Am. 2018;98(6):1211–21. https://doi.org/10.1016/j.suc.2018.07.008. PMID: 30390853
22. Grant MC, Hanna A, Benson A, Hobson D, Wu CL, Yuan CT, Rosen M, Wick EC. Dedicated operating room teams and clinical outcomes in an enhanced recovery after surgery pathway for colorectal surgery. J Am Coll Surg. 2018;226(3):267–76. https://doi.org/10.1016/j.jamcollsurg.2017.12.010. PMID: 29274837